AF869827

THE YEAR IN
ALLERGY

VOLUME 3

THE YEAR IN ALLERGY

VOLUME 3

EDITED BY

S HASAN ARSHAD AND STEPHEN T HOLGATE

CLINICAL PUBLISHING
OXFORD

Clinical Publishing

an imprint of Atlas Medical Publishing Ltd

Oxford Centre for Innovation
Mill Street, Oxford OX2 0JX, UK

Tel: +44 1865 811116
Fax: +44 1865 251550
E mail: info@clinicalpublishing.co.uk
Web: www.clinicalpublishing.co.uk

Distributed by:

Marston Book Services Ltd
PO Box 269
Abingdon
Oxon OX14 4YN, UK
Tel: +44 1235 465500
Fax: +44 1235 465555
E mail: trade.orders@marston.co.uk

© Atlas Medical Publishing Ltd 2006

First published 2006

All rights reserved. No part of this publication may be reproduced, stored in a retrieval system, or transmitted, in any form or by any means, without the prior permission in writing of Clinical Publishing or Atlas Medical Publishing Ltd

Although every effort has been made to ensure that all owners of copyright material have been acknowledged in this publication, we would be glad to acknowledge in subsequent reprints or editions any omissions brought to our attention

A catalogue record for this book is available from the British Library

ISBN 1 904392 60 1
ISSN 1477-8106

The publisher makes no representation, express or implied, that the dosages in this book are correct. Readers must therefore always check the product information and clinical procedures with the most up-to-date published product information and data sheets provided by the manufacturers and the most recent codes of conduct and safety regulations. The authors and the publisher do not accept any liability for any errors in the text or for the misuse or misapplication of material in this work

Project Manager: Rosemary Osmond, Helimetrics Ltd, Chipping Norton, Oxon, UK
Typeset by Hope Services (Abingdon) Ltd, Abingdon, Oxon, UK
Printed by T G Hostench SA, Barcelona, Spain

Contents

Part III

Treatment modalities for allergic diseases

Editors

S Hasan Arshad, DM, FRCP
Senior Lecturer in Respiratory Medicine and Allergy, Schools of Medicine and Life Sciences, Keele University, Keele, Staffordshire, UK

Stephen T Holgate, DSc, FRCP
Medical Research Council Clinical Professor of Immunopharmacology, School of Medicine, University of Southampton, Southampton, UK

Contributors

S Hasan Abid, FCPS
Associate Professor, Department of Otolaryngology, Dow University of Medical Sciences, Karachi, Pakistan

S Hasan Arshad, DM, FRCP
Senior Lecturer in Respiratory Medicine and Allergy, Schools of Medicine and Life Sciences, Keele University, Keele, Staffordshire, UK

K Suresh Babu, DM
Research Fellow, Southampton General Hospital, Southampton, UK

Richard L Baretto, PHD, MRCP, MRCPATH
Consultant Immunologist, Department of Immunology, Leicester Royal Infirmary, Leicester, UK

Taraneh Dean, PHD
Reader in Epidemiology, School of Health Sciences and Social Work, University of Portsmouth, Portsmouth, UK

Gordon Dent, PHD
Lecturer in Pharmacology, Institute of Science and Technology in Medicine, Keele University, Keele, Staffordshire, UK

Susan Ewart, PHD
Associate Professor of Genetics, Michigan State University, East Lansing, Michigan, USA

Sarah Goddard, PhD, MRCP, Dip RCPath
Specialist Registrar, Department of Immunology, Birmingham Heartlands Hospital, Birmingham, UK

Aarnoud Huissoon, PhD, MRCP(I), MRCPath
Consultant Immunologist and Honorary Senior Clinical Lecturer, Department of Immunology, Birmingham Heartlands Hospital, Birmingham, UK

Wilfried Karmaus, MD, Dr.med, MPH
Professor of Epidemiology, University of South Carolina, Columbia, South Carolina, USA

Mamidipudi Thirumala Krishna, PhD, FRCP, MRCPath
Consultant Immunologist and Honorary Senior Clinical lecturer, Department of Immunology, Birmingham Heartlands Hospital, Birmingham, UK

Jaymin Morjaria, MD, MRCP
Research Fellow, Southampton General Hospital, Southampton, UK

John Mucklow, MD, FRCP, FBPharmacolS, DipMedEd
Consultant Physician, Department of Clinical Pharmacology, University Hospital of North Staffordshire, Stoke-on-Trent, UK

Brett Pereira, MD, MRCP
Consultant Physician, Department of Respiratory Medicine, Kent and Canterbury Hospital, Canterbury, Kent, UK

Graham Roberts, DM, MSc, MRCPCH
Clinical Senior Lecturer, Paediatric Allergy and Respiratory Medicine, School of Medicine, University of Southampton, Southampton, UK

Anthony P Williams, PhD, MRCP, MRCPath
Wellcome Trust Clinician Scientist and Honorary Consultant Immunologist, University of Southampton and Department of Immunology, Southampton General Hospital, Southampton, UK

Foreword

N Franklin Adkinson Jr, MD
Professor of Medicine and Allergy
Immunology Training Program Director
Johns Hopkins Asthma and Allergy Center
Baltimore, Maryland, USA

In this 'information age' of medicine, researchers and practitioners have easy access electronically to an ever-increasing portfolio of original research and practice guidelines. Finding recent literature pertinent to almost any medical problem is a skill now taught to most medical students, and definitively in post-doctoral medical education. Finding time to read and digest all we can locate and retrieve with ease is a bigger challenge, but not the biggest one.

After finding and reading a new paper, especially one involving original research, the important facility is the ability to place it in proper context with what has come before. To some degree, authors address this chore in the 'introduction' and 'discussion' section of their papers. But with increasing frequency, authors are not fully aware of the significance (or lack thereof) of their work, the determination of which may require consideration of post-publications dialogues, editorials and public reactions, and integration with what others know is 'in press' or underway.

So the optimal time for trying to assess the merits and heuristic value of published works may be in the year following its publication, preferably by knowledgeable and unbiased observers who are monitoring the 'bigger picture.' Enter now the third volume of *The Year in Allergy* which accomplishes this task admirably for those whose eyes need to be focused on the origins, pathophysiology and treatment of allergic diseases. The authors, backed by skilful editorial oversight, have successfully reviewed some of the most important papers dealing with allergy published over the past eighteen months, and put them into proper perspective scientifically and in most cases clinically as well. Key figures and tables highlight the most important quantitative findings. The *Comment* sections identify the significance of the work and its relationship to previous similar observations, and in some cases to theories under examination. And then each abstracting section author has written a conclusion which attempts to assess what 'progress' has been noted in the topic area in the recent past, and what obstacles are now impeding needed insights or data collection.

All in all, this is a wonderfully stimulating way to review recent reports in each of the major areas of allergic disorders and to get some sense of how the field may have been moved forward in the past year. What I have also found is that these cogent commentaries have primed me appropriately to read new papers coming along with a better sense of importance and potential contribution to the field. I congratulate the Editors on achieving their educational objective, and commend this book to trainees and experts alike, and to both investigators and clinicians. Increasingly, I see efforts like this volume as one of the most fruitful formats for ongoing medical education.

Preface

Stephen T Holgate, DSc, FRCP
Medical Research Council Clinical Professor of Immunopharmacology
School of Medicine
University of Southampton
Southampton
UK

The Year in Allergy series is proving to be a very popular source of recent research findings in allergy. This is the third volume in the series and draws on a research literature over the last 2 years. We have divided the book into 3 main sections with individual subjects within each section dealt with separately. While the concept of allergy has been well accepted since the days of Charles Blackley who first described hay fever or hay asthma (*catarrhus aestevus*) in 1880, and Karl Prausnitz and his assistant Heinz Kustner who are remembered for the first demonstration in humans of reagin (later to be identified as IgE) in 1921, progress since has been relatively slow in determining the role of atopy in disease pathogenesis. Over the last decade, however, there has been an explosion of interest in immunology and immunopharmacology underlying the allergic process through engagement of both B and T lymphocytes and antigen-presenting cells and their subsets involved in subverting the immune response towards an allergic state. The identification of individual chemical substances that contribute to the pathophysiological events of an allergic response has also provided fertile ground for new discovery including the development of novel H_1-antihistamines and cysteinyl leukotriene receptor antagonists.

The clear recognition that all allergic disease and the general state of atopy is progressively increasing in its incidence worldwide in relation to the adoption of a Western-type lifestyle has raised allergy as a public health problem. A better understanding of the cell and molecular basis of allergic mechanisms linked to carefully conducted environmental epidemiology has led to a range of new ideas that might explain these rising trends. In this edition of *The Year in Allergy* there are some new publications that provide a basis for why these diseases are becoming more prevalent and what the underlying environmental factors might be. Allergic diseases, including rhinitis, asthma, food and insect allergy, and atopic dermatitis, are all complex disorders with both environmental and genetic factors playing important roles. The development of modern genetic epidemiology and new ways of exploring human genetics and epigenetics (gene–gene and gene–environment interactions) in complex disease is leading to the discovery of novel molecules, hitherto never thought to be involved in disease mechanisms, let alone allergic disease. Several examples of these are given in this volume including consideration of gene–environmental interactions.

Greater understanding of disease mechanisms has enabled the pharmaceutical and biotechnology industries to develop new treatments that are now entering the clinic. A particularly exciting development has been the ability of manipulating circulating and tissue levels of the allergic antibody, IgE, using monoclonal antibodies and vaccines that target 'upstream' pathways involved in allergic disease. Another field that has expanded considerably is the role of different T-cell subtypes in suppressing allergic responses and targeting vaccines to amplify those that involve activation of toll-like receptors.

Of greater concern to many is the increasing occurrence of 'new' allergic diseases such as sensitization to latex, nuts and exotic fruits. Thirty years ago, these conditions were uncommon, but now they present real problems because their manifestations are often in the young, are severe and life threatening. There has been much speculation as to why these 'new' allergic disorders have arisen but a combination of increased population susceptibility and early life exposure to new allergens seems important. The view that allergic disease progresses over time from birth to adulthood with different clinical manifestations occurring at different stages through life has also provided fertile ground for research, for example milk and eggs allergies which are common in the first year or two of life, often regress later in childhood, only to be replaced by sensitization to aeroallergens, such as grass and tree pollen, dust mite and animal danders linked to rhinoconjunctivitis, atopic dermatitis and asthma. The underlying mechanisms for this 'switch' and why certain allergens are more 'sensitizing' than others are still largely unknown, although the recent identification of intrinsic biological activities or certain allergens (e.g. the proteolytic enzyme activity of dust mite, pollen and fungal allergens) provides one mechanism conferring a 'danger' signal to antigen-presenting cells to redirect the ensuing T-cell response.

While it has not been possible to review every high-quality publication over the last eighteen months, in this volume we hope that, by carefully selecting a range of articles covering different subjects, it has been possible to provide a good overview of the major discoveries and their implications for the mechanisms, diagnosis and treatment of allergic disorders. A unique feature of this series is the identification of major themes introduced by a brief overview followed by a series of abstracts from which we have drawn interpretations and commented upon them. It is our wish that these abstracts complement the new published material and stimulate the reader to find out more about a particular subject of interest. I am especially grateful to my colleague Hasan Arshad as co-editor and a large number of colleagues who have made an enormous investment in time and effort to create this third volume. It is hoped that on reading what we present you will find this a useful compendium for updating your clinical and basic knowledge in allergy as part of your programme in higher professional development.

Part I

Epidemiology and genetics

1

Epidemiology and risk factors

WILFRIED KARMAUS

Introduction

According to the National Survey of Children in the United States ($n = 102\,353$; 2003, age 1–17 years), the prevalence of asthma was 15% (last 12 months), that of hay fever was 12.4%, of skin allergy 9.8% and food or digestive allergy 3.6%. Overall, every fourth child is affected (25.4%). Regarding the diagnosis of asthma in children, the prevalence, for instance in Germany, rose from 1.25% to 2.21% between 1951–1952 and 1964–1965 [1]. For the last 10 years there has been dispute about whether the increase in asthma and allergy has come to a halt. However, the observation period is too short to draw any conclusion. A study of adults went beyond this simple dispute and investigated age and cohort effects for immunoglobulin E (IgE) sensitization from 1992 to 1998–2002 [2]. Approximately 30% of the adults showed any IgE sensitization (house dust mite, grass or cat allergen). The authors concluded that IgE sensitization, particularly to grass, continued to increase and that the prevalence of sensitization to grass was higher in the later cohort (born 1965 and later) compared with the earlier cohort (born 1964–1958).

There is an exceptional burden of allergic disease in children, which is likely to continue into adulthood. Hence, it is of utmost importance to understand the aetiology and development of allergies and asthma, to intervene appropriately, and thus to reduce the prevalence of the disease. However, there is uncertainty regarding risk factors for asthma and allergies. Research has contributed little to better understanding of why some develop the disease and others do not and why in some patients symptoms become chronic whereas other patients grow out of asthma and allergy. There are many controversies, with comparable amounts of supporting evidence for each opposing hypothesis. The hope is that, finally, when the dust settles, we will see a clearer picture.

One predominant group of aetiological explanations gathers around the hygiene hypothesis, which posits that lack of exposure to infectious agents early in life hinders the immune system in switching from an allergic T-helper (Th2) pattern to a Th1 pattern of responses. However, studies on the association between infectious exposures and the outcomes asthma [3] and atopic eczema [4,5], have left a trail of inconsistent findings. Researchers on the other side of the argument have presented credible alternative explanations to some specific aspects of the hygiene hypothesis.

© Atlas Medical Publishing Ltd

However, those in favour of this hypothesis come up with diverging explanations. For instance, the finding that immune susceptibility may be programmed prenatally [6–8], long before the child is exposed to infectious agents, should have initiated a more careful assessment of early childhood responses. However, the focus of the hygiene hypothesis has moved on to other issues without careful evaluation of past findings. Old debates focused on infections, new controversies are about pets and farming. This chapter attempts to balance the discussion by selecting a variety of studies.

Diverging prevalence trends of atopic disorders in Norwegian children: results from three cross-sectional studies

Selnes A, Nystad W, Bolle R, Lund E. *Allergy* 2005; **60**: 894–9

Background. During recent decades there has been extensive epidemiological research to explore the increasing prevalences of asthma and allergy in childhood. The worldwide variations in the prevalences of these diseases necessitate regional rapport. Furthermore, time-trend analyses with comparable methods are important in order to monitor the rapidly changing prevalence of these diseases. Three cross-sectional questionnaire-based studies of asthma and allergy in schoolchildren were conducted in the counties of Troms and Finnmark in northern Norway in 1985, 1995 and 2000. The first two studies included children from randomly selected primary schools (1985, *n* = 1794; 1995, *n* = 1432). The third study was a part of the International Study of Asthma and Allergies in Childhood (ISAAC)-II Europe study (*n* = 3853). Identical items of asthma and allergy were employed. The analyses included only children who were 9–11 years of age.

Interpretation. The prevalence of asthma was 9.3, 13.2 and 13.8% in 1985, 1995 and 2000 respectively. However, great gender differences were detected; the prevalence of asthma increased in males between 1995 and 2000, from 14.1 to 17.0% (risk ratio [RR] 1.2; 95% confidence interval [CI] 1.0–1.5), but decreased in females between 1995 and 2000, from 12.3 to 10.5% (RR 0.9; 95% CI 0.7–1.1). Furthermore, in children with asthma, a changing trend was found in the external factors perceived to cause symptoms, from typical allergens towards other, unspecific agents. The prevalence of self-reported atopic eczema/dermatitis syndrome (AEDS) was 13.4, 21.1 and 20.8% in 1985, 1995 and 2000 respectively. The prevalence of self-reported allergic rhinoconjunctivitis was 16.5, 24.7 and 29.6% in 1985, 1995 and 2000 respectively; the RR (2000/1995) was 1.2 (95% CI 1.1–1.3). The prevalence of asthma in girls reached a plateau, and even decreased from 1995 to 2000. This is in contrast to the prevalence in boys, which tends to increase continuously. The prevalence of AEDS, which increased substantially between 1985 and 1995, did not change from 1995 to 2000. However, the prevalence of allergic rhinoconjunctivitis increased steadily from 1985 to 1995 and 2000.

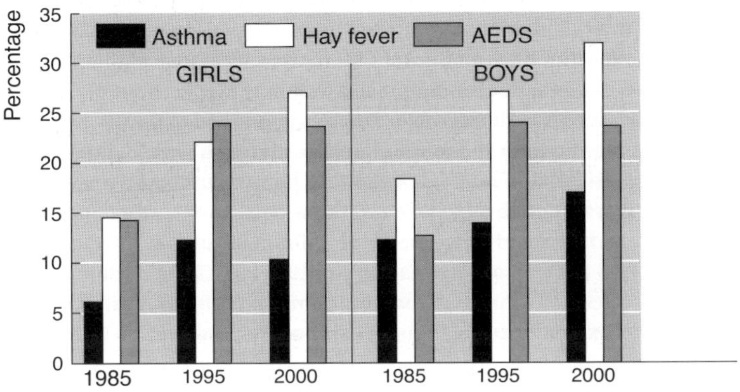

Fig. 1.1 Prevalence (percentage) of self-reported allergic manifestations in children (9–11 years) in Norway. AEDS, atopic eczema/dermatitis syndrome. Source: Selnes *et al.* (2005).

Comment

Three large unselected samples of children, 9–11 years of age, residing in northern Norway, provided an unbiased assessment of self-reported symptoms. The questions in the three surveys varied, but basic comparability was assured. The prevalence of asthma/wheezing was higher than in German studies [**9,10**] but lower than in New Zealand (see below). The results indicate an increase in asthma in boys but not in girls (Fig. 1.1). This is contrary to the findings of surveys of children in Germany, in which girls experienced an increase between 1994/95 and 1999/2000 [**9**]. The Norwegian study also reported a steady increase in hay fever from 1985 to 2000 (Fig. 1.1). Against this, the prevalence of AEDS rose between 1985 and 1995, without any further increase thereafter.

Whereas differences in the worldwide prevalence of allergies cannot be explained by latitude, early infection during the winter months, or the month of first exposure to allergens [**11**], may explain some of the differences. A culturally related behaviour is smoking, which has high prevalence in Norway [**12**] but seems to be declining [**13**]. Thus, future studies on trends in allergic manifestations are warranted.

Asthma and farm exposures in a cohort of rural Iowa children

Merchant JA, Naleway AL, Svendsen ER, *et al. Environ Health Perspect* 2005; **113**: 350–6

Background. Epidemiological studies of farm children are of international interest because farm children are less often atopic, have less allergic disease, and often have

less asthma than do non-farm children—findings consistent with the hygiene hypothesis. The investigators studied a cohort of rural Iowa children to determine the association between farm and other environmental risk factors with four asthma outcomes: doctor-diagnosed asthma; doctor-diagnosed asthma/medication for wheeze; current wheeze; and cough with exercise. Doctor-diagnosed asthma prevalence was 12%, but at least one of these four health outcomes was found in more than a third of the cohort. Multivariable models of the four health outcomes found independent associations between male sex (three asthma outcomes), age (three asthma outcomes), a personal history of allergies (four asthma outcomes), family history of allergic disease (two asthma outcomes), premature birth (one asthma outcome), early respiratory infection (three asthma outcomes), high-risk birth (two asthma outcomes), and farm exposure to raising pigs and adding antibiotics to feed (two asthma outcomes).

Interpretation. The high prevalence of rural childhood asthma and asthma symptoms underscores the need for asthma screening programmes and improved asthma diagnosis and treatment. The high prevalence of asthma health outcomes among farm children living on farms that raise pigs (44.1%; $P = 0.01$) and farms that raise pigs and add antibiotics to feed (55.8%; $P = 0.013$), despite lower rates of atopy and personal histories of allergy, suggests the need for awareness and prevention measures and more population-based studies to further assess the environmental and genetic determinants of asthma among farm children.

Comment

In recent years, there has been a swell of popularity and published reports on the protective effect of growing up on a farm **[14,15]**. Alternative explanations, such as population genetics and centuries of out-selection of allergic individuals from farms, have been ignored in some European studies. This study by Merchant *et al.*, conducted in Iowa, contributes to a more balanced understanding of the farming effect. The proportion of participation was 67.1%. One thousand and four households were included (336 farm, 206 rural non-farm and 462 town households), providing information on 644 children. Farm children in this study were reported by their parents to be exposed as bystanders to farm tasks around livestock as early as 1 year of age. Several studies conducted in Iowa have also reported high levels of occupational exposures to dust, endoxin, hydrogen sulphide and ammonia. The authors reported that children born on a farm had lower IgE levels, but the difference was not significant. For coughing, significant associations were observed between exposure to dogs in the household and addition of antibiotics to feed. In particular, pig production seems to increase the risk of asthma.

Other recent studies raise questions about the protective effect of farm exposures **[16,17]**. There is a need to install a rigorous system of checks and balances and to re-evaluate the idyllic presumptions **[18]** before accepting evidence of protective effects that have emerged from studies conducted in one European region.

Pets and the development of allergic sensitization

Simpson A, Custovic A. *Curr Allergy Asthma Rep* 2005; **5**: 212–20

BACKGROUND. Sensitization to pets remains a risk factor for asthma and rhinitis, and can occur in people who have never lived with a pet. Several reports have indicated that living with a pet reduces the risk of becoming sensitized to that pet. Having a pet in the home gives exposure to more than just allergens. In areas with a high frequency of pet ownership, community exposure to pet allergens is almost certainly sufficient to induce sensitization among non-pet-owners. In this review, the authors examined the results of recent studies that have investigated the relationship between pet ownership, specific sensitization to that pet, and allergic sensitization in general.

INTERPRETATION. For cat ownership, the results are inconsistent between studies of similar design, some studies suggesting an increase in risk and others a decrease in risk among cat-owners. For dogs, results are more consistent, generally suggesting that owning a dog has no effect – or indeed may be protective – against the development of specific sensitization to dogs and allergic sensitization in general.

Comment

This highly informative review focuses on sensitization, not allergic disorders. It distinguishes the type of study (birth cohort, cross-sectional, case–control, and case-only studies), the time of exposure (childhood vs adulthood), and studies in children and adults. A (trans-generational) selection bias limits the conclusions: allergic families will avoid pet exposure but contribute to a higher risk in non-pet-owners. More studies have investigated cat ownership and sensitization to cats than dog ownership and sensitization to dogs. This also may account for the increased heterogeneity of the results found for cats. The results remain confusing and contradictory. However, no study has found that dog ownership is associated with an increased risk of sensitization to dogs. Nevertheless, the authors suggest that, in symptomatic pet-sensitized subjects, the relevant pet should be avoided. It is notable that sensitization to cat dander among non-cat-owners is more prevalent in communities with a high proportion of cat ownership.

A clinical trial in this setting (pet exposure) would be unethical. However, an informative natural experiment may include non-pet-owners moving into neighbourhoods (day-care centres, industries) with a large number of pet-owners.

Risk factors for atopic dermatitis in New Zealand children at 3.5 years of age

Purvis DJ, Thompson JM, Clark PM, *et al. Br J Dermatol* 2005; **152**: 742–9

BACKGROUND. The prevalence of atopic dermatitis (AD) is increasing in Western societies. The hygiene hypothesis proposes that this is due to reduced exposure to environmental allergens and infections during early life. The authors examined factors associated with a diagnosis of AD at 3.5 years of age, especially those factors implicated by the hygiene hypothesis. The Auckland Birthweight Collaborative study is a case–control study of risk factors for small-for-gestational-age babies. Cases were born at term with birth weight at or below the 10th centile; controls were appropriate for gestational age, with birth weight above the 10th centile. The infants were assessed at birth, 1 year and 3.5 years of age. Data were collected by parental interview and examination of the child. AD was defined as the presence of an itchy rash in the past 12 months with three or more of the following: history of flexural involvement; history of generally dry skin; history of atopic disease in parents or siblings; and visible flexural dermatitis according to a photographic protocol. Statistical analyses took into account the disproportionate sampling of the study population.

INTERPRETATION. Analysis was restricted to European subjects. Eight hundred and seventy-one children were enrolled at birth; 744 (85.4%) participated at 1 year and 550 (63.2%) at 3.5 years. AD was diagnosed in 87 (15.8%) children seen at 3.5 years. The prevalence of AD did not differ according to birth weight. AD at 3.5 years was associated with raised serum IgE (above 200 kU/l) and wheezing, asthma, rash or eczema at 1 year. In multivariate analysis, adjusted for parental atopy and breast-feeding, AD at 3.5 years was associated with atopic disease in the parents (maternal atopy only, adjusted odds ratio [OR] 3.83; 95% CI 1.20–12.23; paternal atopy only, adjusted OR 3.59; 95% CI 1.09–11.75; both parents atopic, adjusted OR 6.12; 95% CI 2.02–18.50). There was a higher risk of AD with longer duration of breast-feeding (less than 6 months, adjusted OR 6.13; 95% CI 1.45–25.86; 6 months or longer, adjusted OR 9.70; 95% CI 2.47–38.15) compared with no breast-feeding. These findings remained significant after adjusting for environmental factors and a personal history of atopy. AD at 3.5 years was associated with owning a cat at 3.5 years (adjusted OR 0.45; 95% CI 0.21–0.97) but not with owning a dog at 3.5 years or pets at 1 year, or with older siblings. Furthermore, AD at 3.5 years was not associated with gender, socio-economic status, maternal smoking, parity, damp, mould, immunizations, body mass index (BMI) or antibiotic use in the first year of life. Personal and parental histories of atopic disease are risk factors for AD at 3.5 years. Duration of breast-feeding was associated with an increased risk of AD. No association was found with factors implicated by the hygiene hypothesis. This study suggests that breast-feeding should not be recommended for the prevention of AD.

Comment

This investigation of small-for-gestational-age babies and controls followed to the age of 3.5 years suffers from loss to follow-up (63.2%). Atopic dermatitis was related to a longer duration of breast-feeding. Studies of the association between breast-feeding and AEDS have produced conflicting results [19]. An additional challenge arises when the mother has a history of allergy. Exclusive breast-feeding in children of parents with no allergies, for instance, was related to an increased risk, but not for children of parents with allergies [20]. The best setting to address this question is a randomized prospective study similar to that which Arshad suggested for allergen exposure [21]. However, clinical trials using an intention to breast-feed or not to breast-feed approach have ethical problems. Nevertheless, studies utilizing wet-nurses (Africa) or breast-milk banks (Brazil) are likely to offer new insights.

Breast-feeding, soluble CD14 concentration in breast milk and risk of atopic dermatitis and asthma in early childhood: birth cohort study

Rothenbacher D, Weyermann M, Beermann C, Brenner H. *Clin Exp Allergy* 2005; **35**: 1014–21

BACKGROUND. Breast milk contains a variety of bioactive substances, among them soluble CD14 (sCD14), which plays an important role in innate immunity. The authors analysed data of a large prospective birth cohort study to examine the determinants of sCD14 in breast milk, and investigated whether breast-feeding practice and sCD14 concentrations in breast milk are determinants of the risk of AD and asthma in children. Eight hundred and three mothers and their newborn infants were included in this analysis. They measured sCD14 concentrations in breast milk samples collected 6 weeks post-partum. During a 2-year follow-up the cumulative incidences of AD and asthma were recorded.

INTERPRETATION. Overall, AD was reported for 20.6% of the 2-year-olds and asthma was reported for 19.6%. The lowest incidence of physician-reported AD occurred in children of mothers without a history of atopic diseases if breast-fed for between 6 and less than 9 months. Furthermore, an inverse association between the duration of breast-feeding and the risk of asthma was found, which was especially evident in children with mothers without a history of atopic disease ($P = 0.01$). These patterns persisted after control for other factors by multivariate analysis methods. The protective effect of breast-feeding seemed to be synergistic with sCD14 concentrations in breast milk (P for trend, 0.0005). The results of this prospective birth cohort study suggest that a longer duration of breast-feeding does decrease the risk of asthma in early childhood, especially in children of mothers without a history of atopic disease. The beneficial effects of breast-feeding might be further supported by high levels of sCD14 in breast milk.

Comment

Although there is some evidence that breast-feeding may protect against allergic disease, it is not known whether all breast milk is equally protective. We have not yet identified the protective immune constituents. Other potential mechanisms include a modification of bacterial intestinal colonization or delayed introduction of potential dietary antigens. One protective factor in breast milk may be sCD14, which is part of the lipopolysaccharide recognition complex which binds microbial and other bacterial cell wall components. This study investigated the effect of the duration of breast-feeding on AD and asthma and included information on the sCD14 concentration in breast milk.

The project established a birth cohort of 1066 children (proportion of participation, 67%), of whom 803 were included in the report. Overall, this study also reported that breast-feeding poses a risk of AD (13.2% of the non-breast-fed offspring and 21.3% of the offspring who were breast-fed for 9 months and longer). No additional effect was seen when sCD14 was taken into consideration. For asthma, the cumulative incidence was lower in children who were breast-fed for more than 6 months. In children who were breast-fed for 6 months and longer, the odds ratio was lowest in the category with the highest sCD14 level in mothers' breast milk.

Few studies have investigated the immune constituents of breast milk and their risk for the offspring. To start out with the duration of breast-feeding and a comparative disease approach (AD vs asthma) is the approach future studies should take. The challenge is to determine which constituent(s) in breast milk pose(s) a risk of AD and a protective effect for asthma. However, we have to take into account that allergic disorders are not the only outcome of interest. Breast-feeding is also important in defence against a variety of childhood conditions, including infections, delays in mental development and childhood obesity.

Obesity

Obesity and asthma in 11–12 year old New Zealand children in 1989 and 2000

Wickens K, Barry D, Friezema A, *et al. Thorax* 2005; **60**: 7–12

BACKGROUND. There have been concurrent increases in the prevalences of obesity and asthma in recent years in New Zealand and other countries. Two cross-sectional surveys performed in 1989 and 2000 were used to test this association in children of mean age 11.7 years. BMI was calculated as weight/height^2 (kg/m^2) and obesity and overweight defined according to an international standard. Standard questions were used to measure the prevalence of asthma symptoms.

INTERPRETATION. Significant increases in the prevalence of reported symptoms and disease between 1989 and 2000 were not explained by a concurrent increase in the prevalence of obesity. In 2000, multivariate analysis showed that increasing the BMI standard deviation score was significantly associated with current wheeze ($P = 0.002$), inhaled steroid use ($P = 0.004$) and the use of any medication ($P = 0.001$). None of the associations was significantly different for boys or girls. There is some evidence for an association of obesity with asthma symptoms and treatment, but this does not explain the increasing prevalence of this disease.

Comment

This investigation used two cross-sectional surveys (1989, $n = 871$; 2000, $n = 894$) and the authors determined whether the increase in obesity could explain the rise in prevalence in 2000 compared with 1989. Comparable approaches have shown that the increase in type 2 diabetes mellitus could be explained by obesity of the mother [22]. In addition, the investigation was stratified by sex, which takes into account that the associations may be different in boys and girls. Indeed, in the year 2000, but not in 1989, BMI was associated with wheezing, asthma and asthma medication in girls but not in boys. Reported asthma symptoms and asthma medication increased 2- to 3-fold between 1989 and 2000, but the increase was not explained by a concomitant increase in obesity. The message of this study is that obesity is obviously not the driving force behind the epidemic of asthma. However, we still have to identify the third variable that poses a risk of both obesity and asthma. Possible candidates are maternal smoking, maternal obesity, endocrine factors and breast-feeding.

Sex specificity of asthma associated with objectively measured body mass index and waist circumference: the Humboldt study

Chen Y, Rennie D, Cormier Y, Dosman J. *Chest* 2005; **128**: 3048–54

BACKGROUND. This study investigated the possibility of sex-specificity for the association of obesity and asthma using objective measures of BMI and waist circumference. A cross-sectional study of adults ($n = 2057$) living in Humboldt, Saskatchewan, Canada (a rural community) was performed in 2003. Ever-asthma was defined as lifetime physician-diagnosed asthma, and recent asthma was defined as asthma diagnosed by a physician during the past 12 months. BMI and waist circumference were measured objectively.

INTERPRETATION. Among the participants, 5.6% of men and 10.0% of women reported having ever-asthma, and 2.7 and 6.0% had recent asthma, respectively. Higher levels of both BMI and waist circumference were significantly associated with asthma in women but not in men. The adjusted ORs for women with a BMI of at least 30.0 kg/m^2 relative to women with a BMI of less than 25.0 kg/m^2 were 2.06 (95% CI 1.42–4.05) for ever-asthma and 3.47 (95% CI 1.64–7.32) for recent asthma. This study demonstrated that the increased risk of asthma associated with obesity was significant in women but not in men even when BMI was measured objectively, and this association was robust to the anthropometric measures.

Comment

This community-based cross-sectional investigation was based on 2057 adults (18–79 years of age), 71% of the target population in the rural town of Humboldt. Of the men, 38.2% were obese and 33.7% of the women were obese (BMI at least 30 kg/m^2). Surprisingly, the crude prevalence of asthma showed no relationship with BMI groups in men (<25 kg/m^2, 3.3%; 25–29.9 kg/m^2, 2.1%; ≥30 kg/m^2, 1.9%), but in women a strong and linear association was observed (<25 kg/m^2, 2.6%; 25–29.9 kg/m^2, 6.8%; ≥30 kg/m^2, 8.7%). Wickens *et al.* (see article above) also reported that the association of asthma and BMI was restricted to girls. The reasons for the sex-related associations are not known; however, endocrine effects offer an explanation for the obesity–asthma association. In support of this, a recent study found that hormone replacement therapy in post-menopausal women was associated with increased risk of newly diagnosed asthma |**23**|.

Maternal fish consumption during pregnancy and risk of early childhood asthma

Salam MT, Li YF, Langholz B, Gilliland FD. *J Asthma* 2005; **42**: 513–18

BACKGROUND. Maternal fish consumption during pregnancy may affect children's risk of asthma by modulating early-life immune development. The type of fish consumed may be important because of differences in fatty acid content. To test this hypothesis, the authors conducted a nested case–control study, selecting subjects from the Children's Health Study, a population-based study of school-aged children in southern California. Cases had physician-diagnosed asthma and controls were asthma-free by age 5 years. Mothers or guardians provided information on fish consumption during pregnancy in telephone interviews. They computed the OR and 95% CI by using conditional logistic regression models that accounted for the sampling.

INTERPRETATION. In children born to mothers with a history of asthma, the OR for asthma was 0.20 (95% CI 0.06–0.65) when mothers ate oily fish at least monthly during pregnancy compared with no consumption (*P* for trend, 0.006). Maternal oily fish consumption during pregnancy did not benefit children of non-asthmatic mothers. In contrast, fish stick (a source of *trans* fats) consumption during pregnancy increased the risk of asthma in children (OR 2.04; 95% CI 1.18–3.51). These results suggest that maternal oily fish intake during pregnancy may protect offspring from asthma; however, eating fish sticks during pregnancy may increase the risk of asthma in children.

Comment

This case–control study investigated the relationship between maternal fish consumption during pregnancy and asthma in offspring at age 5. Objective measurements were not available for exposure and outcome. Considering the case–control nature of the study, the lack of objective measurement increases the possibility of recall bias with regard to fish consumption. The sample size was not large enough to see the effect of a higher frequency of fish consumption (for example, weekly). The lack of association in the offspring of mothers without a history of asthma might be the result of different aetiological factors that were not influenced by the consumption of fat fish. On the other hand, some mothers may have avoided fish consumption because of allergic reactions, but their offspring may be at a higher risk. Nevertheless, there are some mechanistic explanations why n-3 fatty acids are protective and n-6 acids are not. The n-3 polyunsaturated fatty acids have anti-inflammatory effects and decrease the synthesis of prostaglandin E_2 and leukotriene B_4 [**24**].

On the other hand, oily fish such as mackerel and salmon contain not only n-3 fatty acids but also dichlorodiphenyldichloroethylene (DDE), the effect of which is reported below. The results warrant future clinical trials in pregnant mothers using fish oil [**25**]. Such trials could further investigate the dose of n-3 fatty acids needed for a beneficial effect and may circumvent the possible confounding effect of other contaminants in fish.

Prevalence and main characteristics of schoolchildren diagnosed with food allergies in France

Rance F, Grandmottet X, Grandjean H. *Clin Exp Allergy* 2005; **35**: 167–72

BACKGROUND. A cross-sectional, descriptive, questionnaire-based survey was conducted in schools in Toulouse, France, to determine the prevalence of food allergies among schoolchildren. The first goal of the survey was to estimate the prevalence of food allergies. The second goal was to determine the main characteristics of the allergies. The questionnaires (3500) were distributed in 150 classes in eight schools. The return rate was 77.6% (2716).

INTERPRETATION. Of the 192 (7.0%) questionnaires with a 'yes' response (report of a food allergy), 182 were retained as reporting true food allergies (6.7%). The cumulative and point prevalences were 6.7% (95% CI 5.8–7.6) and 4.7% (95% CI 3.9–5.5), respectively. The point prevalences were 4.0% for the children aged 2–5 years, 6.8% for the children aged 6–10 years, and 3.4% for the children aged 11–14 years. The main foods reported as causing adverse reactions were cow milk (n = 29; 11.9%), eggs (n = 23; 9.4%), kiwi fruit (n = 22; 9.0%), peanuts (n = 20; 8.2%), fish (n = 19; 7.8%), tree nuts (n = 19; 7.8%) and shrimp (n = 13; 5.3%). The average age at which the allergies were detected was 3.4 ± 2.8 years (range 0.1–12 years). The clinical signs of the food allergies were cutaneous (n = 153; 62.7%), digestive (n = 74; 30.3%), respiratory (n = 17; 6.9%), and anaphylactic shock (n = 12; 4.9%).

Comment

Studies have estimated an overall prevalence of food allergy between 1.4% and 4% in the general population, and 6% in children under the age of 4. Recent studies have suggested that the prevalence of food allergies is on the rise. There is no international study that provides prevalence information on food allergies comparable to the International Study of Asthma and Allergies in Childhood. This French study may be a starting point and the results can be used to determine to what extent food allergies may increase. Of those with food allergy ($n = 182$), 79.7% were allergic to one, 12.6% to two and 7.7% to three or more types of food. In these children, 244 food items were reported to trigger an allergic reaction: 15.5% fish and shellfish, 11.9% cow milk, 11.9% exotic fruit, 9.4% eggs, 8.2% peanuts, and 7.8% tree nuts. Most of the clinical signs were cutaneous (62.7%), followed by gastrointestinal symptoms (30.3%). Of the food-allergic children, 25.4% outgrew their allergies; the proportion doing so was larger for children with milk (58.6%) or egg allergy (39.1%). No information was provided in this cross-sectional study about whether the children developed other allergic manifestations. This study documents the need for more food allergy studies.

Prenatal dichlorodiphenyldichloroethylene (DDE) and asthma in children

Sunyer J, Torrent M, Munoz-Ortiz L, *et al.* *Environ Health Perspect* 2005; **113**: 1787–90

BACKGROUND. The prevalence of asthma increases with increasing levels of DDE. However, the effect of early-life exposure, the fundamental window of exposure, is unknown. The investigators assessed the association of prenatal exposure to DDE and other organochlorine compounds with atopy and asthma during infancy. All women presenting for antenatal care in Menorca (Spain) over 12 months starting in mid-1997 were invited to take part in a longitudinal study; 482 children were subsequently enrolled and 468 (97.1%) provided complete outcome data up to the 4th year of the study. Prenatal exposure to organochlorine compounds was measured in cord serum in 405 (84%) children. Asthma was defined on the basis of wheezing at 4 years of age, persistent wheezing, or doctor-diagnosed asthma. They measured specific IgE against house dust mite, cat and grass in sera extracted at 4 years of age. DDE (median = 1.03 ng/ml) was detected in all children, as were hexachlorobenzene (0.68 ng/ml) and polychlorobiphenyls (0.69 ng/ml).

INTERPRETATION. Wheezing at 4 years of age increased with DDE concentration, particularly at the highest quartile (9% in the lowest quartile [<0.57 ng/ml] vs 19% in the highest quartile [1.90 ng/ml]; RR 2.63 [95% CI 1.19–4.69], adjusting for maternal asthma, breast-feeding, education, social class or other organochlorines). The association was not modified by IgE sensitization and occurred with the same strength among non-atopic subjects and among those with persistent wheezing or diagnosed asthma. DDE was not associated with atopy alone. Prenatal exposure to DDE residues may contribute to the development of asthma.

Comment

This follow-up study of children from birth to age 4 on the Balearic island of Menorca included 405 children, 84% of the children of mothers originally enrolled.

DDE is a metabolite of DDT; exposure occurs mainly through food, in particular fish, and in infants through breast-feeding. The study confirmed findings of a prior cross-sectional study in children [26,27]. However, the time window in this study focused on prenatal exposure. There are two pathways that may explain these associations: immunotoxic and endocrine-disrupting effects. Sex hormones have been related to a number of immune disorders and DDE has an endocrine-disrupting potential. Because the prevalence of asthma and allergies increased during the period when pesticides and organochlorines were accumulating in the food chain, future studies are necessary to evaluate these associations. The challenge, however, is the complex mix of protective and adverse factors, since pesticide exposure is also related to obesity, breast-feeding and farming.

Conclusion

Interesting old and new risk factors include breast-feeding, obesity, fish consumption, farm exposure and endocrine disruption. It is surprising that we do not yet understand why breast-feeding may protect against asthma but not AEDS. What are the protective immune constituents in breast milk? What are risk factors causing some studies to conclude that breast milk may increase the risk of atopic dermatitis? Two articles addressed the risks and benefits of breast-feeding.

Breast-feeding and obesity are related. Whereas there is some evidence that the lack of breast-feeding is a risk factor for obesity [28], to the best of my knowledge no obesity and asthma study has stratified for history of breast-feeding. An important question is whether the concurrent increase in obesity and asthma is just coincidence or whether increasing obesity explains the increasing prevalence of asthma. A study from New Zealand provides evidence that the two processes are independent.

Whereas results of observational studies have provided some evidence that diet and fish consumption, in particular the consumption of oily fish rich in n-3 polyunsaturated fatty acids, may protect against allergies and asthma, the findings of intervention studies are disappointing [24]. Are we misguided in advising the consumption of more fish, in particular during pregnancy?' In a number of countries, fish advisories suggest limiting fish consumption during pregnancy. What about allergies against fish? Should we rather consume non-polluted oil extracted from fish?

And finally, hygiene or hormones [29]? An increasing number of studies in the last year indicate that the endocrine system affects the immune and respiratory systems and subsequently the occurrence and severity of allergy and asthma [30]. Given these findings, the door is open for research on endocrine disruption by persistent organic pollutants such as pesticides and the development of allergy and asthma. However, investigations are only now beginning. Interestingly, this complex of research is related firstly to the farming controversy since the farming industry is a source of pesticides; secondly, it is related to the risk factor of obesity, since these chemical compounds are stored in adipose tissues; and thirdly it is related to the consumption of breast milk and fish, since both are sources of different persistent organic pollutants, as these biomagnify in the food chain. There is hope if explanations other than hygiene- or obesity-related concepts are given equal attention.

References

1. von Berlin-Heimendahl S, Brugge H. [Studies on the effect of environmental factors on the frequency of certain pediatric diseases. Comparative studies (1947–1965)]. *Munch Med Wochenschr* 1968; **110**: 662–9.
2. Jarvis D, Luczynska C, Chinn S, Potts J, Sunyer J, Janson C, Svanes C, Kunzli N, Leynaert B, Heinrich J, Kerkhof M, Ackermann-Liebrich U, Anto JM, Cerveri I, de Marco R, Gislason T, Neukirch F, Vermeire P, Wjst M, Burney P. Change in prevalence of IgE sensitization and mean total IgE with age and cohort. *J Allergy Clin Immunol* 2005; **116**: 675–82.
3. Ramsey CD, Celedon JC. The hygiene hypothesis and asthma. *Curr Opin Pulm Med* 2005; **11**: 14–20.
4. Gibbs S, Surridge H, Adamson R, Cohen B, Bentham G, Reading R. Atopic dermatitis and the hygiene hypothesis: a case–control study. *Int J Epidemiol* 2004; **33**: 199–207.
5. Benn CS, Melbye M, Wohlfahrt J, Bjorksten B, Aaby P. Cohort study of sibling effect, infectious diseases, and risk of atopic dermatitis during first 18 months of life. *BMJ* 2004; **328**: 1223.
6. Karmaus W, Arshad H, Mattes J. Does the sibling effect have its origin in utero? Investigating birth order, cord blood immunoglobulin E concentration, and allergic sensitization at age 4 years. *Am J Epidemiol* 2001; **154**: 909–15.
7. Devereux G, Barker RN, Seaton A. Antenatal determinants of neonatal immune responses to allergens. *Clin Exp Allergy* 2002; **32**: 43–50.
8. van Gool CJ, Thijs C, Dagnelie PC, Henquet CJ, van Houwelingen AC, Schrander J, Menheere PP, van den Brandt PA. Determinants of neonatal IgE level: parity, maternal age, birth season and perinatal essential fatty acid status in infants of atopic mothers. *Allergy* 2004; **59**: 961–8.
9. Maziak W, Behrens T, Brasky TM, Duhme H, Rzehak P, Weiland SK, Keil U. Are asthma and allergies in children and adolescents increasing? Results from ISAAC phase I and phase III surveys in Munster, Germany. *Allergy* 2003; **58**: 572–9.
10. Zollner IK, Weiland SK, Piechotowski I, Gabrio T, von Mutius E, Link B, Pfaff G, Kouros B, Wuthe J. No increase in the prevalence of asthma, allergies, and atopic sensitisation among children in Germany: 1992–2001. *Thorax* 2005; **60**: 545–8.

11. Wjst M, Dharmage S, Andre E, Norback D, Raherison C, Villani S, Manfreda J, Sunyer J, Jarvis D, Burney P, Svanes C. Latitude, birth date, and allergy. *PLoS Med* 2005; **2**: e294.

12. Friestad C, Pirkis J, Biehl M, Irwin CE Jr. Socioeconomic patterning of smoking, sedentary lifestyle, and overweight status among adolescents in Norway and the United States. *J Adolesc Health* 2003; **33**: 275–8.

13. Lund KE, Helgason AR. Environmental tobacco smoke in Norwegian homes, 1995 and 2001: changes in children's exposure and parents attitudes and health risk awareness. *Eur J Public Health* 2005; **15**: 123–7.

14. Riedler J, Braun-Fahrlander C, Eder W, Schreuer M, Waser M, Maisch S, Carr D, Schierl R, Nowak D, von Mutius E. Exposure to farming in early life and development of asthma and allergy: a cross-sectional survey. *Lancet* 2001; **358**: 1129–33.

15. Riedler J, Eder W, Oberfeld G, Schreuer M. Austrian children living on a farm have less hay fever, asthma and allergic sensitization. *Clin Exp Allergy* 2000; **30**: 194–200.

16. Chatzi L, Prokopakis E, Tzanakis N, Alegakis A, Bizakis I, Siafakas N, Lionis C. Allergic rhinitis, asthma, and atopy among grape farmers in a rural population in Crete, Greece. *Chest* 2005; **127**: 372–8.

17. Zekveld C, Bibakis I, Bibaki-Liakou V, Pedioti A, Dimitroulis I, Harris J, Newman Taylor AJ, Cullinan P. The effects of farming and birth order on asthma and allergies in rural Crete. *Eur Respir J* 2006 Feb 15; [Epub ahead of print].

18. Blanc P. End of the idyll: farming and the risk of occupational allergy. *Chest* 2005; **127**: 1087–8.

19. Eigenmann PA. Breast-feeding and atopic eczema dermatitis syndrome: protective or harmful? *Allergy* 2004; **59**(Suppl 78): 42–4.

20. Benn CS, Wohlfahrt J, Aaby P, Westergaard T, Benfeldt E, Michaelsen KF, Bjorksten B, Melbye M. Breast-feeding and risk of atopic dermatitis, by parental history of allergy, during the first 18 months of life. *Am J Epidemiol* 2004; **160**: 217–23.

21. Arshad SH. Primary prevention of asthma and allergy. *J Allergy Clin Immunol* 2005; **116**: 3–14; quiz 15.

22. Dabelea D, Hanson RL, Bennett PH, Roumain J, Knowler WC, Pettitt DJ. Increasing prevalence of Type II diabetes in American Indian children. *Diabetologia* 1998; **41**: 904–10.

23. Barr RG, Wentowski CC, Grodstein F, Somers SC, Stampfer MJ, Schwartz J, Speizer FE, Camargo CA Jr. Prospective study of postmenopausal hormone use and newly diagnosed asthma and chronic obstructive pulmonary disease. *Arch Intern Med* 2004; **164**: 379–86.

24. Devereux G, Seaton A. Diet as a risk factor for atopy and asthma. *J Allergy Clin Immunol* 2005; **115**: 1109–17; quiz 1118.

25. Dunstan JA, Prescott SL. Does fish oil supplementation in pregnancy reduce the risk of allergic disease in infants? *Curr Opin Allergy Clin Immunol* 2005; **5**: 215–21.

26. Karmaus W, Davis S, Chen Q, Kuehr J, Kruse H. Atopic manifestations, breast-feeding protection and the adverse effect of DDE. *Paediatr Perinat Epidemiol* 2003; **17**: 212–20.

27. Karmaus W, Kuehr J, Kruse H. Infections and atopic disorders in childhood and organochlorine exposure. *Arch Environ Health* 2001; **56**: 485–92.

28. Arenz S, von Kries R. Protective effect of breast-feeding against obesity in childhood: can a meta-analysis of observational studies help to validate the hypothesis? *Adv Exp Med Biol* 2005; **569**: 40–8.

29. Rangaraj S, Doull I. Hormones not hygiene? Birth order and atopy. *Clin Exp Allergy* 2003; **33**: 277–8.

30. Forbes L. Asthma and atopy: endocrine or metabolic conditions? *Thorax* 2005; **60**: 793–4.

2

Genetics of asthma and allergy

SUSAN EWART

Introduction

The manifestations of asthma and allergy are the result of both genetic predisposition and environmental factors. This relationship between genes and the environment is complex and has been the subject of intense investigation in recent years. The predisposition to asthma, unlike that to diseases determined by a single gene, is genetically complex. Consequently, it is thought that a number of genes, each with a relatively small contribution, collectively produce an individual's genetic susceptibility profile. This susceptibility profile is then acted upon by environmental factors to result in the phenotypic outcome; that is, the presence or absence of asthma and/or allergy. Because multiple risk factors affect the outcome, the task of identifying each individual genetic and environmental risk factor is daunting. However, in the light of recent advances in molecular techniques, genomics and bioinformatics, progress is being made to this end. Specifically, the ability to conduct large-scale automated genotyping of sequence variants that occur with high frequency, such as single-nucleotide polymorphisms (SNPs), has facilitated this progress.

The initial investigations into the genetics of asthma and allergy focused on asthma and its hallmark components, such as serum immunoglobulin (Ig) E levels, positivity in the skin-prick test, and bronchial hyper-responsiveness. To begin to identify genes contributing to these parameters, a study design commonly employed was that of the genome screen. This required large collections of multi-generation families, and only a limited number of such studies were conducted worldwide. However, these studies served the purpose of identifying genomic regions containing susceptibility genes for asthma. A number of different locations were indicated, and there was some repeatability of linkage to several areas, most commonly on chromosomes 5q, 6p, 11p, 12q and 13q. The next general step in the search for susceptibility genes has frequently been the use of genetic association studies to define specific genes. This study design is population-based and has the advantage of increased power.

This year in the literature a number of asthma and allergy genetic studies were reported. The goal of this article is to provide a representative overview of progress in several areas pertinent to the genetics of asthma and allergy. Novel asthma genes are discussed, and this is followed by a look at a commonly implicated

© Atlas Medical Publishing Ltd

chromosomal region, 5q. Other categories that are examined touch upon asthma and genes implicated in allergy as they relate to treatment methods, the pursuit of genes underlying atopic phenotypes other than asthma, and the influence of environmental factors as they interact with susceptibility genes.

Novel asthma genes

Characterization of a common susceptibility locus for asthma-related traits

Laitinen T, Polvi A, Rydman P, *et al. Science* 2004; **304**: 300–4

BACKGROUND. Genome-wide scans have pointed to a number of genomic regions implicated in asthma. This study used an elegant scheme to investigate chromosome 7p, which had been previously identified as containing susceptibility loci for asthma-related phenotypes. Positional cloning of asthma susceptibility genes was undertaken in the Kainuu subpopulation from Finland and two additional population samples from Quebec, Canada. A hierarchical gene mapping strategy was followed by identification of specific genes on the implicated DNA segment of chromosome 7. The predicted gene in humans was further investigated by RNA expression and immunohistochemical examination of human tissues and in mechanistic studies in a murine model of allergic asthma.

INTERPRETATION. A 133-kilobase risk-conferring segment on chromosome 7p was identified containing two previously undescribed genes, one of which was predicted to belong to the G-protein-coupled receptor family; hence it was named *GPRA* (for G-protein-coupled receptor for asthma susceptibility). Both genes displayed coding polymorphisms in the asthma susceptibility haplotype. *GPRA* RNA was expressed in a variety of tissues; the B isoform was increased in asthmatic bronchial epithelium and smooth muscle compared with controls. Expression of the mouse orthologue of *GPRA* (*Gpra*) was significantly upregulated in mouse lungs after ovalbumin exposure in sensitized mice compared with non-sensitized controls.

Comment

This article is the latest in a series of reports of positional cloning of asthma susceptibility genes, preceded by the positional cloning of the genes *ADAM33*, *PHF11* and *DPP10* [1–3]. The positional cloning approach begins with refined linkage to a defined DNA segment, followed by high-density genotype analyses through the linked region, and then gene identification supported by functional evidence of expression of the gene in appropriate tissues and/or mechanistic relevance. The strength of the positional cloning approach is that the supporting evidence is comprehensive and that gene identification is independent of prior assumptions.

The authors of this study subsequently published a replication study [4]. Replication was done using data from a Western European cross-sectional study and a Swedish birth cohort, with a total of almost 4000 subjects. In these populations they observed associations between childhood allergic disease and *GPR154* (alias *GPRA*) haplotypes. The specific risk haplotypes were not identical to those in the original report, suggesting a general role for this gene, but not specific alleles, in respiratory allergic disease. A replication study was also conducted by Kormann and colleagues in German children. They found that *GPRA* was associated with asthma, bronchial hyper-responsiveness and, to a lesser extent, IgE levels [5]. These replication studies provide an important bolster of the evidence supporting a role for the involvement of *GPRA* (*GPR154*) in asthma and related phenotypes.

Contribution of *ADAM33* polymorphisms to the population risk of asthma

Blakey J, Halapi E, Bjornsdottir US, *et al.* *Thorax* 2005; **60**: 274–6

BACKGROUND. Although *ADAM33* was the first gene identified by positional cloning to underlie the risk of asthma, attempts to replicate the original results have had inconsistent results. In this report, the authors aim to clarify the role of *ADAM33* in asthma by expanding the size of the informative populations and cumulatively analysing data from relevant published studies. *ADAM33* SNPs were genotyped in 60 nuclear families from England recruited from an asthma outpatient clinic, as well as 348 unrelated asthma cases and 262 non-asthmatic controls in an Icelandic population. In addition, data from six previously performed case–control and transmission disequilibrium studies of *ADAM33* and asthma were combined and subjected to meta-analysis.

INTERPRETATION. The total data from the six previous reports and the two populations genotyped in this report included 1299 cases, 1665 controls and 4561 individuals in family studies, collectively a much larger data set than provided by any of the single studies. When taken in isolation, no association of any SNP variant was significant in the Icelandic population. However, four of 13 SNPs were significantly associated with asthma in the combined meta-analysis. Similarly, while no SNPs were significantly over-transmitted in the English population alone, the combined analysis performed on all available family-based data indicated that four SNPs were transmitted more commonly to subjects with asthma. Two *ADAM33* SNPs, F+1 and ST+7, were significantly associated with asthma in both the combined analysis of the case–control and the family-based transmission disequilibrium studies. These two polymorphisms were in tight linkage disequilibrium ($D' = 0.965$).

Comment

This study highlights the issue of sample size in association analyses. Indeed, sample size is one of the driving issues that led to editorial guidelines aimed at ensuring the validity of published genetic association studies [6]. Study populations that contain a small number of subjects may be underpowered to detect genetic associations in complex genetic diseases, such as asthma and allergy. Along with sample size, the relative risk of the disease under study and the allele frequency of each variant examined also affect the required sample size. The concern of an underpowered study is the potential for deriving false-negative conclusions; if power is inadequate to detect an association, true associations may be missed. The authors of this study propose that this occurred in the analysis of data from their Icelandic and English populations, which showed no associations when analysed in isolation. However, it is interesting to note that in the six other populations in their meta-analysis, only two (Puerto Rican and Mexican) reported lack of association in the original studies [7].

Another concern frequently raised regarding methodological approaches to genetic association studies is that of multiple testing [6]. This can have the opposite effect of underpowered studies in that multiple testing can lead to false-positive results. Studies of asthma and related phenotypes frequently involve multiple phenotypes tested for associations with multiple polymorphisms; consequently, corrections in the significance levels for multiple comparisons must be made. Thus, small sample size and multiple testing have surely been factors contributing to the inconsistent results frequently observed in studies on the genetics of asthma. Analysis of combined data sets, as was performed in this study, help to identify genes that truly contribute to susceptibility to asthma.

Chromosome 5q revisited

One of the earliest chromosomal regions to be implicated in asthma and allergy was chromosome 5q31–33. This location is rich in genes that are logical candidates for contributing to asthma and allergy phenotypes, and its original identification in 1994 generated much enthusiasm [8,9]. Genes of interest, termed 'positional candidate genes' when supported by both linkage location and mechanistic relevance, on chromosome 5q were known to include the β_2-adrenergic receptor (*ADBR2*) gene and the cytokine gene cluster containing genes for interleukin (IL)-3, IL-4, IL-5, IL-12 and IL-13. However, further studies of these genes failed to reveal functional sequence variants as definitively causing the phenotypes. Additionally, while over time chromosome 5q has been one of the most consistently replicated regions, its initial identification was followed by reports of asthma linkages to more and different chromosome regions. Thus, enthusiasm for the genes on chromosome 5q suffered with the growing pains of the field of asthma genetics. However, in recent times the focus has returned to chromosome 5q, as is seen in the following reports.

Functional haplotypes of *IL-12B* are associated with childhood atopic asthma

Hirota T, Suzuki Y, Hasegawa K, *et al. J Allergy Clin Immunol* 2005; **116**: 789–95

Background. Increasing evidence demonstrates that cytokines of Th1 and Th2 cells play important roles in allergic disorders. This study examined polymorphisms in the *IL-12B* gene, a primary inducer of the development of Th1 cells with downregulation of the Th2 cytokines. The exons, splice sites and portions of the 5′ and 3′ flanking regions of the *IL-12B* gene were sequenced and 13 polymorphisms identified. A case–control study of Japanese children (297 cases) with asthma stratified by asthma-related phenotypes was conducted on a subset of three of these SNPs. The functional effects of the identified polymorphisms were examined using luciferase and RNA stability assays.

Interpretation. The study shows a significant association between the 3′ untranslated region (UTR) polymorphism of the *IL-12B* gene and childhood atopic asthma. A promoter polymorphism also showed marginal association. Haplotypes constructed from these two SNPs were also associated with atopic asthma. Examination of the expression of the *IL-12B* promoter polymorphism by luciferase reporter constructs revealed that the GC allele had 2.4-fold higher luciferase activity than the alternative allele with potential relevance to differential transcriptional activity between the alleles. Similarly, RNA from the susceptibility allele in the 3′ UTR was more stable than RNA cloned from the alternative variant, suggesting that the 3′ UTR contributes to RNA stability.

Comment

The *IL-12B* gene is located on chromosome 5q31.1–q33.1 and encodes the p40 monomer, which is a component of four secreted proteins (IL-12, IL-23, p80 homodimer and p40 monomer), each having important roles in the development of asthma and the allergy phenotypes. Several groups have recently reported on *IL-12B* gene associations with asthma. Randolph and colleagues examined both adult and paediatric US Caucasian populations and found *IL-12B* associations with asthma, asthma severity and atopy phenotypes [10]. However, the specific variants associating with asthma and related phenotypes were not polymorphic in the above study by Hirota and colleagues. In an earlier study, Morahan *et al.* identified an association of *IL-12B* promoter polymorphism with asthma phenotypes, including asthma severity, in Australians from Perth [11]. Hirota's results confirm this association of promoter polymorphism with asthma, but not its severity. Another study in Melbourne, Australia, that examined this promoter polymorphism, found a relationship between the promoter genotype and lung function in females, but failed to identify an association with asthma severity [12]. In summary, there appear to be multiple studies that support a relationship between the *IL-12B* gene and asthma, but genetic heterogeneity between populations may be an important factor to consider.

Genetic variants of the T-cell immunoglobulin mucin 1 but not the T-cell immunoglobulin mucin 3 gene are associated with asthma in an African-American population

Gao P-S, Mathias RA, Plunkett B, *et al. J Allergy Clin Immunol* 2005; **115**: 982–8

BACKGROUND. The T-cell Ig domain and mucin domain (TIM) proteins, the genes for which are located on chromosome 5q, have been suggested to be involved in allergic disease. This study examined the genetic association of sequence variants of the *TIM1* and *TIM3* genes in an African-American population. Case–control and family-based association analyses were performed for three SNPs each in the *TIM1* and *TIM3* genes, and an insertion/deletion polymorphism in *TIM1*. African-American case–parent trios (*n* = 89) ascertained through asthmatic probands or sib pairs were examined. In the case-control design, 89 unrelated individuals were selected among the African-American families together with 95 randomly selected normal healthy individuals.

INTERPRETATION. In the case–control studies, the minor allele variant of the *TIM1* gene SNP rs2277025 and the deletion variant (157delMTTTVP) were more frequent in patients with asthma than in controls. Variant 157delMTTTVP was also associated with asthma in the family-based analysis, but the SNPs were not. These associations were not dependent on hepatitis A exposure status. None of the three polymorphisms in the *TIM3* gene yielded significant association with asthma or asthma-related phenotypes. This suggests that the genetic variants of *TIM1*, but not *TIM3*, contribute to susceptibility to asthma in the African-American population studied.

Comment

The genetic polymorphisms studied in the *TIM1* gene contributed to asthma susceptibility in this African-American population. TIM-1 is a member of the T-cell immunoglobulin domain and mucin domain family of proteins and it serves as the cellular receptor for the hepatitis A virus. The TIM-1 extracellular mucin-like domain containing the 157ins/delMTTTVP polymorphism is important in both the atopic immune response as well as the uncoating of the hepatitis A virus. Previous evidence suggested a link between these two functions as infection by hepatitis A virus was associated with protection against atopy in individuals with the insertion variant 157insMTTTVP [**13**]. However, the relationship between *TIM1* and asthma in this study was demonstrated to be independent of hepatitis A virus infection status. However, it should be noted that the limited sample size of subjects seropositive for hepatitis A virus (*n* = 28; only two subjects with asthma were seropositive) precludes the complete analysis of the relationship between *TIM1*, hepatitis A exposure and asthma. In addition to the evaluation of individual polymorphisms, haplotype analysis was performed. One *TIM1* haplotype and one *TIM1–TIM3* combined haplotype were associated with asthma in case–control pairs and case–parent trios (Table 2.1). These findings suggest that additional variants in this region or in linkage disequilibrium with this region may also be involved in asthma.

As is common in asthma genetics, several groups have tried to replicate the initial findings of association between *TIM* genes and asthma [14]. Graves and colleagues found *TIM1* polymorphisms to be significantly related to atopy and eczema in the Tucson Children's Respiratory Study in both cross-sectional and longitudinal analyses [15]. Information regarding the seroprevalence of hepatitis A virus was not available in this population. In contrast to the study by Gao and colleagues, Graves *et al.* found significant associations of atopy with SNPs in *TIM3*. They also found an association with the 5' region of the neighbouring gene *ITK*, which was not examined by Gao and colleagues. The identification of an association with the *ITK* gene is interesting in the light of the increased association of a *TIM1–TIM3* haplotype in the African-American population, as *ITK* may be the nearby gene contributing to this result. Although the associations with atopy

Table 2.1 Association of *TIM1*, *TIM3* and *TIM1–TIM3* haplotypes with asthma in an African-American population (89 subjects with asthma, 95 controls)

Gene	Haplotype	Asthma (%)	Control (%)	Odds ratio	*P*-value	Omnibus likelihood ratio test
	C-G-ins-G	40.0	51.6	0.63	0.017	
	T-G-del-G	20.8	9.6	2.48	0.004	
TIM1	T-G-ins-G	9.2	8.9	1.04	0.923	0.073
	C-G-del-G	7.5	8.6	0.87	0.740	
	T-G-del-T	8.0	9.7	0.81	0.528	
	T-T-ins-G	10.1	9.8	1.03	0.925	
	A-C-C	55.6	49.2	1.29	0.139	
	G-C-C	11.5	15.2	0.72	0.421	
TIM3	G-C-T	14.2	15.7	0.89	0.501	0.812
	A-C-T	7.8	9.3	0.82	0.544	
	G-G-C	7.9	6.2	1.29	0.365	
	C-G-ins-G-A-C-C	28.7	34.3	0.77	0.240	
	T-G-del-G-A-C-C	11.2	0	0	0.001	
	T-G-ins-G-A-C-C	3.5	2.6	1.38	0.760	
TIM1–TIM3	C-G-ins-G-G-C-C	1.4	8.1	0.16	0.040	0.406
	C-G-ins-G-G-C-T	6.2	6.1	1.05	0.928	
	C-G-del-G-A-C-C	4.4	6.6	0.66	0.581	
	T-G-del-T-A-C-C	5.1	6.8	0.73	0.565	
	T-G-del-G-G-C-T	5.5	2.5	2.18	0.410	

Haplotypes were analysed for association with asthma in the African-American population. The programme SNPEM was used to generate the haplotypes and their *P*-values, both overall (omnibus likelihood ratio test) and specific. Source: Gao *et al.* (2005).

were consistent across this gene region, no relationships were identified with asthma. Thus, these reports are of associations of related, but not identical, phenotypes.

Positional identification of an asthma susceptibility gene on human chromosome 5q33

Noguchi E, Yokouchi Y, Zhang J, *et al. Am J Respir Crit Care Med* 2005; **172**: 183–8

BACKGROUND. A previous genome-wide screen for mite-sensitive atopic asthma in Japanese families indicated linkage to chromosome 5q33. To identify underlying susceptibility genes, targeted mutational screening and association analyses were performed in this study. Twenty-six genes in a 9.4 Mb region of chromosome 5q were screened. On the basis of finding associations with SNPs in the cytoplasmic fragile X mental retardation protein-interacting protein 2 gene (*CYFIP2*), additional polymorphisms in this gene were analysed, *CYFIP2* tissue expression was examined, and electromobility shift assays were performed to determine the functional significance of *CYFIP2* variants.

INTERPRETATION. A transmission disequilibrium test analysis of 105 polymorphisms in 155 families (538 members) revealed variants in the *CYFIP2* gene associated with asthma. Six variants in *CYFIP2* were in complete linkage disequilibrium, and strong linkage disequilibrium extended to a region containing the *ITK* gene (Fig. 2.1). *CYFIP2* expression was strong in a variety of tissues, including lymph nodes and lymphocytes. Interestingly, expression was higher in resting cells than in activated cells and higher in undifferentiated cells than in differentiated cells. Nuclear protein binding differences were detected associated with a polymorphism of intron 1 of *CYFIP2*.

Comment

While the contributions to susceptibility to asthma of a number of genes in the chromosome 5q region are supported by linkage and association studies, the identification of *CYFIP2* as an asthma susceptibility locus was unexpected. The genetic evidence supporting *CYFIP2* is based on both linkage and association (Fig. 2.1) and is bolstered by the additional gene expression and electromobility shift assay studies conducted. While it is unclear how *CYFIP2* may contribute to

Fig. 2.1 (opposite) (a) Maximum logarithm of the odds score (MLS) plot for asthma on human chromosome 5q33 in 47 families with asthma identified through children with mite-sensitive asthma. (b) Results of a transmission disequilibrium test in the 95% confidence interval for the location of the asthma susceptibility gene for 155 families with asthma. *Y axis*, $-\log_{10}$ (*P*-value); *X axis*, location in megabases (Mb). (c) Pairwise linkage disequilibrium between polymorphisms in a 0.8 Mb region as measured by *D'* in 155 families with asthma. Shaded areas show strong linkage disequilibrium. Source: Noguchi *et al.* (2005).

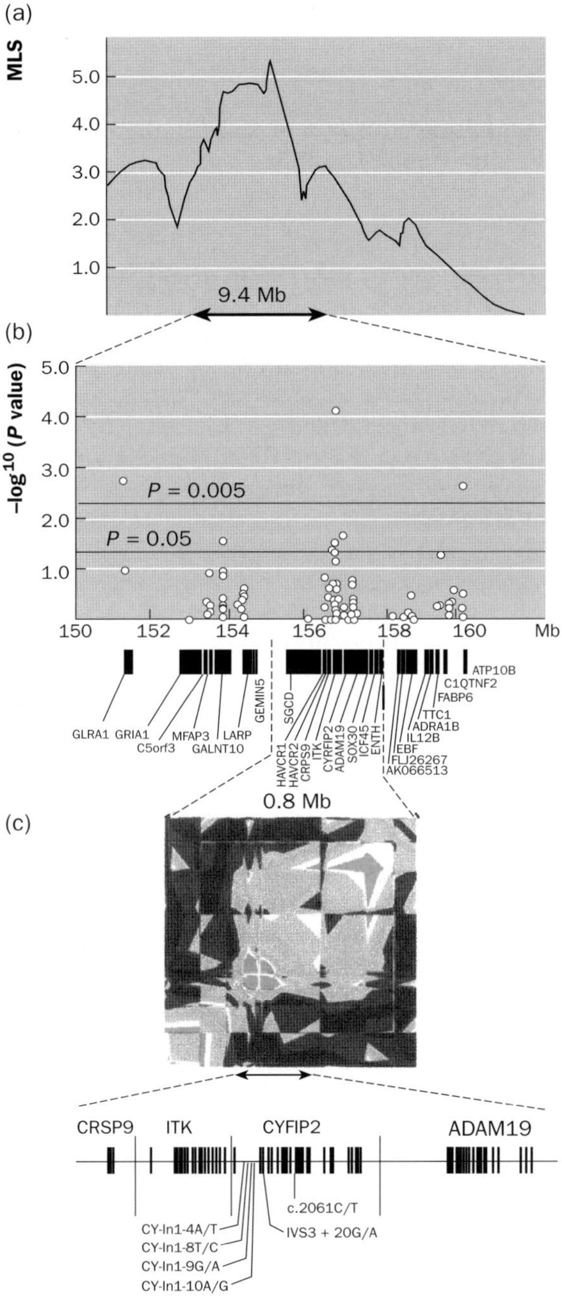
(a)
MLS
5.0
4.0
3.0
2.0
1.0
9.4 Mb
(b)
-log10 (P value)
P = 0.005
P = 0.05
150 152 154 156 158 160 Mb
GLRA1 GRIA1
C5orf3
MFAP3
GALNT10
LARP
GEMIN5
SGCD
HAVCR1
HAVCR2
CRPS9
ITK
CYRFIP2
ADAM19
SOX30
ICF45
ENTH
AK066513
FLJ26267
EBF
IL12B
ADRA1B
TTC1
FABP6
C1QTNF2
ATP10B
0.8 Mb
(c)
CRSP9
ITK
CYFIP2
ADAM19
c.2061C/T
IVS3 + 20G/A
CY-In1-4A/T
CY-In1-8T/C
CY-In1-9G/A
CY-In1-10A/G

asthma, recent positional cloning studies identifying the genes *ADAM33*, *PHF11*, *DPP10* and *GPRA* have underscored the fact that we may not be able to predict accurately all the genes underlying complex phenotypes such as asthma and allergy.

From the studies described in this section, it is clear that the relationship of genes in the chromosome 5q31–33 region with asthma and related phenotypes is complex and there is need for more work to understand these relationships. The genes *TIM1* (alias *HAVCR1*), *TIM3* (alias *HAVCR2*), *ITK* and *CYFIP2* are in close physical proximity (Fig. 2.1) and all have been implicated, individually or in combination, by recent studies. The finding of significant associations with several genes in a block suggests the potential for regional regulation of gene expression relating to asthma. For example, differentially methylated domains may imprint large gene clusters and subsequently exert regional control over gene expression. Further studies in this area are likely to improve our understanding of the interrelationship between the multiple genes in the chromosome 5q region for which there is evidence of involvement in susceptibility to asthma and allergy.

Pharmacogenetics

TBX21: A functional variant predicts improvement in asthma with the use of inhaled corticosteroids

Tantisira KG, Hwang ES, Raby BA, *et al. Proc Natl Acad Sci USA* 2004; **101**: 18099–104

BACKGROUND. The T-bet (T-box 21) gene (*TBX21*) encodes a transcription factor, T-box expressed in T cells, which has been implicated in asthma through its role in Th1 cell induction. Subjects in the Caucasian subset of the Childhood Asthma Management Program (CAMP) were genotyped for a non-synonymous *TBX21* SNP, H33Q. Comparisons between the wild-type and heterozygous H33Q alleles were performed by luciferase activity assay and by studying the ability to control cytokine function in cell culture. The effect of corticosteroids on T-bet expression was determined in human peripheral blood CD4-positive cells.

INTERPRETATION. Children with a copy of the minor allele (glutamine, Q) variant at SNP H33Q who were randomized to the steroid treatment group had improved airway responsiveness (as measured by PC_{20} [provocative concentration of methacholine required to produce a 20% fall in forced expiratory volume in 1 s (FEV_1)]) over time compared with those homozygous for the wild-type (histidine, H) allele (Fig. 2.2). Murine T-bet$^{-/-}$ T cells transfected with wild-type or variant *TBX21* expressed interferon-γ (IFN-γ) and repression of Th2 cytokines, with no difference between the alleles. Furthermore, corticosteroids inhibited the induction of T-bet expression in human CD4-positive T cells.

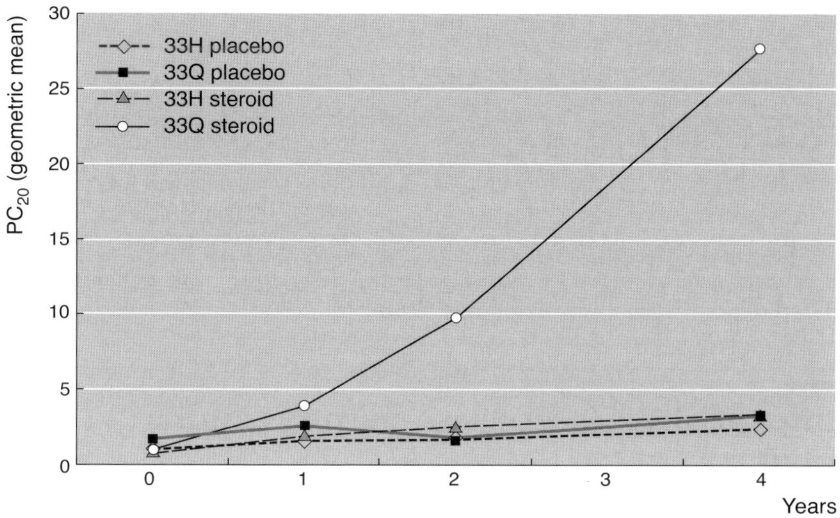

Fig. 2.2 Geometric mean value of PC_{20} at various time points over the 4-year follow-up, stratified by treatment group assignment and H33Q genotype. The mean PC_{20} of individuals on corticosteroids who also possessed a copy of the 33Q variant improved significantly by the end of the first year of the study and continued to improve substantially with time and corticosteroid use. The mean PC_{20} value at 4 years is within the range normally ascribed to individuals without the diagnosis of asthma. Source: Tantisira *et al.* (2004).

Comment

T-bet is a crucial regulator of Th1 lineage cells and IFN-γ production. Murine studies have provided strong evidence that *TBX21* confers susceptibility to asthma-related traits, as T-bet-deficient mice develop spontaneous airway hyper-responsiveness |**16**|. However, less is known about the role of genetic variation in *TBX21*, located on human chromosome 17q21, in the development of human asthma. This pharmacogenetic study examined the relationship between the *TBX21* gene and the response to a common treatment for asthma, inhaled corticosteroids. Such gene–environment interaction studies are important for downstream pharmacogenetic applications. A significant interaction was found to predict improvement in the PC_{20} (a measure of airway responsiveness) in children randomized to the inhaled corticosteroid treatment group (Fig. 2.2). However, the two alleles of the examined variant were equally effective in inducing Th1 characteristics in cell culture. One limitation of this study was the small sample size. The frequency of the minor allele (33Q) was low (4.5%), so the authors observed only a few heterozygotes and no individuals homozygous for the minor allele. Further experiments confirmed the link between *TBX21* and steroids, as the presence of dexamethasone inhibited the expression of *TBX21* in cultured human T cells. The specific role of the T-bet genotype at H33Q was not examined in this experiment.

A subsequent study by this group examined 16 SNP variants in the *TBX21* gene and identified a genetic association between one SNP (c.-7947) and asthma [17]. Airway hyper-responsiveness was also associated with SNP c.-7947 and three others in *TBX21*. This follow-up study also used subjects from the Childhood Asthma Management Program study; however, a family-based association of nuclear families was conducted with replication in a second population of adult males. Associations with atopic phenotypes were not detected. Several other groups failed to demonstrate a relationship between T-bet and asthma or related phenotypes when different populations were examined [18,19].

Genetics of allergic disease—beyond asthma

Most studies of genetic susceptibility to allergic disease have focused on asthma or asthma-related phenotypes, but there has been a growing number of reports on genetic susceptibility to other atopic diseases, such as atopic dermatitis, allergic rhinitis and food allergy, as well as atopy itself. As these outcomes are clearly not entirely independent of one another, the overlap between their genetic underpinnings may lead to interesting results about the basic mechanisms underlying atopy and atopic diseases as a whole.

A genome-wide screen on the genetics of atopy in a multiethnic European population reveals a major atopy locus on chromosome 3q21.3

Kurz T, Altmueller J, Strauch K, *et al. Allergy* 2005; **60**: 192–9

Background. This study examined the genetic basis of sensitization to house dust mite allergens. A genome scan was conducted using 603 microsatellite markers in 82 nuclear families (366 individuals) of German, British and Portuguese origin with at least two affected siblings. Sensitization to *Dermatophagoides pteronyssinus* was assessed by determining specific IgE antibody levels detected by immunochemiluminometric immunosorbent assay and categorized as positive or negative relative to a pre-determined cut-off point.

Interpretation. The population examined in this study had been used previously in a genome screen study. In this study both parametric and non-parametric models for linkage analysis were tested. Three novel regions were significantly associated with dust mite sensitization; chromosomes 2p12, 3q21.3 and 16q21. The 3q21.3 region obtained the highest significance, and has been found by others to be linked to the atopic dermatitis phenotype.

Comment

Through genetic examination of a specific trait, often referred to as an intermediate phenotype such as sensitization to house dust mites, novel chromosomal regions are described. The specific location of the linkages identified herein on chromosomes 2 and 3 had not been reported previously in relation to asthma- or atopy-related traits, although neighbouring chromosomal bands have been linked to specific IgE (2p13) [20], total IgE, atopy and asthma (16q23) [21]. Although the authors propose that the 2p12 and 16q21 linkages may be unique to allergic sensitization, they rightfully consider the possibility that the loci might be the same as those reported on 2p13 and 16q23, respectively. It is interesting to note that the linkage to 3q21 was associated with paternal imprinting, and an atopic dermatitis locus mapping here, reported previously, was also under paternal imprinting [22]. Thus, it seems likely to be the same locus, which underscores the relationship between allergic sensitization, as an intermediate phenotype, and atopic dermatitis. The authors break with tradition in the field of asthma genetic data analysis as they used the MOD score analysis, in which log of the odds (LOD) scores are maximized with respect to disease model parameters. This approach is used more for other complex genetic diseases, such as diabetes, than it has been for asthma. MOD score analysis has the advantage of minimizing type II error, so it is conservative. In summary, the findings reported by Kurz and colleagues support the notion that although atopy, allergic asthma, allergic rhinitis and atopic dermatitis are distinct traits, they are genetically closely related diseases concerning the atopic basis of the traits.

Genome screen in the French EGEA study: detection of linked regions shared or not shared by allergic rhinitis and asthma

Dizier M-H, Bouzigon E, Guilloud-Bataille M, *et al. Genes Immun* 2005; **6**: 95–102

BACKGROUND. Allergic rhinitis and asthma are common comorbidities. Like asthma, the presence of a genetic component in allergic rhinitis has been well established. To identify genetic linkage regions unique to allergic rhinitis, as well as those shared by allergic rhinitis and asthma, a genome screen study was conducted. A total of 295 families in the French Epidemiological Study on the Genetics and Environment of Asthma (EGEA) containing 1317 subjects were genotyped for 396 microsatellite markers. The families included had two siblings with DNA available and at least one asthmatic subject. Three definitions of allergic rhinitis were used, two binary and one categorical. To investigate linkages specific to allergic rhinitis (without asthma), linkage analyses were also conducted in 185 families with at most one asthmatic sib.

INTERPRETATION. A strong relationship was identified between the presence of allergic rhinitis and asthma, as 74 and 82% of subjects with allergic rhinitis (binary definitions 1 and 2, respectively) also had asthma. Genetic linkage to chromosome 1p31 was obtained with the combined phenotype allergic rhinitis and asthma; weaker evidence of linkage to this area was seen when allergic rhinitis and asthma were analysed as separate phenotypes. Linkages for allergic rhinitis alone were identified on chromosomes 2q32 (binary definition) and 3p24 (categorical definition). The allergic rhinitis linkages to chromosomes 2q and 3p were further confirmed by the analysis of 185 families without asthmatic sibships (at most one asthmatic sib). Two additional regions, chromosome 9p22 and 9q22, were linked to allergic rhinitis in the analysis restricted to families without asthma sibships.

Comment

This study is the first genome screen for asthma and allergic rhinitis analysed concurrently. It is the third genome scan for allergic rhinitis and it is applied to a larger sample than previous scans. The linkages observed in this study to chromosomes 9q and 2q replicate findings in previous reports in Japanese |**23**| and Danish populations |**24**|, respectively.

The importance of this study is its concurrent examination of related phenotypes—asthma and allergic rhinitis. It is apparent that the varied manifestations of allergy, such as allergic rhinitis, atopic dermatitis and allergic asthma, are closely tied to one another. The intermediate phenotypes that define atopy, elevated serum IgE or positivity in the skin-prick test, are shared by these diseases, and immune dysregulation in the form of chronic Th2-cell-driven inflammation is a common characteristic. On the basis of these observations it has been postulated that one set of susceptibility genes may underlie the basic immune dysregulation of allergy, while other genes may determine the target organ in which the immune dysregulation is manifested. Thus, studies that identify and compare susceptibility loci between allergic rhinitis, atopic dermatitis and/or asthma are crucial in advancing our understanding of the allergic disease process.

A topic that is of paramount importance in the successful identification of susceptibility loci is the accuracy of the diagnosis or phenotype description. This issue is highlighted in the present study as three questionnaire-based definitions of allergic rhinitis are used and the results vary between the three definitions. The first binary definition is based on the response to questions regarding the diagnosis of allergic rhinitis while the second is based on the presence of symptoms. Scores for the categorical diagnosis of allergic rhinitis were divided into categories, the structure of which was dependent on the number of subjects in each class. On the basis of the significance thresholds applied by the authors, no significant linkage was common to the three allergic rhinitis definitions. These findings underscore the importance of the phenotype definition and indicate the need for careful consideration of classification criteria.

Gene–environment interactions

Although elucidation of the genetic pathways leading to asthma, allergy and atopy is ongoing, perhaps more useful information for today's health professionals may be obtained by studying the relationship between the genes that have been implicated and the environmental exposures that alter the disease risk in genetically susceptible individuals. Any number of factors could conceivably interact with genes to alter asthma and allergy outcomes, including exposure to tobacco smoke (direct and passive), animals, pathogens and allergens, to name a few. Ventures into the area of gene–environment interactions are in their infancy in the field of asthma genetics and arguably it is this area in which the field is poised to make the most rapid progress.

Gene–environment interaction effects on the development of immune responses in the 1st year of life

Hoffjan S, Nicolae D, Ostrovnaya I, *et al. Am J Hum Genet* 2005; **76**: 696–704

BACKGROUND. Asthma is characterized by Th2-dominant cytokine profiles. The risk of developing asthma is lower in children attending day care in the first year of life. Therefore, this study was conducted to assess the interaction between day-care attendance, T-cell cytokine profiles and atopic phenotypes in early childhood. Children ($n = 208$) in the Childhood Onset of Asthma (COAST) study were genotyped for 72 polymorphisms in 45 immune response genes. The COAST cohort was selected on the basis of a high risk of asthma. Measurements of IFN-γ (Th1), IL-5 and IL-13 (Th2), and IL-10 (Treg) were made at birth and at age 1 year and the children were stratified by day-care attendance. Wheeze and atopic dermatitis phenotypes were documented in the first year.

INTERPRETATION. Sixteen polymorphisms at ten loci revealed 22 significant interactions on cytokine profiles and/or atopic phenotypes. Six interactions (at four polymorphisms in three loci) with day care had a significant effect ($P<0.001$) on early-life immune phenotypes; the false discovery rate was 33% for results with $P<0.001$, so four of these six results were predicted to be true. Polymorphisms of the genes *NOS3*, *FECR1B* and *IL-4RA* were significantly associated with multiple phenotypes and had at least one interaction with $P<0.001$. The day-care effect at some loci was due to increased viral infections in subjects attending day care; however, interactions at the *NOS3* locus were independent of viral infections.

Comment

This study is valuable in highlighting the importance of considering environmental risk factors in genetic analysis. It identified significant gene–environment interactions that influence the early patterning of the immune system and perhaps the subsequent development of asthma and atopic phenotypes. Several interactions of interest were identified; for example, children with the Asp/Asp genotype at the *NOS3*-922 polymorphism who attended day care had large *decreases* in Th2 cytokine responsiveness in year 1, whereas Th2 cytokine responsiveness *increased* in children with this same genotype who did not attend day care (Fig. 2.3). Similar interaction results were obtained for the Glu/Gly genotype at *FCER1B* as day-care attendance decreased IL-5 responses and no day care was associated with increased IL-5.

A number of factors common to day-care settings may be responsible for the environmental interaction terms identified in this study. Viral infections occur with increased frequency when young children commingle and a history of early childhood viral respiratory infections is a risk factor for asthma later in life. Thus, covariate analysis was performed to determine the role of viral infections in these interactions; the number of viral infections and the occurrence of respiratory syncytial virus and rhinovirus infections were used as covariates. Additionally, day care or older siblings was also used as a covariate. The effects of day-care attendance on Th2 cytokine profiles of children with specific *NOS3* alleles was not due to increased viral infections of children attending day care. In contrast, the interactive effects of day care and *FCER1B* on IL-5 profiles as well as day care and *IL-4RA* on IFN-γ responses was due to increased numbers of viral infections in children attending day care.

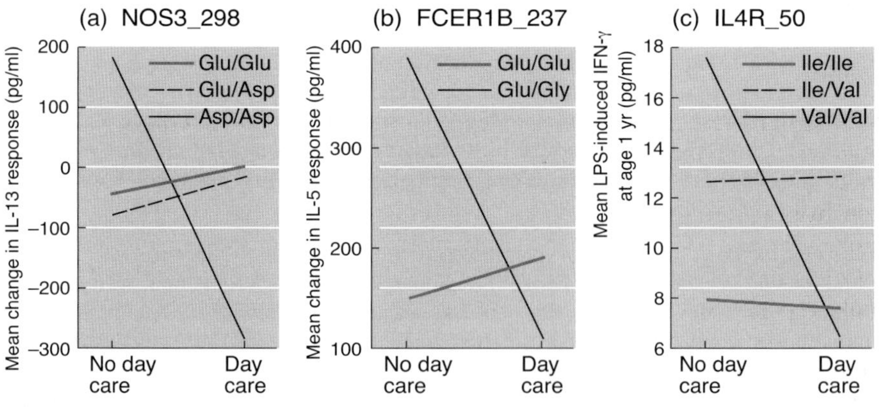

Fig. 2.3 Interaction plots of representative associations between immunological phenotypes, genotypes and day care. Untransformed cytokine values are shown. Source: Hoffjan *et al.* (2005).

Genome screen for asthma and bronchial hyper-responsiveness: interactions with passive smoke exposure

Meyers DA, Postma DS, Stine OC, *et al. J Allergy Clin Immunol* 2005; **115**: 1169–75

BACKGROUND. This study sought to determine the influence of passive exposure to tobacco smoke during childhood on the results of genetic linkage analyses for asthma. A genome-wide linkage screen for asthma and bronchial hyper-responsiveness was performed in 200 families (containing 1183 individuals) from The Netherlands. A set of 266 polymorphic autosomal markers was used. Analyses were performed separately for the entire population and for the smoking-exposed and non-exposed families separately.

INTERPRETATION. Linkages for asthma and bronchial hyper-responsiveness were observed on chromosomes 3p and 5q (Fig. 2.4). The 5q linkages were entirely dependent on exposure to tobacco smoke, with LOD scores of 3.77 for bronchial hyper-responsiveness and 2.54 for asthma in the smoke-exposed families. In contrast, LOD scores in non-exposed families were 0.18 and 0.15 for bronchial hyper-responsiveness and asthma, respectively. The trends were similar but less dramatic on chromosome 3p as the differences in LOD scores between the smoke-exposed and non-exposed groups were smaller. Conversely, chromosome 19 was linked to both asthma and bronchial hyper-responsiveness in non-exposed families, with no evidence for linkage in the smoke-exposed families.

Comment

Significant gene–environment interactions were detected in this study. Indeed, smoke exposure seemed to be crucial for the linkages on chromosome 5q in particular, as there was essentially no relationship between this region and asthma or bronchial hyper-responsiveness phenotypes in the families not exposed to tobacco smoke (Fig. 2.4). The results of this study are consistent with a previous report by Colilla and colleagues in which asthma linkage to chromosome 5q was affected by smoke exposure status in US Caucasian families [25]. These findings are particularly interesting since linkages to chromosome 5q have been detected in numerous studies without regard to smoke exposure status. Based on the strong and consistent results of the studies of Meyers and Colilla, it would be interesting to look more closely at the epidemiological factors that may modulate this gene–environment interaction. Additional factors that could be examined in future studies include the age and extent of environmental tobacco smoke (ETS) exposure during childhood. Specifically, gestational exposure to tobacco smoke via maternal smoking during pregnancy may have a larger impact on the disease outcome. Thus, while extensive work remains to be done in the study of gene–environment interactions in asthma, this report clearly establishes that changes in environment, in this case exposure to smoke, can interact with genetic profiles to alter the risk of the development of disease.

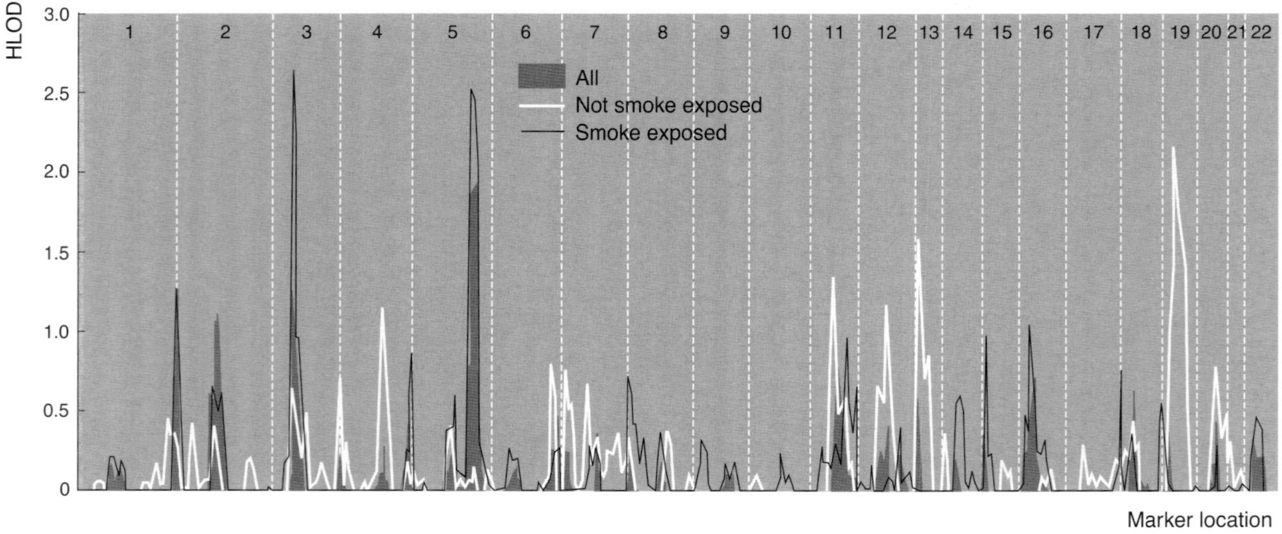

Fig. 2.4 The results of the genome-wide screen for asthma are shown for each chromosome, with the LOD score from the total 200 Dutch families and from the families classified with and without passive cigarette smoke exposure to the children in early life. Source: Meyers *et al.* (2005).

CD14 tobacco gene–environment interaction modifies asthma severity and immunoglobulin E levels in Latinos with asthma

Choudhry S, Avila PC, Nazario S, *et al. Am J Respir Crit Care Med* 2005; **172**: 173–82

BACKGROUND. CD14 is part of the receptor complex for endotoxin, which is a component of tobacco smoke. The *CD14* gene is located on chromosome 5q, a region previously demonstrated to be linked to asthma when stratified for smoke exposure. This study was designed to extend these findings by determining whether polymorphisms in the *CD14* gene are related to this gene–environment interaction on asthma. Puerto Rican (*n* = 362 trios) and Mexican (*n* = 259 trios) families ascertained through a child with asthma were studied. SNPs of the *CD14* gene were sought in Mexican, Puerto Rican and African-American subjects (*n* = 24 each). Three *CD14* SNPs were genotyped in the families and genotypes and haplotypes were assessed for associations with asthma, asthma severity (pre-FEV_1, percentage predicted), bronchodilator responsiveness (relative percentage change in FEV_1) or plasma IgE. Subsequently, analyses were performed after stratifying the data by proband exposure to ETS. A cross-sectional cohort analysis was also conducted to test for association between IgE and the interaction term gene × ETS.

INTERPRETATION. A total of 21 synonymous SNPs were identified in the *CD14* gene, of which A–810C, C–159T and C+1437G were selected for genotyping. When stratified for ETS exposure, asthma severity was associated with *CD14* polymorphisms; SNP +1437 had the most global effect as it was associated in Mexican, Puerto Rican and combined populations, while associations with SNPs –159 and –810 were found in Mexicans only. The –810 polymorphism was associated with plasma IgE levels in ETS-exposed subjects in all populations; this association was also found with –159 in the combined population. In the absence of stratification for smoking, the associations were limited to asthma severity with SNPs –810 and +1437 in Mexicans and with SNP +1437 in the combined population.

Comment

This study demonstrates an interaction between exposure to ETS (environment) and genetic variants in the *CD14* gene that relates to asthma phenotypes of severity and plasma IgE levels. This substantiates the findings of the studies by Meyers (discussed above) and Colilla [**25**], in which linkage to chromosome 5q was dependent on smoke exposure. These results were obtained in populations whose ethnicity was different from the ethnicities in the original gene–environment interaction reports, which further strengthens the overall importance of these findings. The association with IgE was not detected in the absence of stratification for ETS and the association with asthma severity was significantly strengthened by the interaction term. This underscores the importance of gene–environmental interactions in identifying susceptibility loci and probably contributes to the sometimes varied linkage and association results reported for individual genes.

Along with ETS exposure, the data in this study were stratified by other factors, including age, breastfeeding, allergies and exposure to animals. No significant associations between *CD14* genotypes and asthma-related traits were detected in the presence of stratification for these factors. This is somewhat surprising as animal exposure, in particular, is expected to interact with CD14 through animal-derived endotoxin. However, the details relating to these other factors are not provided so these results cannot be assessed critically.

Conclusion

It has been only in recent decades that concerted efforts have been made to begin to reveal the genetic basis of complex genetic diseases, such as asthma and allergy. Much progress has been made in a short time. Genome regions linked to asthma and allergy have been identified and candidate genes have been predicted and interrogated. Issues of study design, such as sample size and statistical significance, have been debated and the overall quality of published reports has visibly matured in the past few years.

While investigators of asthma and allergy genetics are undoubtedly poised to make further significant strides in this field, several points for consideration deserve mention. First, we need to critically evaluate and yet be receptive to novel or controversial findings in the field of asthma genetics. For example, positional cloning results are based on extensive studies and yet in all cases to date these studies have implicated genes not previously considered to be related to asthma and allergy. Such findings lead us to look closely at the methods by which the genes were identified and to examine these novel genes with a mind open to their potential relevance in disease. Similarly, the scientific community must be receptive to discrepant results between studies that are conducted with sound design. Secondly, we need to concentrate on refining methods for data analysis. This will be especially important for studies of complex data sets, gene–environment interactions and gene–gene interactions. Thirdly, the publication of negative findings should be encouraged as these results are extremely valuable in shaping the overall picture of asthma and allergy genetics. Finally, we would benefit from keeping abreast of the literature for other complex genetic diseases, including autoimmunity, as the approaches and even the results are likely to have some relevance to genetic susceptibility to asthma and allergy.

References

1. Van Eerdewegh P, Little RD, Dupuis J, Del Mastro RG, Falls K, Simon J, Torrey D, Pandit S, McKenny J, Braunschweiger K, Walsh A, Liu Z, Hayward B, Folz C, Manning SP, Bawa A, Saracino L, Thackston M, Benchekroun Y, Capparell N, Wang M, Adair R, Feng Y, Dubois J, FitzGerald MG, Huang H, Gibson R, Allen KM, Pedan A, Danzig MR, Umland SP, Egan RW, Cuss FM, Rorke S, Clough JB, Holloway JW, Holgate ST, Keith TP. Association of the ADAM33 gene with asthma and bronchial hyper-responsiveness. *Nature* 2002; **418**: 426–30.
2. Zhang Y, Leaves NI, Anderson GG, Ponting CP, Broxholme J, Holt R, Edser P, Bhattacharyya S, Dunham A, Adcock IM, Pulleyn L, Barnes PJ, Harper JI, Abecasis G, Cardon L, White M, Burton J, Matthews L, Mott R, Ross M, Cox R, Moffatt MF, Cookson WO. Positional cloning of a quantitative trait locus on chromosome 13q14 that influences immunoglobulin E levels and asthma. *Nat Genet* 2003; **34**: 181–6.
3. Allen M, Heinzmann A, Noguchi E, Abecasis G, Broxholme J, Ponting CP, Bhattacharyya S, Tinsley J, Zhang Y, Holt R, Jones EY, Lench N, Carey A, Jones H, Dickens NJ, Dimon C, Nicholls R, Baker C, Xue L, Townsend E, Kabesch M, Weiland SK, Carr D, von Mutius E, Adcock IM, Barnes PJ, Lathrop GM, Edwards M, Moffatt MF, Cookson WO. Positional cloning of a novel gene influencing asthma from chromosome 2q14. *Nat Genet* 2003; **35**: 258–63.
4. Melen E, Bruce S, Doekes G, Kabesch M, Laitinen T, Lauener R, Lindgren CM, Riedler J, Scheynius A, van Hage-Hamsten M, Kere J, Pershagen G, Wickman M, Nyberg F; PARSIFAL Genetics Study Group. Haplotypes of G protein-coupled receptor 154 are associated with childhood allergy and asthma. *Am J Respir Crit Care Med* 2005; **171**: 1089–95.
5. Kormann MS, Carr D, Klopp N, Illig T, Leupold W, Fritzsch C, Weiland SK, von Mutius E, Kabesch M. G-Protein-coupled receptor polymorphisms are associated with asthma in a large German population. *Am J Respir Crit Care Med* 2005; **171**: 1358–62.
6. Hall IP, Blakey JD. Genetic association studies in thorax. *Thorax* 2005; **60**: 357–9.
7. Lind DL, Choudhry S, Ung N, Ziv E, Avila PC, Salari K, Ha C, Lovins EG, Coyle NE, Nazario S, Casal J, Torres A, Rodriguez-Santana JR, Matallana H, Lilly CM, Salas J, Selman M, Boushey HA, Weiss ST, Chapela R, Ford JG, Rodriguez-Cintron W, Silverman EK, Sheppard D, Kwok PY, Gonzalez Burchard E. ADAM33 is not associated with asthma in Puerto Rican or Mexican populations. *Am J Respir Crit Care Med* 2003; **168**: 1312–16.
8. Marsh DG, Neely JD, Breazeale DR, Ghosh B, Freidhoff LR, Ehrlich-Kautzky E, Schou C, Krishnaswamy G, Beaty TH. Linkage analysis of IL-4 and other chromosome 5q31.1 markers and total serum immunoglobulin E concentrations. *Science* 1994; **264**: 1152–6.
9. Meyers DA, Postma DS, Panhuysen CI, Xu J, Amelung PJ, Levitt RC, Bleecker ER. Evidence for a locus regulating total serum IgE levels mapping to chromosome 5. *Genomics* 1994; **23**: 464–70.

10. Randolph AG, Lange C, Silverman EK, Lazarus R, Silverman ES, Raby B, Brown A, Ozonoff A, Richter B, Weiss ST. The IL-12B gene is associated with asthma. *Am J Hum Genet* 2004; **75**: 709–15.

11. Morahan G, Huang D, Wu M, Holt BJ, White GP, Kendall GE, Sly PD, Holt PG. Association of IL-12B promoter polymorphism with severity of atopic and non-atopic asthma in children. *Lancet* 2002; **360**: 455–9.

12. Khoo SK, Hayden CM, Roberts M, Horak E, de Klerk N, Zhang G, Robertson CF, Goldblatt J, Le Souef P. Associations of the IL-12B promoter polymorphism in longitudinal data from asthmatic patients 7 to 42 years of age. *J Allergy Clin Immunol* 2004; **113**: 475–81.

13. McIntire JJ, Umetsu SE, Macaubas C, Hoyte EG, Cinnioglu C, Cavalli-Sforza LL, Barsh GS, Hallmayer JF, Underhill PA, Risch NJ, Freeman GJ, DeKruyff RH, Umetsu DT. Immunology: hepatitis A virus link to atopic disease. *Nature* 2003; **425**: 576.

14. McIntire JJ, Umetsu SE, Akbari O, Potter M, Kuchroo VK, Barsh GS, Freeman GJ, Umetsu DT, DeKruyff RH. Identification of Tapr (an airway hyper-reactivity regulatory locus) and the linked Tim gene family. *Nat Immunol* 2001; **2**: 1109–16.

15. Graves PE, Siroux V, Guerra S, Klimecki WT, Martinez FD. Association of atopy and eczema with polymorphisms in T-cell immunoglobulin domain and mucin domain-IL-2-inducible T-cell kinase gene cluster in chromosome 5 q 33. *J Allergy Clin Immunol* 2005; **116**: 650–6.

16. Finotto S, Neurath MF, Glickman JN, Qin S, Lehr HA, Green FH, Ackerman K, Haley K, Galle PR, Szabo SJ, Drazen JM, De Sanctis GT, Glimcher LH. Development of spontaneous airway changes consistent with human asthma in mice lacking T-bet. *Science* 2002; **295**: 336–8.

17. Raby BA, Hwang ES, Steen KV, Tantisira K, Peng S, Litonjua A, Lazarus R, Giallourakis C, Rioux JD, Sparrow D, Silverman EK, Glimcher LH, Weiss ST. T-bet polymorphisms are associated with asthma and airway hyper-responsiveness. *Am J Respir Crit Care Med* 2006; **173**: 64–70.

18. Ylikoski E, Kinos R, Sirkkanen N, Pykalainen M, Savolainen J, Laitinen LA, Kere J, Laitinen T, Lahesmaa R. Association study of 15 novel single-nucleotide polymorphisms of the T-bet locus among Finnish asthma families. *Clin Exp Allergy* 2004; **34**: 1049–55.

19. Chung HT, Kim LH, Park BL, Lee JH, Park HS, Choi BW, Hong SJ, Chae SC, Kim JJ, Park CS, Shin HD. Association analysis of novel TBX21 variants with asthma phenotypes. *Hum Mutat* 2003; **22**: 257.

20. Wjst M. Specific IgE—one gene fits all? German Asthma Genetics Group. *Clin Exp Allergy* 1999; **29**(Suppl 4): 5–10.

21. Daniels SE, Bhattacharrya S, James A, Leaves NI, Young A, Hill MR, Faux JA, Ryan GF, le Souef PN, Lathrop GM, Musk AW, Cookson WO. A genome-wide search for quantitative trait loci underlying asthma. *Nature* 1996; **383**: 247–50.

22. Lee YA, Wahn U, Kehrt R, Tarani L, Businco L, Gustafsson D, Andersson F, Oranje AP, Wolkertstorfer A, v Berg A, Hoffmann U, Kuster W, Wienker T, Ruschendorf F, Reis A. A major susceptibility locus for atopic dermatitis maps to chromosome 3q21. *Nat Genet* 2000; **26**: 470–3.

23. Yokouchi Y, Shibasaki M, Noguchi E, Nakayama J, Ohtsuki T, Kamioka M, Yamakawa-Kobayashi K, Ito S, Takeda K, Ichikawa K, Nukaga Y, Matsui A, Hamaguchi H, Arinami T. A genome-wide linkage analysis of orchard grass-sensitive childhood seasonal allergic rhinitis in Japanese families. *Genes Immun* 2002; **3**: 9–13.

24. Haagerup A, Bjerke T, Schoitz PO, Binderup HG, Dahl R, Kruse TA. Allergic rhinitis—a total genome-scan for susceptibility genes suggests a locus on chromosome 4q24–q27. *Eur J Hum Genet* 2001; **9**: 945–52.

25. Colilla S, Nicolae D, Pluzhnikov A, Blumenthal MN, Beaty TH, Bleecker ER, Lange EM, Rich SS, Meyers DA, Ober C, Cox NJ; Collaborative Study for the Genetics of Asthma. Evidence for gene–environment interactions in a linkage study of asthma and smoking exposure. *J Allergy Clin Immunol* 2003; **111**: 840–6.

Part II

Pathophysiology and diseases

3

Airway inflammation

GORDON DENT

Introduction

Asthma is a continuing problem for healthcare, particularly in the industrialized world. Some 150 million people are estimated to suffer from asthma worldwide, with 5.2 million sufferers in the UK. Hospital admissions for asthma number 69 000 per annum in the UK, including 28 500 children. Approximately 1400 people die from asthma in the UK annually, of whom over 30% are under the age of 65. Asthma costs the UK National Health Service almost £90 million per annum (statistics from Asthma UK, http://www.asthma.org.uk).

Severe or refractory asthma – which may include inadequately managed as well as pathologically severe disease – is of particular concern. While these cases represent only 5–10% of total asthma cases (approximately 250 000 in the UK), they account for the majority of healthcare spending in this area. Numerous studies in recent years have pointed to the existence of differences in the pathology of mild/moderate and severe asthma. Among these, distinct phenotypes have been proposed which account for differences in neutrophilic–eosinophilic airway inflammation, glucocorticoid responsiveness and airway remodelling [1].

Airway remodelling has acquired increasing acceptance over the past 10 years as a major factor in the development of progressive loss of respiratory function in chronic asthma. The structures involved in remodelling include airway smooth muscle, mucus-secreting epithelial cells and glands, subepithelial basement membrane, and blood vessels, although the nature of their respective contributions to bronchial hyper-responsiveness and declining lung function remains unclear [2]. The apparent importance of remodelling is reflected in an increasing number of published research studies in this area, of which four original contributions are reviewed here.

While changes in the numbers and functions of structural cells in the airways underlie the processes of remodelling, there is increasing evidence that inflammatory cells recruited from the circulation interact with these cells and contribute to the remodelling processes [3]. Cooperativity between inflammatory leucocytes and structural cells in producing survival, proliferation, differentiation and secretory function in both sets of cells may produce an inflammation-driven development of persistent changes in airway structure and function which leads to

© Atlas Medical Publishing Ltd

progression of asthma to more severe forms. These interactions, which are potentially of major importance in asthma pathology, are addressed here in reviews of two papers.

The involvement of inflammation in the pathology of asthma has been recognized for many years [2]. Research continues to explore the mechanisms by which leucocytes are recruited to the airways and become activated in inflammatory lung diseases, such as asthma. Roles for eosinophils and T lymphocytes in the pathogenesis of asthma, while passing in and out of fashion, have been considered important for many years. More recently, however, neutrophils have also come to be regarded as being of importance in some forms of severe asthma, and the recruitment, activation and survival of neutrophils in the airways are being studied extensively. Exploration of the roles of neutrophil chemoattractants, and of molecules which facilitate the movement of leucocytes between vascular, interstitial and airway compartments, is an increasingly important theme. The role of leukotriene B4 and its receptors, which contribute to neutrophil recruitment and other effector functions of the innate and acquired immune systems, are addressed in two of the articles reviewed.

Two important emerging features of asthma and approaches to therapy are also reviewed. Asthma treatment is conventionally guided by targets for normalization of symptom scores, indices of lung function and requirement for bronchodilators [4]. Recently, however, alternative approaches have been proposed, based upon normalization of indices of airway inflammation. The widespread use of measurement of nitric oxide (NO) in exhaled breath as an index of inflammation has been translated into a method for monitoring disease status to guide alteration of treatment regimes.

The involvement of respiratory viral infections in provoking acute exacerbations of asthma has been increasingly recognized in recent years. Here, the identification of a dysfunction in the innate immune system of asthmatic individuals, leading to greater viral infectivity and more severe effects on airway function, is reviewed, along with suggestions for how treatment of at-risk individuals may be adapted.

Overall, the ten original research articles reviewed in the following pages provide a representative view of current emerging or rapidly developing themes in airway inflammation and asthma. While some are of interest in defining new concepts of asthma pathology, others are more directly linked to the identification of distinct forms of the disease and to defining innovative or novel therapeutic approaches.

Airway viral infections in asthma

An important feature of chronic asthma, and one which therapy should seek to minimize, is the occurrence of acute severe episodes or exacerbations. Frequently, these arise as a result of lower respiratory tract infection with the rhinoviruses which cause colds [5]. Asthmatic individuals exhibit increased susceptibility to rhinovirus infections, relative to the general population, suggesting that the ability of their immune systems to clear the virus may be compromised. This has obvious implications, given the risk of exacerbation associated with viral infection in these patients.

Asthmatic bronchial epithelial cells have a deficient innate immune response to infection with rhinovirus

Wark PA, Johnston SL, Bucchieri F, *et al. J Exp Med* 2005; **201**: 937–47

BACKGROUND. Exacerbations of asthma are frequently associated with rhinoviral infection. Rhinoviruses infect respiratory epithelial cells, where they replicate. The presence of viral nucleic acids (DNA and RNA) and the production of new virions provoke an innate immune response, leading to destruction of infected cells through the rapid induction of apoptosis. The lower airways of asthmatic individuals are more susceptible than those of healthy individuals to infection with rhinoviruses, although the basis of this difference has not been understood previously. Using epithelial cells cultured from bronchial brush biopsies of healthy and asthmatic volunteers, rhinovirus 16 (RV16) was found to replicate more rapidly in asthmatic epithelial cells *in vitro*. RV16-infected asthmatic cells exhibited reduced apoptosis, accompanied by increased late virus release. The decrease in virus-induced apoptosis was associated with a suppression of virus-induced secretion of interferon β (IFN-β) but not of a range of other inflammatory cytokines. The addition of exogenous IFN-β reduced the release of infectious virus from infected asthmatic epithelial cells.

INTERPRETATION. The ability of the innate immune system to destroy virus-infected host cells is a vital defence against overwhelming viral infection. Viruses replicate within host cells, leading to the release of new virions and death of the cells by late lysis. Induction of apoptosis through innate immune responses prevents replication of virus within the cells and reduces the overall viral load. The increased susceptibility of asthmatic lower airways to rhinoviral infection may reflect an inability to mount effective innate immune responses to the virus. This has been demonstrated directly by showing that viral replication (measured as viral RNA in, and late virus release from, RV16-infected bronchial epithelial cells) is increased in cells from asthmatic donors. The mechanism by which this increased replication occurs was shown to involve reduced virus-induced activation of the caspase 3/7 enzymes, which promote programmed cell death (apoptosis), leading to prolonged survival of infected cells and increased capacity for viral replication and release. The induction of caspase activity was found to be dependent upon the release of IFN-β from the epithelial cells: asthmatic cells produced less IFN-β following viral infection, while production of other inflammatory cytokines was no different from that in healthy cells. There appears, therefore, to be a dysfunction in the epithelium of the lower respiratory tract of asthmatic individuals which allows rhinoviruses to replicate more extensively.

Comment

The involvement of lower respiratory tract viral infection in the provocation of acute severe asthmatic episodes (exacerbations) is well characterized [5]. The most common exacerbation-provoking viruses – major group rhinoviruses, such as RV16 – enter host cells by binding to intercellular adhesion molecule 1 (ICAM-1) on the host-cell surface. ICAM-1 functions normally as a counterligand for integrins on the surface of leucocytes, mediating adhesion and activation of the leucocytes |**6**|. The expression of adhesion molecules, including ICAM-1, is increased in bronchial epithelial cells from asthmatics |**7**|, suggesting that the infectivity of rhinoviruses is increased in these individuals by the presence of greater numbers of virus 'receptors', leading to more extensive entry of virus into host cells and, consequently, increased viral replication. In the study by Wark *et al.*, however, asthmatic bronchial epithelial cells in culture exhibited increased replication of a range of viruses, including minor-group rhinoviruses, which enter the cell through binding to the low-density lipoprotein receptor, whose expression is not altered in asthmatic cells. These viruses did, however, share the feature of stimulating IFN-β-dependent apoptosis, which was impaired in cells from asthmatic donors owing to reduced virus-induced production of IFN-β.

The ability of exogenous IFN-β to induce epithelial apoptosis and reduce viral replication is taken by the authors as evidence that IFN-β may have a therapeutic use in preventing or treating virus-induced exacerbations of asthma. It remains to be determined, however, whether treatment of uninfected epithelial cells with IFN-β has a potentially deleterious effect. Since IFN-β was most effective in suppressing viral replication when administered both before and during infection, a prophylactic action is likely to be more evident than a remedial action. It would, therefore, be important to determine the effects of the cytokine on the airways in the absence of viral infection.

Nitric oxide monitoring in optimization of asthma therapy

The use of sputum cytology and the measurement of soluble inflammatory mediators in sputum has allowed the monitoring of airway inflammation in numerous clinical research studies without the need for highly invasive procedures such as bronchoscopy and bronchoalveolar lavage (BAL). Monitoring of sputum in this way can assist in the optimization of therapy to control inflammatory processes |**8**|. Measurement of inflammatory indices in exhaled breath is even less invasive than sputum induction, and may represent an alternative, rapid method for monitoring the control of inflammation and minimizing exacerbation frequency.

Use of exhaled nitric oxide measurements to guide treatment in chronic asthma

Smith AD, Cowan JO, Brassett KP, Herbison GP, Taylor DR. *N Engl J Med* 2005; **352**: 2163–73

BACKGROUND. Adjusting the inhaled glucocorticoid dose based on indices of airway inflammation has been proposed as a means of achieving more effective control of asthma than the conventional approach of adjusting steroid dose based on symptoms, lung function and rescue medication use. In a single-blind, placebo-controlled trial, 97 asthmatic patients received fluticasone doses adjusted on the basis either of conventional guidelines or of exhaled nitric oxide fraction (FE_{NO}). The group treated on the basis of FE_{NO} had a lower final required dose of fluticasone and a lower frequency of exacerbation. The use of exhaled NO as an index for the adjustment of inhaled corticosteroid treatment may allow asthma to be controlled more effectively.

INTERPRETATION. Exhaled NO was measured by chemiluminescence analysis. The fluticasone dose was adjusted either according to GINA guidelines (Global Initiative for Asthma; http://www.ginasthma.com/download.asp?intid=188) or on the basis of FE_{NO}; the steroid dose was tapered at 4-week intervals until FE_{NO} rose above 15 parts per billion (ppb) or asthma became uncontrolled, when the dose was increased again to achieve control or a FE_{NO} <15 ppb. Treatment with the optimal dose of fluticasone was maintained for 12 months. The frequency of exacerbation in the group whose fluticasone dose was adjusted on the basis of FE_{NO} was lower (0.49 compared with 0.90 events/patient/year in the control group), while these patients also received a significantly lower mean daily dose of fluticasone (370 μg, compared to 640 μg in the control group; $P = 0.008$). No significant difference was observed between the groups for other indicators of asthma control, including pulmonary function measurements and sputum eosinophil number.

Comment

The definition of markers of asthma severity is necessary both to provide an indication for treatment and to monitor its effectiveness. Current guidelines recommend adjusting the dose of inhaled glucocorticoids to achieve target levels of symptoms, bronchodilator requirement and pulmonary function indices [4]. However, some investigators have suggested that adjusting the steroid dose to achieve target indices of airway inflammation leads to more effective disease control. Treatment strategies based on the normalization of sputum eosinophil numbers have been shown to produce a decrease in exacerbation frequency compared with treatment adjusted according to the symptom-based guidelines of the British Thoracic Society/Scottish Intercollegiate Guidelines Network [8]. Exhaled NO has been proposed and validated as a marker of airway inflammation [9], and allows non-invasive monitoring of inflammatory processes in the lower respiratory tract. While the indices of asthma severity defined in conventional guidelines undoubtedly also reflect airway inflammation, at least in part, there appear to be problems with the cut-off points at which steroid doses are increased. Although patients treated according to the conventional guidelines received higher doses of fluticasone, they were more prone to exacerbation while exhibiting no greater control in terms of symptom score, nocturnal waking or rescue bronchodilator use. It appears, therefore, that inhaled glucocorticoid doses indicated by conventional guidelines are too high and do not provide optimal control of asthma.

Although the measurement of exhaled NO is more rapid and less labour-intensive than the induction, processing, cytology and supernatant analysis of sputum, it requires specialized equipment more at home in a teaching hospital than in a general practitioner's surgery. However, given the healthcare – and other economic – costs of ineffective asthma treatment, the periodic measurement of airway inflammatory indices is likely to provide important benefits for the optimization of therapy. The ability to collect exhaled breath 'offline' for subsequent NO measurement in a central facility [9] may make this an achievable goal.

Leukotriene B_4 in asthma

The recognition of a role for cysteinyl leukotrienes (LTC_4, LTD_4 and LTE_4) in asthma was a major step in the development of a new class of anti-asthma drugs: the $CysLT_1$ receptor antagonists (e.g. montelukast and zafirlukast). Cysteinyl leukotrienes are involved in smooth muscle contraction and proliferation, microvascular leakage and the recruitment of inflammatory cells such as eosinophils. The other major product of the 5-lipoxygenase pathway of arachidonic acid metabolism – the hydroxyleukotriene LTB_4 – has a distinct profile of actions; chief among these is the recruitment of neutrophils, although LTB_4 also has chemotactic activity for other leucocytes, including eosinophils and T lymphocytes. The importance of LTB_4 in exacerbations of chronic obstructive pulmonary disease (COPD) has been demonstrated. It appears, however, that this mediator may also play a role in the pathology of asthma.

Leukotriene B_4 in exhaled breath condensate and sputum supernatant in patients with COPD and asthma

Kostikas K, Gaga M, Papatheodorou G, Karamanis T, Orphanidou D, Loukides S. *Chest* 2005; **127**: 1553–9

BACKGROUND. Some features seem to be common to severe asthma and COPD with reversibility of airflow limitation. The neutrophil chemoattractant leukotriene B_4 (LTB_4) may play a role in COPD and in some forms of asthma. In this study, 55 smokers with no disease, COPD (with or without bronchodilator reversibility of airflow limitation) or asthma underwent measurement of LTB_4 in sputum supernatants and exhaled breath condensate (EBC). Both COPD and asthma patients had higher levels of LTB_4 than control subjects; patients with asthma or reversible COPD exhibited significantly higher levels of LTB_4 than those with irreversible COPD. There

was no correlation between LTB_4 levels and airway obstruction or reversibility in either asthma or COPD. LTB_4 levels correlated with macrophage numbers in COPD (reversible and irreversible) and asthma; correlation with neutrophil numbers, however, was only observed in COPD patients.

Interpretation. A role for LTB_4 in asthma has not been established, and current therapy targeting leukotrienes consists of selective antagonism of the $CysLT_1$ receptor. However, the therapeutic potential of 5-lipoxygenase (5-LO) and 5-LO-activating protein (FLAP) inhibitors – which suppress generation of both LTB_4 and the cysteinyl leukotrienes (LTC4, D_4 and E_4) – in some forms of asthma has been mooted [1]. This study indicates that, when differences in smoking habits are excluded, asthmatic patients have levels of LTB_4 in their airway secretions that are as high as those in COPD and significantly higher than those in healthy smokers. It is suggested that airway inflammation involving LTB_4 is associated with reversible airway obstruction, while the irreversible obstruction in other COPD patients occurs through a different mechanism.

Comment

The cysteinyl leukotrienes play a well-characterized role in asthma, and drugs which target the $CysLT_1$ receptor for these mediators have acquired a place in asthma therapy. The hydroxyleukotriene LTB_4, in contrast, appears to be associated with the neutrophilic airway inflammation characteristic of COPD. There is a range of phenotypes within each disease, however, and some overlap between them: severe asthma with neutrophilia and glucocorticoid insensitivity shares some features with COPD [1]. While neutrophils and their chemoattractants – particularly LTB4 and interleukin 8 (IL-8/CXCL8) – have been implicated in exacerbations of COPD, a role for LTB_4 in asthma has only recently begun to be recognized [10]. Detection of LTB_4 levels has traditionally depended upon semi-invasive and labour-intensive techniques, such as sputum induction, or the relatively insensitive measurement of urinary glucuronide-conjugated LTB_4. The development of EBC analysis has been applied successfully to NO measurements, allowing non-invasive monitoring of airway inflammation (see above). The extension of this approach to include measurement of other inflammatory indices may allow more precise diagnosis and monitoring of respiratory disease.

Requirement for leukotriene B_4 receptor 1 in allergen-induced airway hyper-responsiveness

Miyahara N, Takeda K, Miyahara S, *et al. Am J Respir Crit Care Med* 2005; **172**: 161–7

Background. A role for LTB_4 in the induction of airway hyper-responsiveness was explored through the use of transgenic mice deficient in the BLT1 receptor for LTB_4. Ovalbumin challenge of sensitized wild-type mice resulted in the usual features of experimental asthma, including goblet cell hyperplasia, hyper-responsiveness to inhaled methacholine and elevated BAL fluid concentrations of the Th2 cytokine IL-13.

In contrast, *BLT1*$^{-/-}$ mice (i.e. genetically modified mice lacking the gene coding for the BLT1 receptor) exhibited significantly lower responses. *BLT1*$^{-/-}$ mice also exhibited lower numbers of IL-13-positive T lymphocytes of both the helper (CD4$^+$) and cytotoxic/suppressor (CD8$^+$) types. Adoptive transfer of T cells from *BLT1*$^{+/+}$ (i.e. BLT1-expressing) sensitized mice fully restored hyper-responsiveness following ovalbumin challenge in sensitized *BTL1*$^{-/-}$ mice.

Interpretation. The development of lung responses to inhaled antigen was suppressed in sensitized animals lacking BLT1. Responsiveness to inhaled methacholine was reduced (an approximate 5-fold decrease in bronchoconstrictor response to 10 mg/ml methacholine; P <0.05) and the development of goblet cell hyperplasia was significantly reduced (32 cells/mm basement membrane, compared with 51 cells/mm in *BLT1*$^{+/+}$ mice; P <0.05). Other indices of inflammation, including extravascular eosinophils, showed no difference between *BLT1*$^{+/+}$ and *BLT1*$^{-/-}$ mice. Levels of IL-13 in BAL and in the supernatants of *ex vivo* antigen-stimulated lung cells were significantly reduced in *BLT1*$^{-/-}$ mice. T lymphocytes were isolated from sensitized *BLT1*$^{+/+}$ mice and transferred to sensitized *BLT1*$^{-/-}$ mice: airway hyper-responsiveness in the recipient mice following antigen challenge was no different from that in *BLT1*$^{+/+}$ mice (Fig. 3.1), indicating that BLT1 expression on primed T cells is required for the development of hyper-responsiveness.

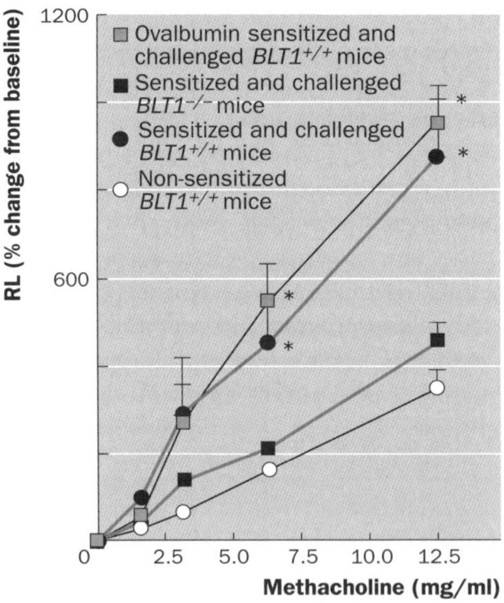

Fig. 3.1 Adoptive transfer of allergen-induced airway hyper-responsiveness with *BLT1*$^{+/+}$ T lymphocytes. Ovalbumin-sensitized and -challenged *BLT1*$^{+/+}$ mice (*grey squares*) exhibited hyper-responsiveness to inhaled methacholine compared with sensitized and challenged *BLT1*$^{-/-}$ (*solid squares*). Hyper-responsiveness was restored by transfer of T cells from sensitized and challenged *BLT1*$^{+/+}$ mice (*solid circles*) but not from non-sensitized *BLT1*$^{+/+}$ mice (*open circles*). *P <0.05 compared with non-sensitized *BLT1*$^{+/+}$ mice. Source: Miyahara *et al.* (2005).

Comment

Some studies have revealed a beneficial action of 5-LO inhibitors on exercise and adenosine-induced bronchoconstriction in asthma, suggesting a role for leukotrienes in general in these responses |**11**|. However, the proven efficacy of $CysLT_1$ receptor antagonists, in the absence of positive results for BLT_1 antagonists, has led to the assumption that suppression of LTB_4 synthesis does not play a role in the actions of 5-LO inhibitors in asthma. Focus upon LTB_4 as a chemoattractant for neutrophils has led to its being considered more important in COPD than in asthma, where an involvement of neutrophils has only recently been appreciated. However, LTB_4 also exerts actions – including chemoattraction – on T lymphocytes, cells whose contribution to asthma pathology is well established |**12**|.

The study by Miyahara *et al.* is supported by a similar study by Terawaki *et al.* in which sensitized $BLT1^{-/-}$ mice exhibited reduced airway hyper-responsiveness following allergen challenge |**13**|. The latter study also showed reduced immunoglobulin E production and BAL IL-5 levels, which, in combination with Miyahara and co-workers' finding of reduced IL-13 production, indicates that Th2-mediated mechanisms are affected by the absence of BLT1. Surprisingly, no differences in BAL neutrophil numbers were reported in either study. This may reflect either redundancy of neutrophil attractants, the lack of LTB_4 response being compensated for by levels of IL-8 and other chemoattractants (including other chemokines – such as Groα/CXCL1 and Ena78/CXCL5 – and complement anaphylatoxin C5a), or a greater dependence of lung neutrophil numbers upon prolonged survival than stimulated migration.

Factors effecting T-cell trafficking in the lungs are poorly understood but vitally important, since T cells are at the centre of the cytokine network which regulates immune responses in the lung. The identification of an LTB_4-dependent involvement of T cells in the inflammatory changes in allergen-challenged airways provides a useful indication of the therapeutic potential of suppressing LTB_4 in asthma.

Cell–cell interactions in asthma

Our understanding of the roles of the various cell types in the airway has had to be revised with evidence of unexpected functions of many structural cells. The cytokine-secreting activity of epithelial cells, fibroblasts and smooth muscle cells contributes to the regulation of the tissue environment, including the populations of infiltrating cells such as leucocytes. Moreover, it is increasingly apparent that the resident structural cells and the transient inflammatory cells exert mutual influences; inflammatory cells may control their own accumulation through the regulation of the release of chemotactic and survival factors from structural cells, while the structural cells, in turn, may effect repair of the tissue through the stimulation of cytokine and growth factor secretion from inflammatory cells.

Two characteristic infiltrating cells of asthmatic airways – eosinophils and T lymphocytes – interact in potentially important ways with structural cells.

Induction of IL-6 in coculture of bronchial epithelial cells and eosinophils is regulated by p38 MAPK and NF-κB

Wang CB, Wong CK, Ip WK, Li MLY, Tian YP, Lam CWK. *Allergy* 2005; **60**: 1378–85

BACKGROUND. Eosinophil infiltration of the mucosa is a feature of asthmatic airways. Their adhesion to bronchial epithelial cells has been proposed to lead to the generation of inflammatory mediators which may contribute to asthma pathology. Bronchial epithelial cells (BEAS-2B cell line) and peripheral blood eosinophils were cultured alone or in combination and the production of an inflammatory cytokine, IL-6, was measured. IL-6 was produced principally by epithelial cells and the production was enhanced more than 10-fold in the presence of eosinophils. Significant augmentation of epithelial IL-6 production persisted even when eosinophils were fixed with paraformaldehyde. The eosinophil-induced IL-6 production was extensively inhibited by inhibitors of p38 mitogen-activated protein (MAP) kinase or nuclear factor κB (NFκB).

INTERPRETATION. BEAS-2B bronchial epithelial cells and eosinophils showed time-dependent release of IL-6, epithelial cells releasing approximately 6 times more IL-6 than eosinophils. In the presence of eosinophils, however, bronchial epithelial cell IL-6 production was increased more than 10-fold (Fig. 3.2a). Fixation of epithelial cells – to prevent secretion while maintaining cell-surface adhesion molecule expression – abolished the augmentation of IL-6 release (Fig. 3.2c), indicating that the upregulated IL-6 secretion was exclusively from the epithelial cells. In contrast, fixation of eosinophils caused only an approximate 60% decrease in the enhancement of IL-6 secretion (Fig. 3.2b), suggesting that a proportion of the upregulation was due entirely to ligation of epithelial adhesion molecules by counterligands on the eosinophil cell surface. Coculture with eosinophils led to increased activity of p38 MAP kinase and NFκB in epithelial cells; upregulation of IL-6 secretion was abolished by incubation of the epithelial cells with inhibitors of p38 MAP kinase (SB 203580) or NFκB (BAY 11-7082). The authors conclude that interaction between eosinophils and bronchial epithelial cells may contribute to inflammatory processes in the airways through the p38 MAP kinase- and NFκB-dependent release of cytokines.

Comment

The precise functional significance of eosinophils within asthmatic airways remains open to question. While the abilities of eosinophil-derived mediators to effect bronchoconstriction and to damage epithelial cells have been demonstrated, there is evidence that non-destructive interactions of eosinophils with the bronchial epithelium may make an important contribution to airway inflammation [14]. Eosinophils and bronchial epithelial cells in coculture exhibit elevated secretion of both eosinophil-derived LTC_4 and eosinophil- and/or epithelium-derived chemokines [15,16]. These interactions appear to be largely dependent upon direct contact

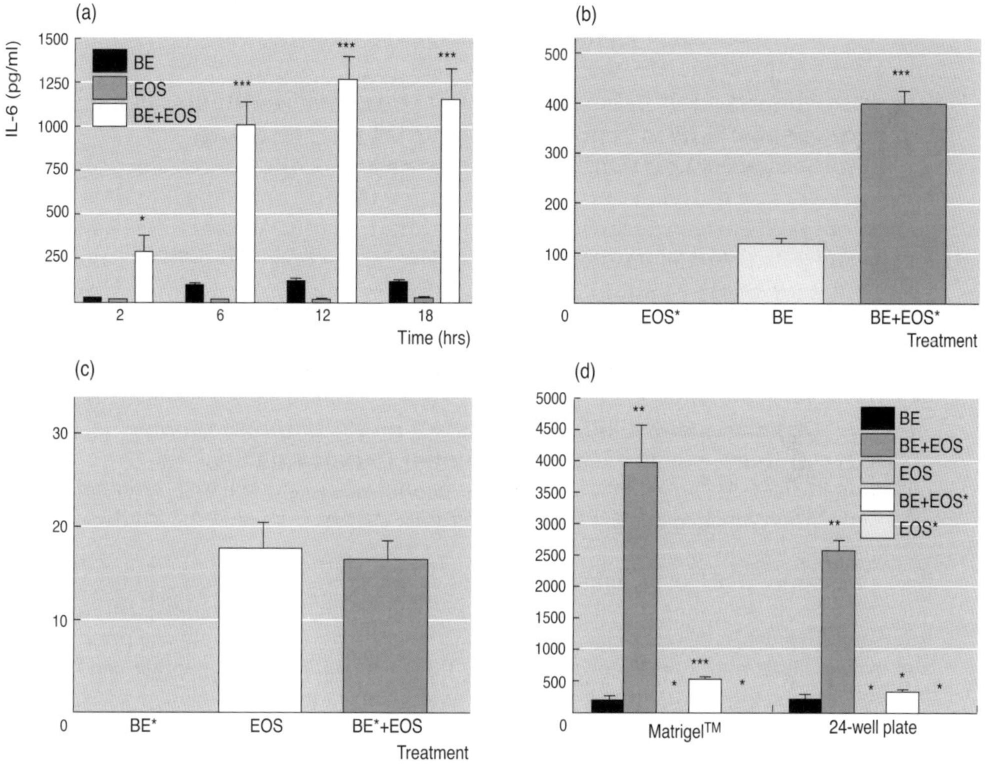

Fig. 3.2 IL-6 generation in cocultures of bronchial epithelial cells and eosinophils. (a) Human blood eosinophils and BEAS-2B bronchial epithelial cells were cultured alone or in combination for various times; IL-6 was measured in the supernatants by ELISA (enzyme-linked immunosorbent assay). (b, c) Experiments were repeated at the 12 h time-point using paraformaldehyde-fixed eosinophils (EOS*) or epithelial cells (BE*). (d) Experiments were repeated with cells cultured in bare plastic or Matrigel™ (solubilized basement membrane preparation)-coated tissue-culture plates. Source: Wang *et al.* (2005).

– and presumably, therefore, upon mutual ligation of cell surface adhesion molecules – between the two cell types, since, in most cases, the augmentation of cytokine release could be abolished by separating eosinophils and epithelial cells with permeable membranes but not by blocking secretory activity of the eosinophils |**16**|. These findings suggest that factors secreted from eosinophils cannot, by themselves, enhance epithelial cytokine secretion. While the augmentation of epithelial cytokine secretion may be due simply to the ligation of epithelial adhesion molecules (e.g. ICAM-1) by counterligands on eosinophils (e.g. CD44, Mac-1), the possibility also exists that adherence of eosinophils to epithelial cells promotes secretion of eosinophil soluble factors, so that adequate concentrations are achieved to stimulate the epithelial cells. The partial inhibition of the cooperative IL-6 secretion by eosinophil fixation suggests that a combination of the two mechanisms is likely to be involved.

The role of intracellular signalling pathways, including the activation of protein kinases (including MAP kinases) and transcription factors (including NFκB) is the subject of much current research. The identification of crucial roles for p38 MAP kinase and NFκB in the eosinophil–epithelium interaction may indicate therapeutic roles for selective inhibition of these factors in suppressing asthmatic airway inflammation.

Agonists of toll-like receptors 2 and 4 activate airway smooth muscle via mononuclear leukocytes

Morris GE, Whyte MKB, Martin GF, Jose PJ, Dower SK, Sabroe I. *Am J Respir Crit Care Med* 2005; **171**: 814–22

BACKGROUND. Toll-like receptors (TLRs) act as receptors for numerous stimuli of immune cells, including bacterial cell wall constituents (lipopolysaccharide [LPS] from Gram-negative bacteria and lipopeptides from Gram-positive species), plasma proteins and extracellular matrix breakdown products. TLR2 and TLR4 bind lipopeptide and LPS respectively, mediating responses of alveolar macrophages and other immune cells to bacterial infection in the lungs. Exposure of lungs to LPS leads to pro-inflammatory responses of a number of cell types, including airway smooth muscle, which secretes a number of cytokines involved in leucocyte recruitment and the Th2 polarization of immune responses. Human airway smooth muscle cells were cultured with LPS in the absence and presence of peripheral blood mononuclear cells to determine direct and leucocyte-dependent TLR-mediated responses. LPS had little direct effect on smooth muscle cells. Although treatment with inflammatory cytokines (IL-1, and tumour necrosis factor α) induced expression of TLR2 and TLR4, this was not associated with significantly enhanced responses to LPS. In contrast, in the presence of mononuclear cells (particularly when enriched with monocytes), smooth muscle cells showed a marked cooperative response to LPS, which was mimicked by stimulating smooth muscle cells with supernatants of LPS-activated mononuclear cells.

INTERPRETATION. Addition of mononuclear cells (as few as 100 cells/well) to airway smooth muscle cell cultures facilitated responses to TLR agonists – the lipopeptide tripalmitoyl-Cys-Ser-Lys$_4$ (Pam$_3$CSK$_4$, TLR2) and purified LPS (pLPS, TLR4) – quantified as secretion of IL-6 and IL-8/CXCL8 (Fig. 3.3). Cooperativity was enhanced by enrichment of mononuclear cell preparations with monocytes, but not T lymphocytes. Stimulation of cytokine secretion could be achieved by treatment of smooth muscle cells with supernatants of LPS-stimulated mononuclear cells. However, cooperative cytokine secretion was reduced when cocultured smooth muscle and mononuclear cells were separated by permeable membranes. Cooperative responses to TLR agonists were

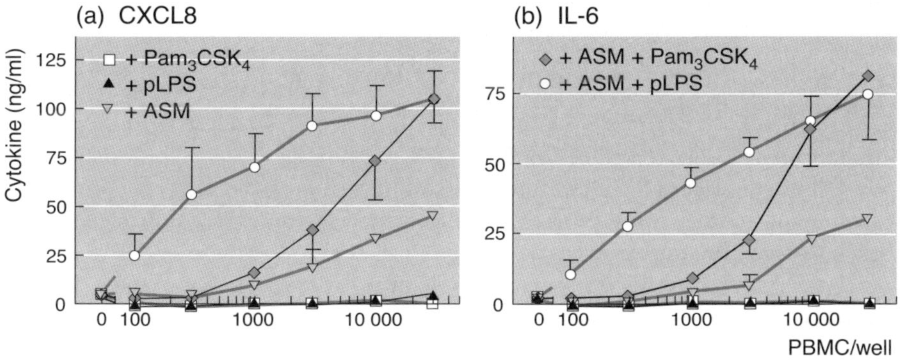

Fig. 3.3 Cooperative responses of airway smooth muscle cells and mononuclear cells to TLR agonists. Airway smooth muscle (ASM) cells were cultured alone or in the presence of increasing numbers of peripheral blood mononuclear cells (PBMC) in the absence or presence of the TLR2 agonist Pam_3CSK_4 or the TLR4 agonist pLPS (purified LPS). Cytokine concentrations were measured in 24 h culture supernatants by ELISA (enzyme-linked immunosorbent assay). Source: Morris *et al.* (2005).

abolished by the IL-1 receptor antagonist (IL-1ra), although the concentration of IL-1β in the supernatants (mean 3.5 ng/ml) was insufficient to account by itself for the stimulation of IL-6 and IL-8 secretion. The authors conclude that mononuclear cells – particularly monocytes – amplify inflammation produced by TLR agonists, such as LPS, through cooperation with airway smooth muscle cells.

Comment

Morris *et al.* demonstrate cooperation between monocytes and airway smooth muscle cells which may contribute to amplification of inflammatory signals in the airway. Increasingly, airway structural cells are seen as having accessory functions in the direction of the immune responses in the lung |**17**|. Thus, when inflammatory stimuli such as bacterial endotoxins are encountered by monocytes, these recognition cells trigger a response in the smooth muscle which leads to the recruitment (through secretion of IL-8), differentiation and proliferation (through secretion of IL-6) of T cells and neutrophils. These cytokines drive the local inflammatory response.

The authors suggest that the action of monocytes upon smooth muscle cells is dependent upon the build-up of high local concentrations of IL-1β, since physical separation of the cells results in a diminution of the cooperative response. The direct cell-to-cell contact required for interaction between airway smooth muscle cells and T lymphocytes is recognized |**18**| but the dependence of the interaction upon secreted IL-1β suggests an indirect activation of the smooth muscle. By an argument similar to that advanced above for eosinophil–epithelium interactions, however, contact-dependent augmentation of LPS-induced IL-1β may contribute to the stimulation of smooth muscle cells.

The role of bacterial products in asthmatic reactions is unclear, both chronic protective and acute exacerbating actions being attributed to LPS. Understanding the role of LPS in pulmonary immune reactions requires a clear definition of its mechanisms of action within the lung. The identification of an LPS-dependent cell–cell interaction in the airway provides an important indication of a process by which inflammatory responses are amplified and may, therefore, suggest a target at which they can be suppressed.

Airway remodelling in asthma

Airway remodelling is of major importance in the development and progression of chronic asthma. Numerous factors involved in producing the changes in tissue architecture which characterize asthma have been identified. However, phenotypic differences in the sources and quantities of the factors which drive remodelling, as well as the responsiveness of airway structural cells to these factors, are only beginning to be understood. Recent work in the area of airway remodelling has produced exciting evidence of the relationship between inflammatory processes and remodelling. Interestingly, these long-term changes in the airway seem largely to be dependent upon the same kind of cell–cell interactions that are involved in homeostasis of the tissue environment.

Antigen-specific CD4$^+$ T cells drive airways smooth muscle remodeling in experimental asthma

Ramos-Barbón D, Presley JF, Hamid QA, Fixman ED, Martin JG. *J Clin Invest* 2005; **115**: 1580–9

BACKGROUND. Airway hyper-responsiveness in asthma may involve smooth muscle growth, a manifestation of airway remodelling. The involvement of inflammatory cells in the induction of airway smooth muscle growth was studied *in vivo* and *ex vivo* in a brown Norway rat model of asthma. Transfer of CD4$^+$ T lymphocytes from ovalbumin-sensitized animals induced an increase in airway smooth muscle mass in naive animals upon repeated ovalbumin challenge. *Ex vivo*, coculture of antigen-stimulated CD4$^+$ T cells and airway smooth muscle cells led to myocyte proliferation and prolonged T-cell survival.

INTERPRETATION. Adoptive transfer of T-helper (CD4$^+$) lymphocytes from sensitized rats to naive rats led the recipients to mount an inflammatory response to inhaled specific allergen (ovalbumin), mimicking the response to allergen challenge in sensitized animals. Repeated challenge of these recipient rats led to an increase in airway smooth muscle mass (index = 3.25, compared with 1.42 for sham-challenged sensitized rats; $P < 0.001$), which represented a combination of increased proliferation and decreased apoptosis of myocytes. Coculture of airway smooth muscle cells and cervical lymph-node T cells from sensitized rats produced contact- and T-cell activation-dependent proliferation of the myocytes (measured as incorporation of 5-bromo-2-deoxyuridine [BrdU], Fig. 3.4). Neither contact culture with unactivated T cells nor transwell coculture (in which the two cell types are separated by a permeable membrane, allowing free diffusion of soluble factors but no direct cell–cell contact) produced any significant proliferation of myocytes. Reciprocally, direct cell contact with myocytes prevented apoptosis in the ovalbumin-activated T cells, indicating a prolongation of survival. The data support a direct contribution of activated CD4$^+$ T cells to airway smooth muscle remodelling in asthma.

Comment

Airway hyper-responsiveness in asthma has been regarded largely as resulting from inflammatory processes leading to epithelial damage and mucosal oedema. The results of several studies in experimental animal models of asthma, however, have suggested a lack of direct association between short-term inflammation and hyper-responsiveness, while the importance of airway remodelling in this phenomenon

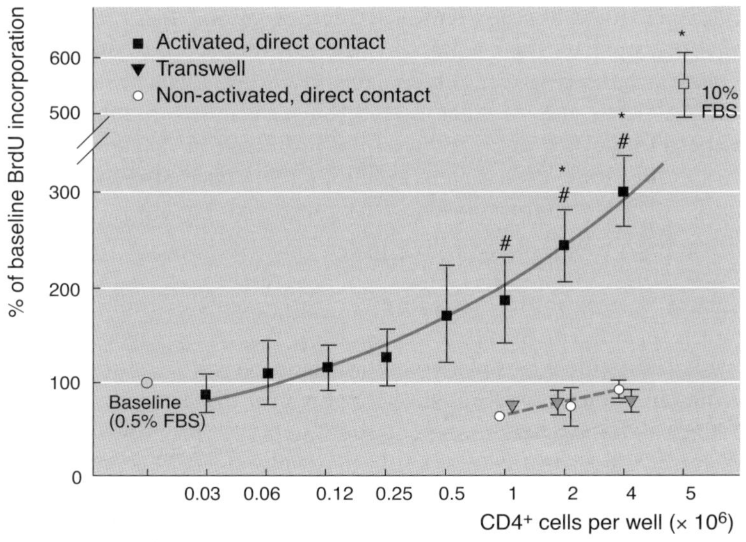

Fig. 3.4 Induction of airway smooth muscle cell proliferation by activated CD4$^+$ T lymphocytes. Primary airway smooth muscle cells (99% smooth muscle α-actin positive) from ovalbumin-sensitized brown Norway rats were cultured in the absence or presence of lymph-node T cells from the same animals, either in direct contact or separated by transwells. T cells were activated with ovalbumin (200 μg/ml). BrdU (5-bromo-2-deoxyuridine) incorporation was measured over the final 24 h of a 48 h coculture. $*P < 0.05$ compared with baseline; $\dagger P < 0.05$ compared with transwells or non-activated T cells. Source: Ramos-Barbón *et al.* (2005).

has been increasingly indicated [2]. Among the changes constituting the overall picture of remodelling, increases in airway smooth muscle mass are likely to contribute most directly to increased bronchoconstriction in response to a stimulus [19]. In common with other features of airway remodelling (see below), the relationship of smooth muscle hyperplasia to inflammation has been poorly understood for many years. Although *in vitro* studies have suggested that activated T-helper ($CD4^+$) lymphocytes may stimulate airway myocyte proliferation [18,20], the study by Ramos-Barbón *et al.* is the first to demonstrate that this action translates to an induction of remodelling *in vivo*. While remodelling in the airways of actively sensitized and antigen-challenged animals has been reported (see below), the role of specific cell populations in these systems cannot be dissected. The authors addressed this issue by transferring $CD4^+$ T cells from sensitized rats to non-sensitized recipients, thereby providing the recipient rats with a population of antigen-specific T cells which could drive cell-mediated immune responses in these animals, notably in the absence of transferred humoral (antibody-dependent) immunity.

Using *in vitro* coculture techniques, the authors were able to show a direct interaction between airway myocytes and $CD4^+$ T cells. While this interaction was dependent upon direct cell–cell contact, the mechanisms by which myocyte proliferation and T-cell survival are enhanced remain unclear. The cells express surface proteins which mediate their adhesion; smooth muscle CD44 and T-cell integrins have been proposed as candidates [20] but other myocyte adhesion molecules, including CD40 and vascular endothelial cell adhesion molecule 1 (VCAM-1), have been implicated in the induction of proliferation via activation of MAP kinase, phosphoinositide 3-kinase and cyclin D_1 [19]. These adhesion events may evoke responses in cells via direct 'inside-out' signalling and by stimulating the secretion of soluble factors, such as cytokines, which promote the survival and/or differentiation of both cell populations.

T cells and airway smooth muscle cells form a tightly regulated unit in which T cells, in response to antigen, stimulate production of IL-6 by myocytes (see above), which evokes systemic acute-phase reactions and recruits and activates T cells within the airway. Prolonged stimulation of this unit drives an increase in muscle mass which may underlie the development of bronchial hyper-responsiveness. Clearly, therefore, the interaction between these cells is potentially central to asthma pathology.

Airway fibroblasts exhibit a synthetic phenotype in severe asthma

Lewis CC, Chu HW, Westcott JY, *et al. J Allergy Clin Immunol* 2005; **115**: 534–40

BACKGROUND. Airway remodelling is considered to be of major importance in the pathology of asthma, with subepithelial basement membrane thickening in particular

being indicative of early development of the disease and characteristic of its progression. Airway fibroblasts are central cells in the processes of remodelling: increased deposition of fibroblast-derived connective tissue proteins and differentiation of fibroblasts into contractile myofibroblasts are consistent observations in morphological studies of moderate to severe asthmatic airways. The secretory function of fibroblasts is under the control of locally produced growth factors such as vascular endothelial cell growth factor (VEGF, see below) and platelet-derived growth factor (PDGF). Airway fibroblasts were cultured from healthy volunteers and subjects with asthma of various degrees of severity; their responses to PDGF were determined in order to ascertain whether heightened sensitivity of fibroblasts to growth factor stimulation is characteristic of any asthmatic group. PDGF significantly enhanced procollagen I expression in fibroblasts from severe asthmatic subjects compared with mild/moderate asthmatics and healthy controls. This was associated with elevated expression of the PDGFR, receptor for the growth factor on fibroblasts from asthmatic subjects.

INTERPRETATION. PDGF consists of homo- or heterodimers of A and B subunits, and may therefore exist as PDGF-AA, PDGF-AB and PDGF-BB isoforms. These interact with dimeric receptors, which are formed when the PDGF A and B chains bind to PDGFRα and β receptor subunits. PDGFRα recognizes either chain, while PDGFR recognizes only the B chain; therefore, PDGF-AA may bind only to $\alpha\alpha$ homodimers, PDGF-AB may bind to $\alpha\alpha$ homo- or $\alpha\beta$ heterodimers, and PDGF-BB may bind to any dimer. In this study, PDGF-BB was used as a stimulus for airway fibroblast secretory function and its actions were related to the expression of its specific receptor subunit, PDGFRβ. Fibroblast PDGFRβ expression was found to be elevated in both mild/moderate and severe asthmatic groups (healthy control, 3.7 ng/100 μg total protein; mild/moderate asthma, 13.3 ng/100 μg; severe asthma, 15.2 ng/100 μg; $P = 0.0024$). Strikingly, however, PDGF-BB (5 ng/ml)-stimulated secretion of procollagen I – a precursor of type-I collagen (deposited at elevated levels in the submucosa of asthmatic airways) – was increased only in fibroblasts from severe asthmatics (Fig. 3.5). The data show an alteration in fibroblast phenotype – to a synthetic/secretory type – in severe asthma which may contribute to airway remodelling. This is not exclusively dependent upon altered PDGF receptor expression but may involve alterations in the PDGFR signalling pathway.

Comment

The hallmark pathological features of asthma include tissue eosinophilia and subepithelial basement membrane thickening [21,22]. The contribution of eosinophilia to subepithelial collagen deposition, via production of the profibrotic agent transforming growth factor β (TGFβ) has been explored recently; airway tissue eosinophils express higher levels of the TGFβ2 isoform in severe asthma than in milder forms of the disease [23]. The other side of the remodelling equation is the phenotype (proliferative, synthetic/secretory, contractile) and responsiveness to endogenous stimuli of subepithelial structural cells, including smooth muscle and fibroblasts. PDGF has been suggested to play a predominant role in airway remodelling in asthma on the basis of its actions (fibroblast chemotaxis, proliferation and collagen production) and its cellular sources (including activated

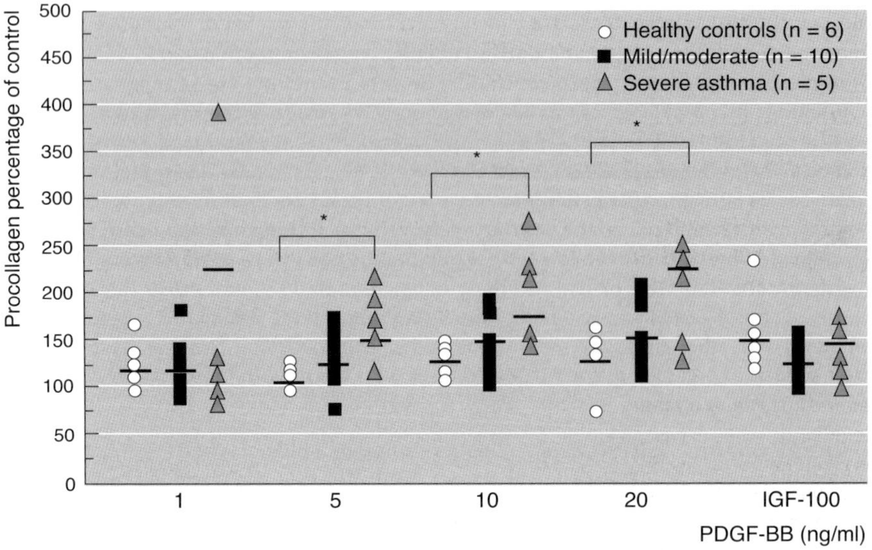

Fig. 3.5 PDGF-BB-induced procollagen-1 expression in cultured airway fibroblasts from healthy, mild/moderate asthmatic and severe asthmatic donors. Fibroblasts obtained by bronchial biopsy were cultured through one to four passages prior to stimulation with PDGF-BB at the indicated concentrations. Procollagen-1 was measured in culture supernatants by ELISA (enzyme-linked immunosorbent assay). *P <0.05. Source: Lewis *et al.* (2005).

macrophages and eosinophils) |**21,24**|. However, the lack of any significant difference in PDGF isoform levels in BAL fluid or expression of PDGF receptor subunits in airway biopsies between asthmatic subjects and healthy controls has detracted from the perceived importance of this family of growth factors |**25**|. With the demonstration that fibroblasts isolated from the airways of severe asthmatic subjects exhibit heightened procollagen secretion in response to PDGF, Lewis *et al.* have added to the evidence supporting a central role for the fibroblast in effecting remodelling in the airways in severe asthma.

The mechanism underlying the increased synthetic/secretory activity of severe asthmatic fibroblasts remains unclear. Evidently, it cannot be accounted for by increased expression of growth factor receptors, since elevated PDGFR, expression in mild/moderate asthmatic fibroblasts was not accompanied by any significant change in PDGF-induced procollagen secretion. An alternative possibility is that the intracellular signalling pathway mediating responses to PDGF receptor activation, which involves activation of phosphoinositide 3-kinase (PI3K)/Akt |**26**|, might be altered in severe asthma |**27**|. The role of specific isoforms of PI3K in the regulation of activity of various inflammatory cells, including T lymphocytes and eosinophils, is under investigation. The growth-factor-induced differentiation and activation of fibroblasts represents an interface between the previously poorly connected features of inflammation and remodelling in asthmatic airways. The existence of common signalling pathways in inflammatory and structural cells may present novel therapeutic targets which affect remodelling at both the stimulator and the effector level.

Vascular endothelial growth factor (VEGF) induces remodeling and enhances T_H2-mediated sensitization and inflammation in the lung

Lee CG, Link H, Baluk P, *et al. Nat Med* 2005; **10**: 1095–103

BACKGROUND. VEGF, originally described as a vascular permeability factor generating tissue oedema, has been found to exert a range of angiogenic actions, including epithelial cell proliferation, blood vessel formation and endothelial cell survival. Elevated levels of VEGF have been detected in bronchial tissues and secretions of asthmatic individuals, raising questions regarding its possible pathogenetic role in asthma. Using transgenic mice in which local overexpression of VEGF could be induced in the lungs by administration of a tetracycline antibiotic, Lee *et al.* demonstrated induction of an asthma-like phenotype with airway inflammation and oedema, hyper-responsiveness and remodelling (airway, parenchymal and vascular). Antigen-induced airway inflammation was accompanied by VEGF production by epithelial cells and Th2 cells, with production by Th1 cells markedly lower. Inhibition of VEGF suppressed Th2 airway inflammation and hyper-responsiveness in antigen-sensitized/challenged mice.

INTERPRETATION. VEGF is a stimulator of inflammation and of airway and vascular remodelling. Production of VEGF is a critical event in Th2-dependent airway inflammation in an experimental model of asthma: it is produced by Th2 cells in the allergen-challenged lung and is also required for the heightened elaboration of Th2 cytokines, possibly through a shift in the population of antigen-presenting dendritic cells in the lung from Th1-specific DC1 to Th2-specific DC2 cells. In addition to these roles in airway inflammation, VEGF contributes to the long-term lung remodelling characteristic of severe asthma. Mucous metaplasia, angiogenesis and smooth muscle hyperplasia are induced by VEGF, and their induction by repeated allergen challenge is at least partly dependent upon VEGF. These findings indicate a possible role for regulation of VEGF in the therapy of Th2-driven conditions, including asthma.

Comment

Numerous endogenous factors – inflammatory mediators, cytokines, proteases, antibody/soluble receptor complexes, etc. – have been proposed to play major roles in the pathology and/or pathogenesis of asthma. In many cases, the importance of these factors has been difficult to demonstrate owing to their potential involvement at several stages in the process of pathogenesis: development, sensitization, chronic inflammation with remodelling, and acute airway inflammation and bronchoconstriction. The ability to delete or induce specific genes at various stages in the life-cycle of an animal has presented opportunities to make more detailed study of the role of the proteins encoded by these genes at various critical stages in development of a disease. To date, the use of genetic deletion (knockout) has allowed roles to be demonstrated for various cytokines and other factors in a range of features of experimental models of asthma [28]. This recent study from Dr Elias's group at Yale University has revealed a number of important roles for VEGF, a growth factor which has been found previously to be associated with asthma but whose involvement in the disease process was undefined [29]. The ability of VEGF to mimic all of the characteristic features of asthma is reinforced by the ability of VEGF deletion to prevent the induction of several features in a conventional model of allergen sensitization and challenge. VEGF appears to be involved in the well-characterized processes of Th2 lymphocyte-mediated inflammation; one important action of VEGF – the induction of mucous metaplasia (differentiation of epithelial cells into mucus-secreting goblet cells) – is secondarily dependent upon the Th2 cytokine IL-13, as VEGF failed to induce the change in IL-13 knockout animals. Curiously, while overexpression of VEGF induced inflammation, vascular remodelling, mucous metaplasia, dendritic cell population shift, smooth muscle hyperplasia and airway hyper-responsiveness, the withdrawal of the overexpression failed to reverse the increase in smooth muscle and airway responsiveness, although all other features were readily reversed. Several experimental models of asthma have revealed dissociation between airway inflammation and hyper-responsiveness; this may reflect the involvement of distinct – and irreversible – mechanisms in the induction of hyper-responsiveness.

Airway remodeling and inflammation in symptomatic infants with reversible airflow obstruction

Saglani S, Malmström K, Pelkonen AS, *et al. Am J Respir Crit Care Med* 2005; **171**: 722–7

BACKGROUND. Thickening of the reticular basement membrane has been identified as an early change occurring in the airways of asthmatic individuals, with significant thickening observable from the age of 6. However, no data are available to indicate when basement membrane thickening begins or whether thickening shows any relationship to symptoms, lung function or airway inflammation. Fifty-three infants (aged 3.4–26 months, with symptoms including dyspnoea, cough and wheeze) undergoing clinically indicated bronchoscopy provided biopsies for histological study. Analysis revealed no difference in basement membrane thickness between symptomatic and non-symptomatic infants, or between these infants and healthy children (6–16 years) or adults (21–42 years). All of these groups, however, had thinner basement membranes than asthmatic children (6–16 years). There was no difference in basement membrane thickness between atopic and non-atopic infants.

INTERPRETATION. Subject groups were as follows: group A, 15 symptomatic infants with decreased specific airway conductance (sG_{aw}) and bronchodilator reversibility (mean

46% increase in sG_{aw}); group B, 22 symptomatic infants with decreased sG_{aw} but without bronchodilator reversibility; group C, 15 symptomatic infants with normal sG_{aw}; group D, 17 children with difficult asthma; group E, ten children without asthma; Group F, nine adults without asthma. There were no significant differences in basement membrane thickness or tissue eosinophil, neutrophil, mast cell or plasma cell numbers among groups A, B and C. Basement membrane thickness in these groups (group A, median 4.3 μm; group B, 4.2 μm; group C, 3.8 μm) was not significantly different from those in groups E (5.0 μm) and F (4.3 μm); group D (8.3 μm), however, showed significantly greater basement membrane thickness than all other groups (Fig. 3.6). The authors conclude that the basement membrane thickening and eosinophilic inflammation of the airways characteristic of asthma in childhood are not present in symptomatic infants with reversible airflow obstruction.

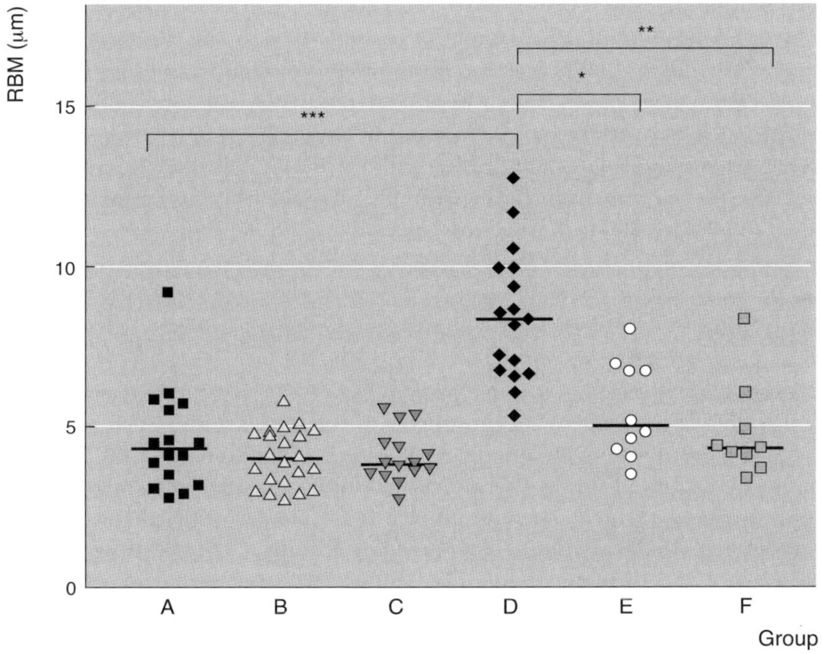

Fig. 3.6 Lack of association of reticular basement membrane (RBM) thickness with asthma symptoms in infants. RBM thickness was measured in symptomatic infants (groups A–C; see text), asthmatic children (group D) and healthy children (group E) and adults (group F). No difference in basement membrane thickness was observed among the three groups of symptomatic infants, and these did not differ from healthy children or adults. *P <0.05; **P <0.01; ***P <0.001. Source: Saglani *et al.* (2005).

Comment

The importance of airway remodelling in asthma pathology was highlighted by the finding that significant basement membrane thickening is observable in children as young as 6 years with difficult asthma. This pathognomic change was observed independently of lung function or airway eosinophilia and it was suggested that it may precede the development of chronic inflammation |**30**|. Longitudinal studies of pre-school-age children were recommended to determine whether basement membrane thickening in early childhood may be predictive of the development of persistent asthma, which cannot be predicted from early symptoms. In their study, Saglani *et al.* measured basement membrane thickness in airway sections from children up to 26 months old in order to determine whether remodelling was apparent in symptomatic infants. No association was apparent between membrane thickness and symptoms; moreover, no association could be observed between symptoms and inflammatory cell numbers. A dependence of basement membrane thickening upon eosinophilic inflammation might explain the absence of this aspect of remodelling in infants who have not developed airway eosinophilia |**3**|. It is clear, however, that symptoms such as recurrent wheeze and cough may occur independently of these processes. The authors of this study propose to follow up their cohort of patients to determine which children develop asthma at school age. Longitudinal measurements in these children may identify inflammatory or remodelling indices which are predictive of disease onset and progression.

Conclusion

The effort expended on basic scientific research in airway inflammation is increasingly returning valuable understanding of the disease processes which underlie asthma. Several common themes emerge from a study of the recent literature. First, the homeostatic control of the local environment in the airways is dependent upon interactions between resident structural cells and transient inflammatory cells. These interactions, when the set-point is altered by chronic allergen exposure or by genotypic/phenotypic differences in one of the cell populations, may lead to outcomes which produce changes in the airways associated with the pathology of asthma. Thus, these cell–cell interactions are likely to prove vital in the pathogenesis of the disease and, consequently, to offer targets for therapeutic intervention in the development and/or progression of asthma.

Secondly, some specific molecules arise in several contexts. Interleukin 13, for example, is elevated in the inflammatory exudates of allergen-challenged lungs and the levels of this cytokine, as well as the numbers of IL-13$^+$ T lymphocytes, are dependent upon BLT_1-mediated actions of LTB_4. IL-13 is also essential for the production of mucous metaplasia in the airways in response to VEGF, one of the major remodelling stimuli. As a Th2 cytokine, IL-13 appears to play a role in the development of hyper-responsiveness that is dependent upon LTB_4 and involves

VEGF. Pathways originating in the acute generation of inflammatory mediators and resulting in chronic changes in airway structures, regulated by T-cell-derived cytokines, thus begin to be formed.

The identification of very early events which direct the development of asthma remains difficult. Remodelling changes which are observable even in young children are not observed in infants with respiratory symptoms that indicate the potential for development of asthma. Longitudinal studies of these infants may help to define key changes in early life which do signal the beginning of the processes leading to asthma.

The monitoring of airway inflammation by the measurement of factors in exhaled breath condensate is proving to be valuable. As well as aiding in the optimization of treatment, these measurements should prove useful in further mechanistic studies. The ability to measure LTB_4 in exhaled breath condensate, for example, permits further study of the importance of this mediator in asthma. The apparent requirement for LTB_4 in the development of hyper-responsiveness suggests that its production might be a useful target for therapeutic control. Being able to measure airway levels of LTB_4 over very short periods could be useful in determining the relationship between its production in response to allergen challenge and the long-term changes which may result.

Several promising programmes of research are under way which have the potential to offer greater understanding of the fundamental processes which produce asthma. As each produces new results, the possibilities for new therapies based on this understanding continue to emerge.

References

1. Wenzel S. Severe asthma in adults. *Am J Respir Crit Care Med* 2005; **172**: 149–60.
2. Bousquet J, Jeffery PK, Busse WW, Johnson M, Vignola AM. Asthma: from bronchoconstriction to airways inflammation and remodeling. *Am J Respir Crit Care Med* 2000; **161**: 1720–45.
3. Jeffery PK, Holgate S, Wenzel S. Methods for the assessment of endobronchial biopsies in clinical research: application to studies of pathogenesis and the effects of treatment. *Am J Respir Crit Care Med* 2003; **168**: S1–S17.
4. British Thoracic Society. The British Guidelines on Asthma Management; 1995 Review and Position Statement. *Thorax* 1997; **52**(Suppl 1): S1–20.
5. Message SD, Johnston SL. Host defense function of the airway epithelium in health and disease: clinical background. *J Leukoc Biol* 2004; **75**: 5–17.

6. Burke-Gaffney A, Hellewell PG. A CD18/ICAM-1-dependent pathway mediates eosinophil adhesion to human bronchial epithelial cells. *Am J Respir Cell Mol Biol* 1998; **19**: 408–18.
7. Papi A, Johnston SL. Rhinovirus infection induces expression of its own receptor intercellular adhesion molecule 1 (ICAM-1) via increased NF-κB-mediated transcription. *J Biol Chem* 1999; **274**: 9707–20.
8. Green RH, Brightling CE, McKenna S, Hargadon B, Parker D, Bradding P, Wardlaw AJ, Pavord ID. Asthma exacerbations and sputum eosinophil counts: a randomised controlled trial. *Lancet* 2002; **360**: 1715–21.
9. Kharitonov SA, Gonio F, Kelly C, Meah S, Barnes PJ. Reproducibility of exhaled nitric oxide measurements in healthy and asthmatic adults and children. *Eur Respir J* 2003; **21**: 433–8.
10. Luster AD, Tager AM. T-cell trafficking in asthma: lipid mediators grease the way. *Nat Rev Immunol* 2004; **4**: 711–24.
11. Reid JJ. ABT-761 (Abbott). *Curr Opin Investig Drugs* 2001; **2**: 68–71.
12. Busse WW, Lemanske RF Jr. Asthma. *N Engl J Med* 2001; **344**: 350–62.
13. Terawaki K, Yokomizo T, Nagase T, Toda A, Taniguchi M, Hashizume K, Yagi T, Shimizu T. Absence of leukotriene B_4 receptor 1 confers resistance to airway hyper-responsiveness and Th2-type immune responses. *J Immunol* 2005; **175**: 4217–25.
14. Sexton DW, Walsh GM. Eosinophil–epithelial cell interactions: an important facet of asthmatic inflammation. *Clin Exp Allergy* 2002; **32**: 811–13.
15. Dent G, Rühlmann E, Bodtke K, Magnussen H, Rabe KF. Upregulation of human eosinophil leukotriene C_4 generation through contact with bronchial epithelial cells. *Inflamm Res* 2000; **49**: 236–9.
16. Wong CK, Wang CB, Ip WK, Lam CW. Role of p38 MAPK and NF-kB for chemokine release in coculture of human eosinophils and bronchial epithelial cells. *Clin Exp Immunol* 2005; **139**: 90–100.
17. Hirst SJ. Airway smooth muscle as a target in asthma. *Clin Exp Allergy* 2000; **30**(Suppl 1): 54–9.
18. Hakonarson H, Kim C, Whelan R, Campbell D, Grunstein MM. Bi-directional activation between human airway smooth muscle cells and T lymphocytes: role in induction of altered airway responsiveness. *J Immunol* 2001; **166**: 293–303.
19. Lazaar AL, Panettieri RAJ. Airway smooth muscle: a modulator of airway remodeling in asthma. *J Allergy Clin Immunol* 2005; **116**: 488–95.
20. Lazaar AL, Albelda SM, Pilewski JM, Brennan B, Pure E, Panettieri RAJ. T lymphocytes adhere to airway smooth muscle cells via integrins and CD44 and induce smooth muscle cell DNA synthesis. *J Exp Med* 1994; **180**: 807–16.
21. Muro S, Minshall EM, Hamid QA. The pathology of chronic asthma. *Clin Chest Med* 2000; **21**: 225–44.
22. Synek M, Beasley R, Frew AJ, Goulding D, Holloway L, Lampe FC, Roche WR, Holgate ST. Cellular infiltration of the airways in asthma of varying severity. *Am J Respir Crit Care Med* 1996; **154**: 224–30.
23. Balzar S, Chu HW, Silkoff P, Cundall M, Trudeau JB, Strand M, Wenzel S. Increased TGF-β2 in severe asthma with eosinophilia. *J Allergy Clin Immunol* 2005; **115**: 110–17.

24. Ross R, Raines EW, Bowen-Pope DF. The biology of platelet-derived growth factor. *Cell* 1986; **46**: 155–69.

25. Chanez P, Vignola M, Stenger R, Vic P, Michel FB, Bousquet J. Platelet-derived growth factor in asthma. *Allergy* 1995; **50**: 878–83.

26. Reif S, Lang A, Lindqvist JN, Yata Y, Gabele E, Scanga A. The role of focal adhesion kinase-phosphatidylinositol 3-kinase-Akt signaling in hepatic stellate cell proliferation and type I collagen expression. *J Biol Chem* 2003; **278**: 8083–90.

27. Dube J, Chakir J, Laviolette M, Martin SS, Boutet M, Desrochers C, Auger F, Boulet LP. In vitro procollagen synthesis and proliferative phenotype of bronchial fibroblasts from normal and asthmatic subjects. *Lab Invest* 1998; **78**: 297–307.

28. Moffatt JD. What targets have knockouts revealed in asthma? *Pharmacol Ther* 2005; **107**: 343–57.

29. Lee YC, Lee HK. Vascular endothelial growth factor in patients with acute asthma. *J Allergy Clin Immunol* 2001; **107**: 1106–8.

30. Payne DN, Rogers AV, Adelroth E, Bandi V, Guntupalli KK, Bush A, Jeffery PK. Early thickening of the reticular basement membrane in children with difficult asthma. *Am J Respir Crit Care Med* 2003; **167**: 78–82.

4

Atopic dermatitis

HASAN ARSHAD

Introduction

Atopic dermatitis (AD) is a chronic inflammatory condition of the skin which usually starts in infancy. It is sometimes called 'atopic eczema' or even simply 'eczema'. Recently, the term 'atopic eczema dermatitis syndrome' has also been proposed to indicate the varied nature of this disease. The diagnosis is based on clinical features of a chronic itchy dermatitis with typical morphology and distribution and a relapsing and remitting course. For a more formal diagnosis, the criteria of Hanifin and Rajka [1] or the UK Working Party [2] have been commonly used.

As the name implies, AD is often an atopic condition, especially in early childhood. It is commonly associated with food allergy and both conditions tend to improve in the majority of young children. It has been suggested that nearly half of these children develop asthma. In a minority, AD persists into later childhood and adult life. However, even in early childhood no evidence of atopy can be found in some children. The proportion of non-atopic individuals is even higher in older children and adults with AD. The clinical manifestations are similar but aetiologically these might be two different conditions. There is some suggestion of different risk factor profiles for extrinsic (atopic) AD and intrinsic (non-atopic) AD [3]. Extrinsic AD is an allergic condition that is associated with food allergy and asthma, usually first presents in infancy and has a male preponderance, whereas intrinsic AD is a non-allergic condition and presents later in childhood.

AD is a multifactorial heritable disorder, genes as well as the environment playing a role in its development. Parental atopy in general, and parental AD in particular, increases the risk of AD in the offspring. Genome-wide screens have identified several susceptibility regions, with some overlap with susceptibility regions for psoriasis but not asthma. Among the environmental factors, infant feeding and socio-economic status have been found to be associated with the development of AD but factors related to hygiene, such as daycare attendance and the number of older siblings, have not.

Triggers for AD include allergens, irritants and infections. Food allergens are common triggers in early childhood, and inhalant allergens may play a role in older children and adults. *Staphylococcal aureus* infections and their associated bacterial products and toxins are important exacerbating factors at all ages and in all forms

© Atlas Medical Publishing Ltd

of AD. Colonization by *S. aureus* is common in AD skin and correlates with disease activity. *S. aureus* toxins act as superantigens, stimulating lymphocytes and monocytes to produce pro-inflammatory cytokines.

The standard treatment of AD is topical corticosteroids. They are effective but prolonged use may cause skin atrophy and suppression of the hypothalamic–pituitary–adrenal axis. Systemic corticosteroids, phototherapy and immunosuppressants are effective but their use is limited by significant adverse effects. Thus, novel, effective but non-toxic treatments are needed. In the last few years, calcineurin inhibitors such as topical tacrolimus and pimecrolimus have been investigated. Both are topical immune modulators which suppress T-cell activation, inhibit antigen-presenting cells and reduce the release of inflammatory cytokines. In clinical trials they have proved effective and are well tolerated.

There has been significant improvement in our understanding of the natural history and pathophysiology of AD in recent years. The papers reviewed in this chapter reflect these developments. The central role played by *S. aureus* infection in promoting inflammation in AD is discussed as the main theme of pathogenesis in AD. At the end of the chapter, three papers discuss new treatments as replacements for, or additional to, therapy with topical corticosteroids.

Natural history

AD is very common in infancy and early childhood, with a prevalence approaching 20% or more, but improves or remits in the majority of these children. At this stage many acquire aeroallergen sensitization and develop asthma and/or rhinitis. This progression from AD and associated food sensitization to asthma/rhinitis and associated aeroallergen sensitization is called the 'atopic march'. However, the natural history of AD has rarely been studied in long-term unselected birth cohort studies. We also know very little about the natural history of AD in adults. Two papers published in the last couple of years aimed to establish the natural history of AD in children and adults.

The natural course of atopic dermatitis from birth to age 7 years and the association with asthma

Illi S, von Mutius E, Lau S, *et al.*; Multicenter Allergy Study Group. *J Allergy Clin Immunol* 2004; **113**: 925–31

BACKGROUND. AD is considered to be one of the first manifestations in the atopic march. The aim of this study was to investigate prospectively the natural course of AD to determine factors influencing its prognosis and to analyse the relationship of AD with childhood asthma. The Multicenter Allergy Study, a German birth cohort, followed 1314 children from birth to age 7 years. Physical examinations, parental interviews on atopic symptoms and diagnoses, and determination of specific immunoglobulin (Ig)E levels were performed regularly.

INTERPRETATION. The cumulative prevalence of AD in the first 2 years of life was 22%. Of these patients, 43% were in complete remission by age 3 years, 38% had an intermittent pattern of disease and 19% had persistent symptoms every year. Severity and atopic sensitization were major determinants of prognosis. Early wheeze and a specific sensitization pattern, but not AD, were significant predictors of wheezing at school age. Early AD, without these cofactors, conferred no increased risk of subsequent wheeze or bronchial hyper-reactivity. Early AD is associated with asthma at school age, but in many of these asthmatic children wheezing manifests before or with the onset of AD. Children with AD and wheeze have a marked loss in lung function, suggesting a distinct phenotype rather than a progressive development from AD to asthma.

Comment

The Multicenter Allergy Study is a prospective study of 1314 infants recruited at birth to investigate the epidemiology, prognosis and risk factors for asthma and allergy development. The importance of studying these children from birth cannot be overstated as more than 60% of AD cases start in the first year of life. The cohort was followed up extensively every year for the first 7 years using questionnaires and measurement of specific IgE, and the presence or absence of allergic disease and sensitization was determined.

This study confirms previous observations that AD is common in early childhood but improves in the majority of children during the first 7 years of life. However, the prognosis was less favourable than previously believed. Nearly 20% had persistent disease and another 40% continued to have intermittent symptoms. Parental AD was a stronger risk factor than parental asthma or rhinitis, indicating disease specificity in the heritability of atopy.

The paper also explores the relationship of AD with wheeze during childhood. Nearly half of the children with moderate to severe AD had associated wheeze in early childhood; the risk of wheeze persisted to age 7 and wheeze was 3 times more likely than in those without early AD. However, early AD without concomitant wheeze was not a risk factor for the development of asthma. This challenges the prevalent concept of the atopic march (AD followed by asthma). It seems that AD and wheeze develop concomitantly, and in this phenotype wheeze persists with early loss of lung function.

Prognosis and prognostic factors in adult patients with atopic dermatitis: a long-term follow-up questionnaire study

Sandstrom MH, Faergemann J. *Br J Dermatol* 2004; **150**: 103–10

BACKGROUND. AD is a chronic relapsing skin disease. Several investigations concerning the long-term prognosis of AD among children and teenagers have been performed but there are few data for adults. The aim of this study was to investigate the prognosis and prognostic factors in adult patients with AD using a long-term follow-up (25–38 years). A follow-up questionnaire was sent to 922 AD patients

examined in an out-patient clinic between 1960 and 1973 among 1366 registered patients with AD. The patients were aged 20 years or older when they visited the clinic and 45 years or older when they answered the follow-up questionnaire.

Interpretation. The response rate was 90.4%. The age range at the time of follow-up was 45–86 years (mean 55 years). Of the 833 patients who responded, 59% reported AD at some time during the last 12 months, which was defined as persistent AD. The mean clearance rate per person-year was 18%. One of the most important factors associated with the persistence of AD was dermatitis of the head and neck with or without other AD locations at the time of examination, according to the old patient records. This study showed that the majority of adults with AD still had AD when they became older. This was particularly so if negative prognostic factors existed.

Comment

The characteristics of AD, including morphology, distribution and prognosis, may vary according to age. For instance, AD in adults is often non-atopic and the hands, head and neck are commonly involved. AD commonly starts in early childhood but remission occurs frequently. In adults the long-term prognosis is less clear. Therefore, this was an important study as it assessed the outcome of AD in adults after 25–38 years. However, the first assessment was retrospective, based on hospital records. The disadvantage of this approach is that the data are limited by the information recorded at the time. Moreover, the reliability, accuracy and consistency of diagnosis cannot be guaranteed. The strengths of the study included adequate numbers and a credible response rate.

This study shows that remission in adults is relatively infrequent. Even after 25–30 years, 60% of subjects had persistent AD. Adverse prognostic factors included hand and neck involvement, a sibling with AD, allergic sensitization to pollen and sensitivity to animals and nickel (Table 4.1). Nearly 70% of subjects with

Table 4.1 Importance of certain factors in persistent atopic dermatitis

Factors	No. of patients with the factor in persistent AD (%)	No. of patients with the factor in healed AD (%)	*P*-value: bivariate analysis	*P*-value: logistic regression analysis
Head/neck localization*	274/487 (56)	151/341 (44)	0.001	0.03
Asthma	122/484 (25)	45/342 (13)	<0.0001	NS
AR	262/480 (55)	114/337 (34)	<0.0001	NS
Parent with AD	113/490 (23)	57/342 (17)	0.017	NS
Siblings with AD	128/433 (30)	60/301 (20)	0.006	0.04
Allergy to furred animals	274/480 (57)	128/338 (38)	<0.0001	0.01
Pollen allergy	254/476 (53)	111/336 (33)	<0.0001	0.01
OAS	230/486 (47)	89/341 (26)	<0.0001	0.001
Eczema worsened by food	253/475 (53)	131/320 (41)	<0.0001	NS
Nickel sensitivity	161/486 (33)	71/341 (21)	<0.0001	0.004

AD, atopic dermatitis; AR, allergic rhinoconjunctivitis; OAS; oral allergy syndrome; NS, not significant.
*With or without other locations at the time according to the old patient record.
Source: Sandstrom *et al.* (2004).

persistent AD had a history of asthma and/or rhinitis, highlighting the importance of atopy even in adults with AD.

Pathophysiology of AD

AD is a chronic inflammatory skin disease characterized by highly pruritic, eczematous lesions. Most (70–80%) AD patients exhibit atopic diathesis with high IgE levels and allergen sensitization (atopic or extrinsic AD). The skin is infiltrated by $CD4^+$ lymphocytes and T-helper (Th) 2 cytokines such as interleukin (IL)-4, IL-5 and IL-13 are in abundance, although in chronic lesions Th1 cells secreting interferon γ (IFN-γ) are also present. In AD skin lesions, T cells express skin homing receptor, the cutaneous lymphocyte antigen (CLA). In a significant minority (20–30%) there is no evidence of atopy (non-atopic or intrinsic AD). Clinical features are, however, similar and T lymphocytes play a critical role in both forms of AD.

The skin of AD subjects is often colonized by *S. aureus*, which is important in the causation and exacerbation of inflammation [4]. The presence and number of bacteria correlate with disease activity. *S. aureus* toxins have superantigen properties and may attract and activate T lymphocytes. The mechanism of increased susceptibility to skin colonization by *S. aureus* in AD is not clear, but it may be related to decreased endogenous antimicrobial peptides (AMP) in atopic skin. Four papers, reviewed in this section, focus on mechanisms underlying the infiltration of AD skin with T lymphocytes and their interaction with toxins produced by *S. aureus.*

CCL18 is expressed in atopic dermatitis and mediates skin homing of human memory T cells

Gunther C, Bello-Fernandez C, Kopp T, *et al. J Immunol* 2005; **174**: 1723–8

Background. CCL18 is a human chemokine secreted by monocytes and dendritic cells. The receptor for CCL18 is not yet known and the effects of this chemokine on immune cells are not fully elucidated.

Interpretation. CCL18 was present in skin biopsies of AD patients but not in normal or psoriatic skin. CCL18 was specifically expressed by antigen-presenting cells (APCs) in the dermis and by Langerhans and inflammatory dendritic epidermal cells in the epidermis. In addition, the serum levels of CCL18 and the percentages of CCL18-producing monocyte/macrophages and dendritic cells were significantly increased in AD patients compared with healthy controls. Furthermore, it was demonstrated that CCL18 binds to CLA^+ T cells in peripheral blood of AD patients and healthy individuals and induces the migration of AD-derived memory T cells *in vitro* and in severe combined immune deficient (SCID) mice that had received transplants of human skin. These findings highlight a unique role of CCL18 in AD and reveal a novel function of this chemokine in mediating the skin homing of a subpopulation of human memory T cells.

Comment

Chemokines are a group of proteins that attract leucocytes to the site of inflammation. The homing of lymphocytes to AD skin is attributed to various chemokines, such as CCL17, CCL22 and CCL27. This study focuses on CCL18, which is a chemokine secreted by APC. It suggests that CCL18 may be a key chemoattractant factor in AD. CCL18 was strongly expressed in AD skin but not in normal or psoriatic skin; the percentage of CCL18 producing mononuclear cells (in response to IL-4) was significantly higher than normal in peripheral blood in AD patients, and serum levels of CCL18 were 3-fold higher in AD patients compared with healthy controls. The authors then investigated the specific function of CCL18 in AD. Their *in vitro* and *in vivo* (mouse) experimental models demonstrated that CCL18 induced migration of both naive and memory T cells. Its precise function may be to specifically attract Th2 cells, as CCL18 was not expressed in the skin in psoriasis, which is a Th1-mediated disease. This study very nicely demonstrates the role of CCL18 in the pathogenesis of AD.

T regulatory cells in atopic dermatitis and subversion of their activity by superantigens

Ou LS, Goleva E, Hall C, Leung DY. *J Allergy Clin Immunol* 2004; **113**: 756–63

BACKGROUND. AD is a chronic inflammatory skin disease involving colonization by superantigen-secreting *S. aureus*. $CD4^+CD25^+$ T regulatory (Treg) cells are thought to play an important role in controlling inflammatory responses. It was hypothesized that Treg cells might be deficient in patients with AD. $CD4^+CD25^+$ and $CD4^+CD25^-$ T cells were isolated from peripheral blood mononuclear cells (PBMCs) and cultured with anti-CD3 or superantigens (staphylococcal enterotoxin B [SEB]) for 72 h. $CD4^+$, $CD8^+$, $CD25^+$ cells were isolated and CLA expression on PBMCs was assessed by means of flow cytometry. RNA was extracted from isolated subsets of T cells and a real-time polymerase chain reaction for FoxP3 mRNA was performed.

INTERPRETATION. Surprisingly, $CD4^+CD25^+$ T cells were significantly ($P<0.01$) increased in patients with AD ($6.68 \pm 0.99\%$; $n = 15$) compared with asthmatic patients ($3.42 \pm 0.58\%$; $n = 12$) and non-atopic healthy control subjects ($3.34 \pm 0.43\%$; $n = 14$). Patients with AD also had greater expression of $CD25^+$ in skin-homing, $CD4^+$, CLA-positive T cells than asthmatic and non-atopic subjects (35.95, 22.44 and 23.03% respectively; $P<0.006$). Only $CD4^+CD25^+$ cells expressed FoxP3; $CD4^+CD25^-$ T cells and $CD4^-$ cells did not. Consistently with known properties of Treg cells, $CD4^+CD25^+$ cells were anergic to anti-CD3 stimulation. When $CD4^+CD25^+$ cells from each study group were mixed with $CD4^+CD25^-$ cells, proliferative responses were equally suppressed after anti-CD3 stimulation. In contrast, after SEB stimulation, $CD4^+CD25^+$ cells were no longer anergic. Furthermore, when $CD4^+CD25^+$ cells were mixed with $CD4^+CD25$ cells and stimulated with SEB, the suppressive function of Treg cells was reversed. In conclusion, patients with AD had significantly increased numbers of peripheral blood Treg cells with normal immunosuppressive activity. However, after superantigen stimulation Treg cells lose their immunosuppressive activity. These data suggest a novel mechanism by which superantigens could augment T-cell activation in patients with AD.

Comment

Treg cells constitute 5–15% of peripheral blood $CD4^+$ T cells. The significance of Treg cells in modifying immune responses has been recognized increasingly in recent years. They suppress T-cell proliferation and immune responses and have been shown to inhibit airway eosinophilia in animal models [5]. In view of their inhibitory properties, it was hypothesized that Treg cells might be deficient in number or function in AD. To the investigators' surprise, Treg cells constituted a higher proportion of $CD4^+$ T cells, including those expressing skin-homing receptor (CLA), in subjects with AD compared with subjects with asthma and non-atopic subjects. If Treg cells were functional, the inflammatory responses should have been suppressed. However, AD is a chronic inflammatory condition. These Treg cells are either non-functional or have altered properties. To assess the functional properties of Treg cells, the investigators carried out proliferative responses to anti-CD3. As expected, Treg cells were themselves non-responsive, and actively suppressed the stimulation of other $CD4^+$ cells by anti-CD3 in both AD patients and healthy subjects. In view of the staphylococcal colonization of skin in more than 90% of AD patients, the investigators went on to assess the response of Treg cells to staphylococcal toxin, SEB or superantigen. Treg cells not only responded to SEB stimulation but also lost their suppressive effect on other $CD4^+$ T cells in both AD and healthy subjects. This important finding indicates that Treg cell function is altered by exposure to staphylococcal toxins or superantigens in AD skin. Superantigens are potent stimulators of T cells and macrophages. They are also known to increase the expression of CLA, thus facilitating the infiltration of T cells in AD skin. This, combined with the demonstration in this study that superantigen can reverse the suppressive function of Treg cells, highlights the significance of *S. aureus* infection in promoting chronic inflammation in AD.

Interleukin-10 downregulates anti-microbial peptide expression in atopic dermatitis

Howell MD, Novak N, Bieber T, *et al. J Invest Dermatol* 2005; **125**: 738–45

BACKGROUND. Recurrent skin infections in extrinsic atopic dermatitis (EAD) may occur because of the suppression of AMP expression by IL-4 and IL-13. Twenty to

thirty per cent of cases of AD, however, are classified as intrinsic atopic dermatitis (IAD). These patients exhibit normal serum IgE levels, no allergen-specific sensitization, and lower levels of IL-4 and IL-13 than EAD. Both forms of AD have increased propensity to skin infection, suggesting a novel mechanism for infection in IAD.

INTERPRETATION. Significantly decreased expression of the human β-defensin (HBD)-2 gene was found in the skin of both IAD ($P = 0.010$) and EAD patients ($P = 0.004$) compared with psoriasis patients. Conversely, IAD ($P = 0.019$) and EAD ($P = 0.002$) skin lesions exhibited elevated IL-10 gene expression when compared with psoriasis. Using primary keratinocytes, it was shown that the deficiency in AMP expression is an acquired rather than a constitutive defect. Interestingly, neutralizing antibodies to IL-10 augmented the production of tumour necrosis factor-α (TNF-α) and IFN-γ by PBMCs from AD patients. Additionally, treatment of AD skin explants with anti-IL-10 augmented the expression of HBD-2. Thus, increased levels of IL-10 may contribute to the AMP deficiency in both IAD and EAD by reducing cytokines that induce AMP.

Comment

AD presents as two distinct phenotypes: atopic or extrinsic (high total IgE and evidence of allergen sensitization) and non-atopic or intrinsic (normal IgE and no specific allergen sensitization). A prominent feature of both forms of AD is susceptibility to staphylococcal infections. In extrinsic AD it was thought that this susceptibility stems from the downregulation of AMP by Th2 cytokines (IL-4 and IL-13). However, intrinsic AD is not associated with high IL-4 and IL-13. β-Defensin is one of the AMPs the expression of which was reduced in both forms of AD. As levels of Th2 cytokines are not high in IAD (this would suppress AMP), another mechanism must exist. These investigators suggest that an increased level of IL-10, found in both intrinsic and extrinsic AD, mediates AMP deficiency by reducing the secretion of TNF-α and IFN-γ by PBMCs. Given the importance of staphylococcal infection in the pathogenesis of AD, this study contributes significantly to our understanding of the mechanisms of susceptibility to infection in both forms of AD.

Alpha-toxin is produced by skin colonizing *Staphylococcus aureus* and induces a T helper type 1 response in atopic dermatitis

Breuer K, Wittmann M, Kempe K, *et al. Clin Exp Allergy* 2005; **35**: 1088–95

BACKGROUND. ***S. aureus*** **is a well-known trigger factor for AD. Besides the superantigens, further exotoxins are produced by** ***S. aureus*** **and may have an influence on the disease. This study was designed to explore the impact of staphylococcal α-toxin on human T cells, as these represent the majority of skin-infiltrating cells in AD. Adult patients with AD were screened for cutaneous colonization with α-toxin-producing** ***S. aureus.*** **As α-toxin may induce necrosis,** $CD4^+$ **T cells were incubated with sublytic α-toxin concentrations. Proliferation and upregulation of IFN-γ**

at the mRNA and protein levels were assessed. The induction of t-bet translocation in $CD4^+$ T cells was detected with the electrophoretic mobility shift assay.

Interpretation. Thirty-four per cent of the patients were colonized with α-toxin-producing *S. aureus* and α-toxin was detected in lesional skin of these patients by immunohistochemistry. Sublytic α-toxin concentrations induced a marked proliferation of isolated $CD4^+$ T cells. Microarray analysis indicated that α-toxin induced particularly high amounts of IFN-γ transcripts. Upregulation of IFN-γ was confirmed at both the mRNA and the protein level (Fig. 4.1). Stimulation of $CD4^+$ T cells with α-toxin resulted in DNA binding of t-bet, known as a key transcription factor involved in primary Th1 commitment. This study shows that sublytic α-toxin concentrations activate T cells in the absence of

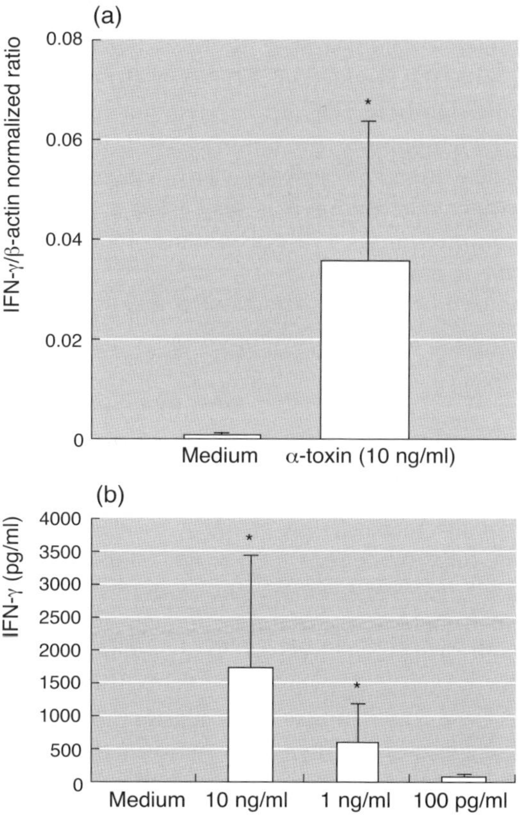

Fig. 4.1 Upregulation of IFN-γ after incubation with α-toxin. (a) $CD4^+$ T cells were incubated with 10 ng/ml α-toxin for 24 h. mRNA for IFN-γ was detected by real-time polymerase chain reaction (PCR). $P = 0.025$ ($n = 5$). (b) $CD4^+$ T cells were incubated with α-toxin for 4 days. IFN-γ protein concentrations in the cell culture supernatants were measured by ELISA (enzyme-linked immunosorbent assay). $P < 0.05$ ($n = 6$). Source: Breuer *et al.* (2005).

APCs and are relevant for the induction of a Th1-like cytokine response. In AD, this facilitates the development of Th1-cell-dominated chronic eczema.

Comment

The role of *S. aureus* in promoting chronic inflammation in AD has been investigated extensively in recent years and the significance of the production of enterotoxins with superantigenic properties has become clearer. Superantigens stimulate APCs to produce IL-12, which in turn promotes Th1 responses and contributes to ongoing inflammation. However, not all *S. aureus* strains produce enterotoxins and it is known that treatment of non-enterotoxin-producing bacteria with antimicrobials also improves AD. Some strains of *S. aureus* isolated from patients with AD produce α-toxin. This study shows that a significant number of patients with AD are colonized by α-toxin-producing *S. aureus*, and the toxin was shown to be present in the lesional skin. They further demonstrated the role of α-toxins in activating $CD4^+$ T lymphocytes to induce the production of IFN-γ, a Th1 cytokine.

The inflammation of AD is supported by both Th1 and Th2 cytokine responses. In acute lesions and exacerbations, Th2 lymphocytes predominate, while in chronic lesions there is evidence of Th1-cell activation and typically a Th1 cytokine milieu exists. α-toxins produced by some *S. aureus* strains may play a key role in the chronicity of AD by stimulating and promoting $CD4^+$ T cells and the production of Th1 cytokines, especially IFN-γ. *S. aureus* is a known trigger for exacerbation of AD and there may be other toxins, produced by different strains of *S. aureus*, responsible for acute exacerbation and promoting Th2 cytokine responses.

Investigations

In many patients with AD, exposure to food and aeroallergens causes exacerbation of AD lesions. An important part of the management of AD is to identify and remove allergenic triggers. While the measurement of specific IgE (sIgE) and the skin-prick test (SPT) can detect allergic sensitization, the relevance of this sensitization to AD is not always straightforward. For example, the significance of a positive SPT to grass pollen or moulds in patients with AD is uncertain unless a clear history of an exacerbation on exposure is available. Many patients show positive sIgE or SPT to foods such as egg or cows' milk without a history to support their clinical relevance. In general, correlation is often poor between these tests and the clinical manifestation. Application of allergens, such as house dust mite (HDM), on the skin can induce eczematous lesions in certain AD patients. This epicutaneous patch test, with application of food or aeroallergens and evaluation of eczematous reaction 24–72 h later, is termed the 'atopy patch test' (APT). In recent years, several studies have suggested that the APT is a useful addition to the SPT and sIgE measurement in the assessment of AD. However, results from these studies show wide variation, possibly because of methodological differences |**6**|.

The prevalence of positive reactions in the atopy patch test with aeroallergens and food allergens in subjects with atopic eczema: a European multicenter study

Darsow U, Laifaoui J, Kerschenlohr K, *et al. Allergy* 2004; **59**: 1318–25

BACKGROUND. The APT was proposed to evaluate IgE-mediated sensitizations in patients with AD. The prevalence and agreement with the clinical history and sIgE of positive APT reactions was investigated in six European countries using a standardized method. A total of 314 patients with AD in remission were tested in twelve study centres on clinically uninvolved, non-abraded back skin with HDM, cat dander, grass, and birch pollen allergen extracts with defined major allergen contents in petrolatum. Extracts of egg white, celery and wheat flour with defined protein content were also patch-tested. APT values were evaluated at 24, 48 and 72 h according to the European Task Force on Atopic Dermatitis guidelines. In addition, SPT and sIgE results and a detailed history of allergen-induced eczema flares were obtained.

INTERPRETATION. Previous eczema flares, after contact with specific allergens, were reported in 1% (celery) to 34% (HDM) of patients. The frequency of clear-cut positive APT reactions ranged from 39% with HDM to 9% with celery. All reactions were observed after 48 and 72 h. Positive SPT (16–57%) and elevated sIgE (19–59%) results were more frequent. A clear-cut positive APT with all negative SPT and sIgE results was seen in 7% of the patients, whereas a positive APT without a positive SPT or sIgE for the respective allergen was seen in 17% of the patients. APT, SPT and sIgE results showed significant agreement with the history for grass pollen and egg white ($P = 0.01$). With regard to the clinical history, the APT had a higher specificity (64–91% depending on the allergen) than the SPT (50–85%) or sIgE (52–85%). Positive APT results were associated with longer duration of eczema flares. In ten non-atopic controls, no positive APT reaction was seen. The authors concluded that aeroallergens and food allergens are able to elicit eczematous skin reactions after epicutaneous application and the relevance of aeroallergens for AD flares may be evaluated by the APT in addition to the SPT and sIgE.

Comment

This large multinational, European study was designed to assess the value of the APT with standardized methodology. They used standardized biological preparations in a petrolatum vehicle, applied to non-abraded, non-lesional, untreated skin. Most common food allergens (egg white, celery and wheat) and aeroallergens (HDM, cat, grass and birch pollen) were included, except cows' milk. All reactions were assessed after 24, 48 and 72 h and graded with conventional contact allergy patch-testing rules. Weaknesses of this study were its reliance on the history to establish the clinical relevance of allergic sensitization and the fact that provocation tests – the gold standard – were not performed.

The commonest positive reactions were to HDM (39%), followed by reactions to pollen; food reactions were relatively uncommon (10%). It should be noted that

Table 4.2 Sensitivity and specificity of different test procedures with regard to the patient's history

Test	Sensitivity			Specificity		
	SPT	sIgE	APT	SPT	sIgE	APT
Dermatophagoides pteronyssinus	68*	72*	45	50*	53*	64*
Cat dander	79*	80*	14	71*	69*	91
Grass pollen	80*	84*	28*	54*	53*	91*
Birch pollen	69*	73*	15	57*	52*	83
Egg white	68*	59*	32*	78*	85*	91*
Celery	100*	50	33	81*	71	91
Wheat flour	30	78	30	85	63*	91

The APT shows a higher specificity than classical tests for IgE-mediated hypersensitivity with regard to the allergen-specific history.
All values are percentages.
*Agreement with history (two-sided Pr >|Z| ≤0.01); refers to the predictive history of eczema exacerbations in the pollen season, in direct contact with allergen or after food ingestion ($n = 314$).
Source: Darsow *et al.* (2004).

most reactions were observed at 48 or 72 h, pointing to the fact that AD is not a type I, immediate hypersensitivity reaction. Interestingly, in a small subgroup of AD patients the ATP was positive but the SPT and sIgE were negative to common allergens. These patients would otherwise be regarded as non-atopic or intrinsic. This raises the interesting possibility that all AD patients could be proven extrinsic or 'atopic' if highly sensitive tests were available. However, a positive test is meaningless unless it is clinically relevant. In this respect the results were encouraging as APT showed high specificity (Table 4.2). Unfortunately, the sensitivity was too low for this to be used as the main diagnostic tool. Perhaps it is best used as a follow-up to the SPT or sIgE—either to investigate the clinical relevance of a positive SPT or sIgE result, or in those AD patients in whom clinically there is a strong suspicion of atopy but SPT or sIgE has turned out to be negative.

Treatment

Topical corticosteroids are the mainstay of treatment of AD. However, concerns regarding local and systemic (following absorption through the skin) adverse effects of steroids have led to the discovery of alternative anti-inflammatory treatments. In recent years, a number of clinical trials have evaluated the efficacy and safety of topical tacrolimus and pimecrolimus in AD. Both drugs inhibit calcineurin in the skin, which regulates the activity of several transcription factors involved in the proliferation and activation of T cells. This systemic review and meta-analysis by Ashcroft *et al.* is a timely effort to provide an overall view of the efficacy and safety of these topical treatments. The other two papers reviewed in this section evaluate additional immunosuppressive and anti-inflammatory treatments that might become available in the near future.

Efficacy and tolerability of topical pimecrolimus and tacrolimus in the treatment of atopic dermatitis: meta-analysis of randomised controlled trials

Ashcroft DM, Dimmock P, Garside R, Stein K, Williams HC. *BMJ* 2005; **330**: 516

BACKGROUND. This systematic review and meta-analysis was performed to determine the efficacy and tolerability of topical pimecrolimus and tacrolimus compared with other treatments for AD. Electronic searches of the Cochrane Library, Medline and Embase were carried out. Randomized, controlled trials of topical pimecrolimus or tacrolimus reporting efficacy outcomes or tolerability were included. Efficacy was assessed by investigators' and patients' global assessments of response, proportions of patients with flares of AD, and improvements in quality of life. Tolerability was assessed from overall rates of withdrawal, withdrawal due to adverse events, and proportions of patients with burning of the skin and skin infections.

INTERPRETATION. Of the 6897 participants in 25 randomized controlled trials, 4186 received topical pimecrolimus or tacrolimus. Both drugs were significantly more effective than a vehicle control. Tacrolimus 0.1% was as effective as potent topical corticosteroids at 3 weeks and more effective than hydrocortisone acetate 1% alone or combined treatment with hydrocortisone butyrate 0.1% (potent, used on trunk) plus hydrocortisone acetate 1% (weak, used on face). Direct comparisons of tacrolimus 0.03% and tacrolimus 0.1% consistently favoured the higher-strength formulation, but efficacy differed significantly between the two strengths only after 12 weeks of treatment. Pimecrolimus was far less effective than betamethasone valerate 0.1% (moderate-potency steroid). Pimecrolimus and tacrolimus caused significantly more skin burning than topical corticosteroids. Rates of skin infections did not differ in any of the comparisons. In conclusion, both topical pimecrolimus and topical tacrolimus are more effective than placebo. Topical tacrolimus is similar in efficacy to potent topical corticosteroids but seems to be safer. In the absence of key comparisons with mild corticosteroids, the clinical need for topical pimecrolimus is unclear.

Comment

This is a thorough and well-performed meta-analysis. Topical pimecrolimus was assessed in eleven trials that included a total of 2688 subjects and tacrolimus was evaluated in 14 trials (4209 subjects), and in one trial ($n = 141$) the two drugs were compared with each other. Overall, both drugs were superior to placebo (vehicle) in several outcome variables and were found to be safe, with burning sensation of the skin as the main adverse effect. Pimecrolimus was less effective than moderate-potency topical steroids, while tacrolimus 0.1% was more effective than mild steroids and equally effective when compared with potent steroids.

Adverse effects from mild corticosteroids are rare but long-term use of potent steroids is associated with local and systemic adverse effects, such as thinning of the skin and adrenal suppression. Thus, tacrolimus offers a useful and safe alternative to potent topical steroids in AD. It may be indicated (i) in those cases of AD in which adverse effects are likely with repeated applications, such as treatment of the face, or (ii) in treatment failures with potent steroids. Pimecrolimus may be an alternative to mild-potency steroids in mild to moderate AD but this needs to be proven in randomized trials.

Efficacy and tolerability of three different doses of oral pimecrolimus in the treatment of moderate to severe atopic dermatitis: a randomized controlled trial

Wolff K, Fleming C, Hanifin J, *et al.*; Multicentre Investigator Group. *Br J Dermatol* 2005; **152**: 1296–303

BACKGROUND. Adult AD can seriously affect the quality of life of patients and their families, and the patient's disease is frequently not satisfactorily controlled with topical therapy. There is a need for alternatives to topical treatment in patients with moderate to severe AD. These authors investigated the efficacy and safety of three different doses of oral pimecrolimus in the treatment of AD. In a double-blind, placebo-controlled, parallel-group, dose-finding study, patients with moderate to severe AD were randomized to receive either placebo or oral pimecrolimus 10, 20 or 30 mg twice daily. The study consisted of a pre-treatment phase, a 12-week double-blind treatment phase, and a 12-week post-treatment phase.

INTERPRETATION. In total, 103 patients were randomized. A clear, dose-dependent therapeutic effect of pimecrolimus treatment was observed, with a statistically significant difference in efficacy at week 2 and the greatest reduction from baseline of the Eczema Area and Severity Index of 66.6% at week 7 in the group given 30 mg twice daily (Fig. 4.2). Oral pimecrolimus was well tolerated and there were no signs of nephrotoxicity or the induction of hypertension.

Comment

For severe AD, the available systemic treatments include systemic corticosteroids, established immunosuppressive agents such as azathioprine and ciclosporin, and ultraviolet phototherapy. There is considerable risk of adverse effects with these drugs and close monitoring is needed. There is therefore a need for safe, effective and convenient therapy for severe AD. The new calcineurin inhibitors may offer some hope. Pimecrolimus inhibits T-cell activation and the production of pro-inflammatory cytokines. Topical ointment is licensed for AD and oral pimecrolimus is effective in psoriasis.

This was a well-designed study of patients with moderate to very severe AD. A significant improvement was demonstrated in the objectively assessed severity of AD and a dose–response relationship was evident (Fig. 4.2). Importantly, pimecrol-

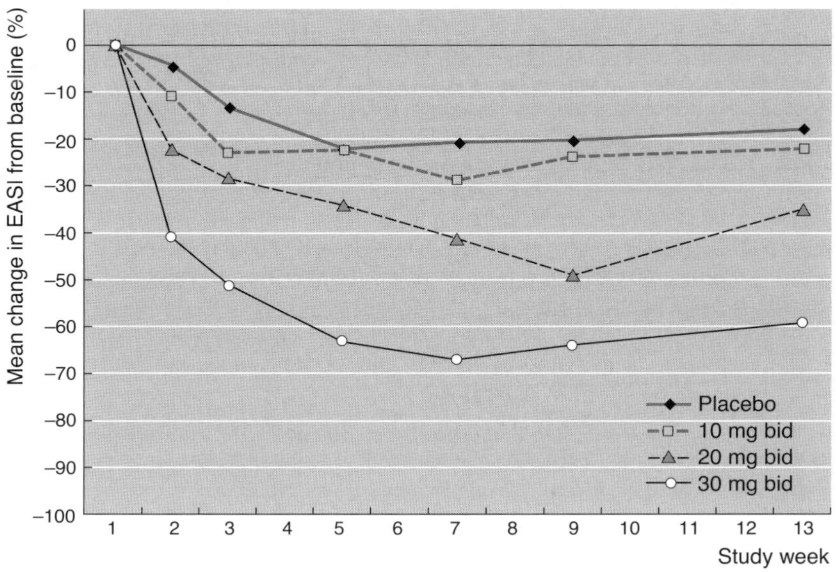

Fig. 4.2 Mean percentage change from baseline in Eczema Area and Severity Index (EASI) score. Source: Wolff *et al.* (2005).

imus was well tolerated and there were no serious adverse effects. Specifically, there was no evidence of nephrotoxicity or development of hypertension. This initial study shows promising results. However, further longer-term studies are required in larger samples to confirm efficacy and, importantly, to evaluate the longer-term safety.

Efficacy and acceptability of a new topical skin lotion of sodium cromoglicate (Altoderm) in atopic dermatitis in children aged 2–12 years: a double-blind, randomized, placebo-controlled trial

Stainer R, Matthews S, Arshad SH, *et al. Br J Dermatol* 2005; **152**: 334–41

Background. AD is a common inflammatory allergic disease of children. The primary anti-inflammatory therapy is topical steroids. An effective treatment without the topical and systemic adverse effects of corticosteroids would be useful. Topical formulations of sodium cromoglicate have been researched in the past, but without consistent results. A new aqueous skin lotion of sodium cromoglicate was developed and assessed for efficacy and safety in children with AD. This was a double-blind, controlled study in which children aged 2–12 years with moderately severe AD were randomized to 12 weeks of treatment with a lotion containing 4% sodium cromoglicate

(Altoderm) or the lotion base. The two groups were compared for changes in the severity of AD, objectively using the Scoring Atopic Dermatitis (SCORAD) index. Secondary outcome measures included parents' assessment of symptoms, the use of topical steroids recorded on daily diary cards, and final opinions of treatment by the parent and clinician.

INTERPRETATION. Fifty-eight children were randomized to Altoderm and 56 to placebo and all were included in the intention-to-treat analysis. The SCORAD scores at baseline (mean ± SD) were 41.0 ± 9.0 for Altoderm and 40.4 ± 8.73 for placebo. These scores were reduced after 12 weeks by 13.2 (36%) with Altoderm and by 7.6 (20%) with placebo. The difference of 5.6 (95% confidence interval [CI] 1.0–10.3) was statistically significant ($P = 0.018$). Diary card symptoms and topical steroid use were reduced in both groups but the improvement was significantly greater in the Altoderm-treated patients. However, improvement in itching and sleep loss were not significantly different. Altoderm was well tolerated with no serious adverse effects. Most treatment-related adverse events referred to irritation, redness and burning at the site of application. The authors conclude that Altoderm gives a clinically useful benefit in children with moderately severe AD.

Comment

Sodium cromoglicate has been used in inhaled powder formulation for more than 30 years as an effective treatment in asthma, especially in children. It is also available as topical therapy for rhinitis and conjunctivitis. It is extremely well tolerated, with few concerns, if any, regarding its safety profile. This makes it an attractive therapeutic option, especially for children. However, previous attempts at making a topical skin formulation for AD have yielded inconsistent results. Altoderm is an aqueous skin lotion of 4% sodium cromoglicate in an emollient base containing emulsifying ointment. This particular formulation was constructed to enhance absorption through the eczematous skin. The mechanism of action of sodium cromoglicate is ill understood but it may involve inhibition of the release of inflammatory mediators from mast cells.

The trial itself was well designed and appropriately conducted and confirmed the effectiveness of Altoderm in reducing the severity of AD (Fig. 4.3) and reducing steroid use. There was a significant placebo effect, possibly attributable to the regular use of the emollient base. Overall, Altoderm was well tolerated with few adverse effects. However, it did cause irritation, redness and burning at the site of application in approximately 15% of patients. Although, Altoderm was found to be safe and effective in moderately severe AD patients, further information is needed, especially about its efficacy and safety compared with other available treatment options, such as mild- to moderate-potency topical steroids and calcineurin inhibitors.

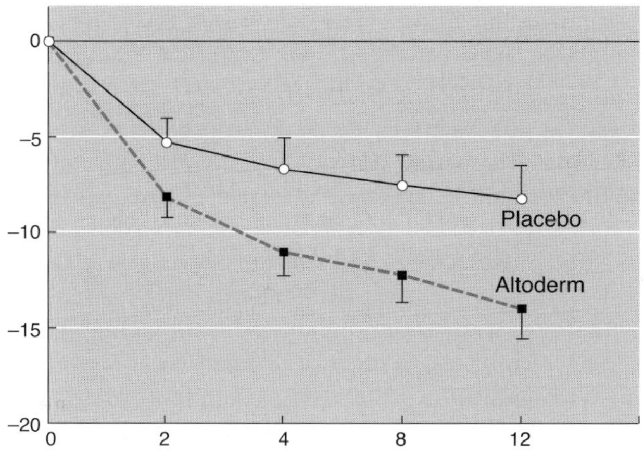

Fig. 4.3 Change in SCORAD score from the end of baseline (visit 2): *x*-axis, weeks of treatment; *y*-axis, change in SCORAD score. Results are shown as mean ± SEM. SCORAD at baseline: Altoderm 41.0 ± 1.2; placebo 40.4 ± 1.2. Difference in change in SCORAD at 12 weeks = 5.6 (95% CI 1.0–10.3; $P = 0.018$). Source: Stainer *et al.* (2005).

Conclusion

The first two papers, studying the natural history of AD, concluded that remission is not as common as was previously assumed. In children, AD and wheeze often start together in infancy and nearly 40% have some problem with AD after 7 years. The presence of AD increases the risk of persistence of wheeze and abnormal lung function, but AD is not followed by the later development of wheeze (the atopic march), as was previously thought. In adults, nearly 60% had persistent AD after a long follow-up of 25 years or more.

Atopic (Th2) immune responses with $CD4^+$ T-cell infiltration and infection with *S. aureus* are two main features of AD pathogenesis. Studies reviewed in this chapter improve our understanding of the skin homing of T cells by CCL18, the mechanism of increased susceptibility of AD patients to *S. aureus* infection, and how staphylococcal toxins influence the immune system to promote inflammation of the skin in AD. The importance of Treg cells in controlling and suppressing immune-related inflammation has been increasingly recognized in recent years. The finding that *S. aureus* toxin is capable of reversing the function of Treg cells explains the chronic nature of inflammation in AD, which is associated with staphylococcal colonization in more than 90% of these patients. The paper by Howell *et al.* describes the role of IL-10 in increasing susceptibility to staphylococcal infection by inhibiting AMP. This was shown in both forms of AD but may be the major mechanism in those with intrinsic AD, as they lack Th2 cytokines, which have also been shown to inhibit AMP. α-toxin is yet another staphylococcal toxin with pro-inflammatory activity. Bacterial colonization with *Staphylococcus* is an integral part of the disease; not only does it cause exacerbation but it is also critical in the continuation of the inflammatory process in both acute and chronic lesions. The paper by Breuer *et al.* suggests that the predominance of Th1 cytokines in chronic lesions of AD may be due partly to the α-toxin-producing strains of *S. aureus*. Thus, the eradication of superinfection with *S. aureus* with antiseptic cleaning agents and antibiotics should be an essential part of the management of AD.

APT has the potential to be a useful, clinically relevant test in AD if the procedure can be standardized. Darsow *et al.* attempted to fill this gap by assessing the role of APT in a large multinational study with standardized methodology. It seems that APT cannot be used as a screening test to identify allergens because of its poor sensitivity. However, it might aid in the process of assessing the clinical relevance of allergens identified with the SPT or sIgE.

The meta-analysis by Ashcroft *et al.* confirms that both tacrolimus and pimecrolimus, when applied topically, are effective and relatively safe treatments for AD. However, their long-term safety has yet to be fully assessed. Their place in clinical practice has not yet evolved fully. Tacrolimus may be used in place of moderate potency or potent corticosteroids. Further trials comparing pimecrolimus with mild topical steroids are required. The initial study by Wolff *et al.* suggests that oral pimecrolimus could be used in severe AD, which has failed to respond to topical therapy. Stainer *et al.* reformulated sodium cromoglicate in an aqueous formulation and showed that it is safe and effective in moderately severe AD. However, further information is needed regarding its efficacy in comparison with mild- to moderate-potency steroids before its use can be recommended.

References

1. Hanifin JM, Rajka G. Diagnostic features of atopic dermatitis. *Acta Derm Venereol Suppl (Stockh)* 1980; **92**: 44–7.
2. Williams HC, Burney PGJ, Pembroke AC, Hay RJ. The UK Working Party's diagnostic criteria for atopic dermatitis. III Independent hospital validation. *Br J Dermatol* 1994; **131**: 406–16.
3. Kusel MMH, Holt PG, de Klerk N, Sly PD. Support for 3 variants of eczema. *J Allergy Clin Immunol* 2005; **116**: 1067–72.
4. Morishita Y, Tada J, Sato A, Toi Y, Kanzaki H, Akiyama H, Arata J. Possible influences of Staphylococcus aureus on atopic dermatitis—the colonizing features and the effects of staphylococcal enterotoxins. *Clin Exp Allergy* 1999; **29**: 1110–17.

5. Oh JW, Seroogy CM, Meyer EH, Akbari O, Berry G, Fathman CG, Dekruyff RH, Umetsu DT. CD4 T-helper cells engineered to produce IL-10 prevent allergen-induced airway hyperreactivity and inflammation. *J Allergy Clin Immunol* 2002; **110**: 460–8.

6. Kerschenlohr K, Darsow U, Burgdorf WH, Ring J, Wollenberg A. Lessons from atopy patch testing in atopic dermatitis. *Curr Allergy Asthma Rep* 2004; **4**: 285–9.

5

Allergic rhinitis

HASAN ABID

Introduction

Allergic rhinitis (AR) is a high-prevalence disease. This high prevalence translates into a high cost to society in terms of overall healthcare utilization, and also a high cost in terms of the quality of life of those who suffer from moderate or severe disease.

AR has traditionally been divided into seasonal allergic rhinitis (SAR) and perennial allergic rhinitis (PAR). This classification is helpful in indicating the season of maximum symptoms and the likely causative allergens. However, it has been found to be less helpful in indicating the severity of the condition, and thus the need for treatment. A new classification has been proposed by the Allergic Rhinitis and its Impact on Asthma (ARIA) workgroup. The usefulness of this classification in everyday practice has yet to be fully evaluated.

It has recently been suggested that asthma and AR are different manifestations of the same disease—AR and asthma syndrome (ARAS) [1]. Indeed, there is considerable epidemiological, pathogenetic and therapeutic evidence supporting the one airway–one disease approach. Asthma and AR coexist in a significant proportion of allergy sufferers [2]. Even those children with AR who do not have overt symptoms of cough and wheeze often exhibit bronchial hyper-responsiveness [3]. AR is a strong risk factor for the development of adult-onset asthma [4]. The nature and mechanism of airway inflammation are also similar [5]. This inflammation is manifested in hypersecretion, obstruction, hyper-reactivity, respectively causing rhinorrhoea, nasal obstruction and sneezing in the nose, and sputum production, wheeze and cough in the lung. The evidence outlined above supports a common management approach to asthma and AR. Apart from environment control and immunotherapy, drugs which counteract inflammation by inhibiting proinflammatory cytokines and mediators may be effective in both diseases. Treatment of AR with topical corticosteroids has been shown to improve asthma outcomes [6]. Conversely, treatment of asthma with leukotriene receptor antagonists may improve rhinitis.

AR is diagnosed and assessed on clinical grounds. The level of symptoms generally dictates the type and intensity of treatment. Should we be making an effort to assess rhinitis more objectively with the use of rhinomanometry, nasal peak flow

© Atlas Medical Publishing Ltd

or nasal provocation tests [7]? At present, these methods are confined to research and clinical trials. The use of these devices and procedures is cumbersome and a definite advantage in terms of improved prognosis, monitoring or choice of treatment must be shown before these methods can be recommended for clinical use.

Advances in pharmacotherapy in recent years have been reflected in better treatment choices. Leukotriene antagonists are now licensed for the treatment of AR. Drugs such as omalizumab and sublingual immunotherapy have been shown to be effective in AR. Innovative methods of immunomodulation are being developed, with the aim of optimizing efficacy and reducing the risk of adverse effects.

Prevalence of allergic rhinitis

There is little doubt that the prevalence of allergic diseases, including AR, increased several-fold between the 1960s and the 1990s, at least in the developed world. In the 1990s, for the first time there were indications of a levelling of the prevalence of asthma and AR. A recent report from Germany and Switzerland investigated the prevalences of asthma, hay fever and atopy on three occasions between 1992 and 2000, using the same standardized questionnaires and showed that the prevalence of allergy remained constant throughout the 1990s in these countries [8]. This is encouraging but further research is needed in different countries and populations to confirm that the rising trend in the prevalence of allergy has finally plateaued.

Trends in prevalence of asthma and allergy in Finnish young men: nationwide study, 1966–2003

Latvala J, von Hertzen L, Lindholm H, Haahtela T. *BMJ* 2005; **330**: 1186–7

BACKGROUND. These investigators have previously reported the prevalence of asthma and allergy in young Finnish men examined for military service. A significant and linear rise in the prevalence of asthma was convincingly documented between 1966 and 1989. Whether similar trends in the prevalences of asthma, AR and eczema have continued since 1990 was investigated and the periods before and after 1990 were compared.

INTERPRETATION. Figure 5.1 shows the prevalence trends for asthma, rhinitis and eczema. Overall, the prevalence of asthma increased 12-fold between 1966 (0.29%) and 2003 (3.45%), showing a continuous rising trend during this period. The average annual increment in prevalence during this period was 0.1%. The prevalence of allergic rhinitis remained low (<0.1%) until 1970 but increased steadily thereafter. The rise in prevalence of allergic rhinitis has been particularly striking since 1991, with the peak in 2000 (8.9%), and the trend is still upwards. The prevalence of atopic eczema, however, has remained fairly constant (about 1.2%) since the early 1980s. The authors concluded that the prevalences of asthma and AR continue to rise in a linear fashion.

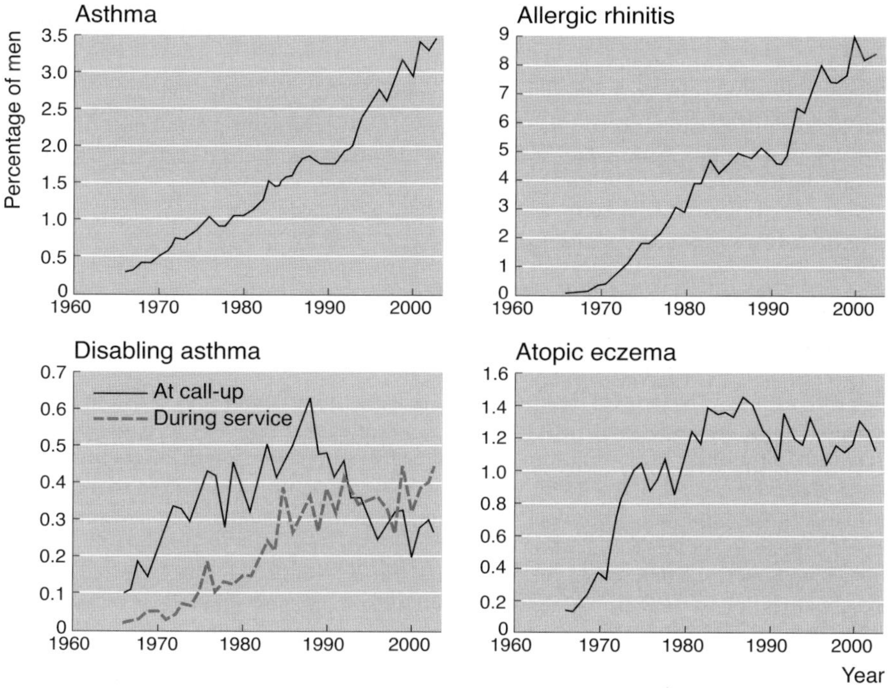

Fig. 5.1 Prevalences of asthma, allergic rhinitis, and atopic eczema in young Finnish men during 1966–2003. Source: Latvala *et al.* (2005).

Comment

Several studies from European countries and Canada have reported a levelling off in the prevalences of asthma and allergic rhinitis after several decades of relentless rise. In Finland, 98% of men are examined for their fitness for military service and diagnostic codes for any diseases are recorded. This gives an excellent opportunity to examine changes in the prevalence of disease over a number of years or decades. In 1990, these authors reported a linear increase in the prevalence of asthma in Finland since the 1960s. No signs of a reduction in the prevalences of asthma and allergic rhinitis in young Finnish men by 2003 were found, although asthma seems to have become milder and better controlled during the last 13 years.

Natural history

Allergic diseases are chronic conditions, but it is well known that long periods of remission (cure?) commonly occur. This is characterized by a typical sequence of progression of atopic diathesis, some clinical disorders developing while others subside. This atopic march is the recognized natural history of allergic manifestations. It is generally agreed that atopic dermatitis and food allergy peak in the first years of life and then decline, whereas asthma and allergic rhinitis increase over time as sensitization to aeroallergens develops. The peak incidence of allergic rhinitis occurs during adolescence. Subsequently, a significant proportion of adults experience a remission but few studies have investigated the natural history of AR in adult life.

Remission of allergic rhinitis: an 8-year observational study

Bodtger U, Linneberg A. *J Allergy Clin Immunol* 2004; **114**: 1384–8

BACKGROUND. These investigators estimated the rate of remission of AR and sensitization to aeroallergens with two cross-sectional assessments 8 years apart. They also determined factors that might predict this remission. Participants in a population-based study of 15- to 69-year-old patients in 1990 were invited to a follow-up in 1998. Questionnaires on respiratory symptoms were administered and serum for specific immunoglobulin E (IgE) was collected at both visits in 734 subjects. Remission of AR was defined as AR at baseline but no rhinitis symptoms at follow-up, and sensitization as specific IgE level class ≥2 at baseline and class <2 at follow-up.

INTERPRETATION. Remission of AR occurred in 12% (pollen AR), 19% (animal AR) and 38% (house dust mite AR), with an overall remission of 17%. A decrease in specific IgE level was observed in only 22% of remitting subjects, but this was significantly greater than in non-remitting subjects (7.4%). Remission of sensitization occurred in 6% (house dust mite) to 11% (pollen, furred animals). Remission to both AR and sensitization was predicted by low specific IgE levels. Age, sex, asthma, predisposition to atopy, age at AR onset and AR duration had no predictive value. The authors concluded that remission of AR was relatively infrequent and that remission of both symptoms and IgE sensitization was rare.

Comment

Repeated assessments of the same population using the same method provide an opportunity to study the outcome of disease. However, these studies are difficult to perform as loss to follow-up is often significant. Of 1581 subjects who were selected randomly at baseline, the eventual participation in both assessments was less than 50% (734). This may underestimate remission as subjects with disease remission are less likely to be enthusiastic about participating in a second assessment. However, the remission rate of 17% is similar to that reported previously [9].

Our understanding of the natural history of AR dictates that young adults with AR tend to improve. It is interesting to note that, in this study, age had no bearing on the induction of remission. It is possible that the number of subjects in this age group was not sufficient to identify this, or that the period of follow-up (8 years) was not adequate.

Remission of pollen-related AR was significantly less common then that of AR caused by house dust mite allergy. The authors argue that avoiding house dust mite may have facilitated remission. This is an interesting and important hypothesis to test in future intervention studies. Treatment with allergen-specific immunotherapy had no effect on the remission rate but the numbers were too small for a definitive conclusion to be drawn.

New classification

The traditional classification of AR into seasonal and perennial forms is useful in terms of defining the period of symptoms and the types of allergens likely to be involved, such as pollen for SAR and house dust mite, other animals or moulds for PAR. However, the clinical usefulness of this classification has been challenged because (i) seasonality in symptoms has been observed in those with PAR, (ii) it gives no information on the severity of the disease, and (iii) importantly, patients are often sensitized to several allergens. The ARIA group, in conjunction with the World Health Organization (WHO), has revised the classification of AR to make it more useful for practising allergists. According to the new classification, AR should be classified as intermittent or persistent according to predefined criteria, and a severity index should be assigned to each type (Fig. 5.2). Thus, a person could have mild intermittent, mild persistent, moderate–severe intermittent or moderate–severe persistent rhinitis.

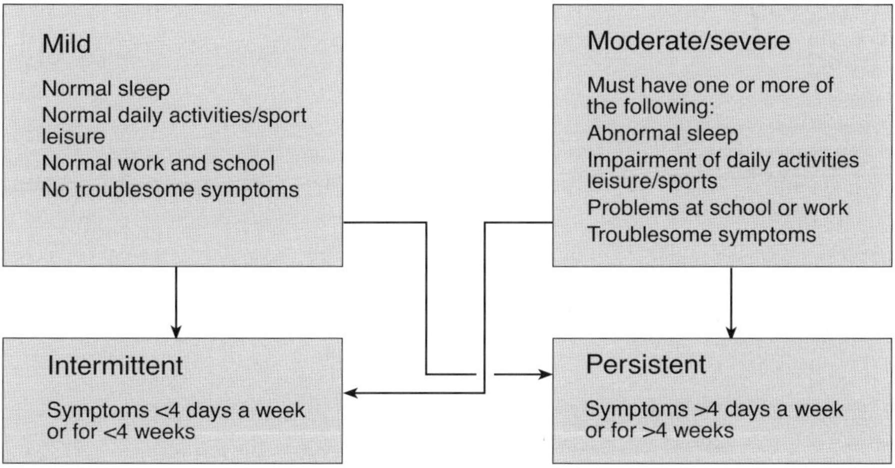

Fig. 5.2 The new classification for allergic rhinitis proposed by the Allergic Rhinitis and its Impact on Asthma (ARIA) workgroup. Source: Bousquet *et al.* (2001) |**10**|.

Seasonal and perennial allergic rhinitis: is this classification adherent to real life?

Ciprandi G, Cirillo I, Vizzaccaro A, *et al.* *Allergy* 2005; **60**: 882–7

BACKGROUND. This study assessed the validity of the traditional classification in a large group of young males attending for routine assessment for military service fitness. They were screened for symptoms of AR. Those with AR were further characterized for the severity of symptoms, allergen sensitization, spirometry and methacholine challenge. They were classified, according to sensitization, into SAR (pollen), PAR (perennial allergens only) or mixed AR (both pollen and perennial allergens).

INTERPRETATION. Of 19 325 subjects, 2347 (12 %) had AR. Seventy-two per cent of the subjects had mixed AR, 17% SAR and 11% PAR. Patients with SAR had a higher level of symptoms and airway obstruction during summer and frequent ocular involvement; irritative symptoms were common, such as itching, sneezing and rhinorrhoea. In PAR, nasal obstruction was more prominent and symptoms and airway obstruction occurred in autumn and winter (Table 5.1). Pulmonary function abnormalities indicating airway obstruction and bronchial hyper-reactivity were more common in patients with PAR. Patients with mixed AR had no seasonal variation in symptoms or airway obstruction; they had overlapping characteristics but behaved overall more like patients with PAR (Table 5.1).

Table 5.1 Clinical and functional features in patients with seasonal allergic rhinitis (SAR), perennial allergic rhinitis (PAR) and mixed allergic rhinitis

Features	SAR	PAR	Mixed AR
Prevalence	17%	11%	72%
Ocular involvement	64.9%	46.4%	47.9%
'Irritative' symptoms	2.7	1.2	1.8
'Obstructive' symptoms	1.4	2.8	2.2
TSS, seasonal variation	Yes	Yes	No
FEV_1 <80%	4.2%	12%	7.8%
FEV_1, seasonal variation	Yes	No	No
FEF_{25-75} <80%	14%	21%	22.5%
FEF_{25-75} seasonal variation	Yes	Yes	No
BHR, percentage of patients	53.6%	82.2%	73.6%
BHR, seasonal variation	Yes	No	Yes

TSS, total symptom score; FEV_1, forced expiratory volume in 1 s; FEF, forced expiratory flow; BHR, bronchial hyper-reactivity. Source: Ciprandi *et al.* (2005).

Comment

This study confirms that SAR and PAR have specific characteristics, including seasonal variation, but most patients cannot be classified into one of these groups. The vast majority (>70%) were sensitized to a number of seasonal and perennial allergens, a condition that was termed 'mixed AR'. This severely affects the usefulness of this classification in real life. Evidence of airway obstruction on testing for pulmonary function and in the bronchial provocation test was surprisingly high in patients reporting nose symptoms alone.

Epidemiological characterization of the intermittent and persistent types of allergic rhinitis

Bauchau V, Durham SR. *Allergy* 2005; **60**: 350–3

BACKGROUND. The validity of the new classification of AR proposed by the ARIA group is still largely unknown, especially the extent to which it differs from the classical SAR/PAR classification, and how and whether intermittent and persistent types of AR differ from each other. These investigators carried out a telephone survey of 9646 subjects. At the second step, 726 subjects attended the clinic for a clinical diagnosis of AR, including measurement of specific IgE.

INTERPRETATION. Self-reported AR was 19%. Among these, 30% of cases were persistent and 70% intermittent AR. Nearly half of those with intermittent AR and persistent AR would have been classified as having PAR. Thus, there was no association between the intermittent/persistent and the SAR/PAR classifications. Among those with a diagnosis of AR, 29% were classified as having persistent AR. Subjects with persistent AR had more severe symptoms and regular use of medication. Interestingly, subjects with persistent AR were more often sensitized to pollen and less often to house dust mite. In conclusion, the classic terms of SAR/PAR cannot be used interchangeably with the new classification of intermittent/persistent.

Comment

The new classification proposed by ARIA group needs to be validated. This study answered some of the questions. First, they were able to show that 'intermittent' and 'persistent' are not simply different names for SAR and PAR. These are distinct groups with specific characteristics. Especially, persistent AR is a more severe disease with a specific allergen sensitization pattern and a higher level of medication use. These results support the validity of the new ARIA classification.

Assessment of nasal inflammation

Allergic rhinitis is an inflammatory disorder which involves the recruitment and activation of various structural cells and circulatory leucocytes, including eosinophils and mast cells. Allergic inflammation is orchestrated by T lymphocytes, with secretion of Th2-type cytokines (interleukin [IL] 4, IL-5, IL-13) causing endothelial cell activation, upregulation of adhesion molecules and recruitment, and activation and increased survival of eosinophils in the mucosal layers. Mediator release from mast cells, basophils and eosinophils accounts for the pathophysiological processes leading to symptom expression. Monitoring of nasal inflammation is important in testing the anti-inflammatory effects of new drugs and may be used clinically to assess prognosis and guide treatment.

Objective monitoring of nasal airway inflammation in rhinitis

Howarth PH, Persson CG, Meltzer EO, Jacobson MR, Durham SR, Silkoff PE. *J Allergy Clin Immunol* 2005; **115**: S414–41

BACKGROUND. Allergic rhinitis is an inflammatory nasal disorder in which a range of different cells participate. A variety of approaches has been used to monitor nasal inflammation objectively to investigate disease processes and to evaluate the effect of therapeutic intervention. These approaches include nasal lavage, nasal cytology and nasal biopsy, together with the more recently established measurement of nasal nitric oxide (NO) concentration. Although all provide information about nasal mucosal inflammation, the extent of information that can be obtained by each approach, the ease of sampling, and the complexity of sample handling differ.

INTERPRETATION. Nasal lavage is simple and rapid to perform, is well tolerated, and provides a sample that yields information about luminal cell recruitment, cell activation and plasma protein extravasation. Nasal cytology involves sampling and recovering mucosal surface cells. It is also easy to perform and is well tolerated in general, although some find that the procedure causes a transient unpleasant sensation. A differential cell count from the sample provides information about relative cell population sizes. The handling of nasal cytology samples is easier, but nasal lavage offers the advantage of providing considerably greater information from the sample. Nasal biopsy is an invasive procedure and requires expertise not only in tissue sampling but also in biopsy processing. Therefore, it is applicable only in specialist centres. However, nasal biopsy is the only sampling technique that informs directly about tissue cellular events, although these may be implied, in part from the other sampling approaches. Measurement of nasal NO involves expensive equipment but provides an instantaneous result, unlike the other approaches, all of which require sample processing and analysis. The limitations of nasal NO are that it reflects only a certain aspect of allergic mucosal inflammation, and that because a proportion of nasally measured NO is derived from the sinuses under normal circumstances, nasal NO is not specific for nasal disease.

Comment

This review provides an excellent summary of the current status of objective assessment of nasal inflammation. Common approaches include nasal lavage to recover cells and mediators, nasal cytology to assess the nature of epithelial and luminal cells, nasal biopsy to examine mucosal inflammation, and biomarkers in exhaled breath to evaluate the nature and degree of inflammation.

During nasal lavage, fluid is introduced into the nasal cavity and the recovered fluid is evaluated for soluble factors (cytokines, mediators), and some of the fluid is centrifuged for microscopic examination of the cell pellet to study the nature of cellular inflammation. It has been used widely to study nasal inflammation following provocation with a variety of stimulants, including allergens, capsaicin, cytokines and occupational sensitizers. The technique is relatively non-invasive and easy to perform. However, it has so far been confined to research and has not found a place in everyday clinical practice.

Nasal cytology can help in distinguishing between inflammatory and infective rhinitis and in gaining insight into the type of infective (bacterial/viral) or inflammatory (allergic/non-allergic) process. It can also be used to follow the course of disease and the response to treatment. Thus, it can be a useful procedure in the diagnosis, prognosis and management of difficult cases of rhinitis. However, the usefulness of nasal cytology depends on adequate sampling, processing (preparation and staining) and interpretation. Neutrophils are the predominant cells in nasal secretions in normal subjects and those with rhinitis. However, eosinophils and basophils are seen in increasing numbers in cytology specimens from subjects with allergic rhinitis, whereas nasal cytology from those with non-allergic (vasomotor) rhinitis is characterized by the absence of eosinophils.

Nasal biopsy has been used to study nasal structure and cell population in health and disease. It is an invasive procedure but good-quality biopsies can be taken with little discomfort to the patient. It is primarily used in research to study disease pathogenesis and to assess the effect of novel anti-inflammatory treatment.

Nitric oxide is a mediator of inflammatory response. Inducible NO synthase (iNOS) is expressed at a higher level in nasal mucosa in allergic rhinitis. The large amounts of NO produced by iNOS promote inflammation through tissue damage, the recruitment of eosinophils and an increase in vascular congestion and nasal secretion. Nasal NO has the potential to act as a marker of nasal inflammation. Nasal NO has been shown to be increased in subjects with allergic rhinitis, with further increase during the pollen season and a decrease following treatment with intranasal corticosteroids. However, it has not been convincingly shown to correlate with symptoms or nasal obstruction. Its place in the diagnosis and monitoring of allergic rhinitis remains to be determined.

In summary, this review describes a number of approaches to the evaluation of inflammatory changes within the nose. There is some overlap but these techniques can be complementary to each other as each may depict a specific aspect of the inflammatory process. The choice of method depends on the specific question asked and the availability of expertise and equipment. Nasal NO is a non-invasive marker and further studies are needed to establish its place in the monitoring of nasal inflammation in the clinical and research settings.

Analysis of exhaled leukotrienes in non-asthmatic adult patients with seasonal allergic rhinitis

Cap P, Pehal F, Chladek J, Maly M. *Allergy* 2005; **60**: 171–6

BACKGROUND. Leukotrienes are present in increased amounts in exhaled breath condensate (EBC) in patients with asthma. So far, no data have been reported about leukotriene levels in non-asthmatic patients with SAR. The aim of the study was to find out whether the leukotriene levels in EBC were increased in the non-asthmatic adult patients with SAR both during and after the pollen season in comparison with healthy controls, and to assess changes in leukotriene levels after the pollen season. Twenty-nine non-asthmatic adult patients with SAR and 50 healthy non-smoking controls underwent measurement of exhaled leukotrienes in the EBC during and after the pollen season. Spirometry, skin-prick tests and total IgE were also evaluated.

INTERPRETATION. Leukotriene concentrations (B4, E4 but not D4) were significantly increased in and after the pollen season in patients with SAR in comparison with healthy controls. In most of the samples, LTC_4 was undetectable. The values of all exhaled leukotrienes were significantly decreased after the pollen season compared with the seasonal baseline: LTB_4, $P = 0.023$; LTD_4, $P = 0.020$; LTE_4, $P = 0.047$. In conclusion, levels of exhaled LTB_4 and LTE_4 were higher in SAR patients than in healthy controls and decreased after the pollen season.

Comment

Collection of EBC is a non-invasive way of obtaining samples from airways. Various mediators and cytokines can be measured in EBC as biomarkers of airway inflammation. Leukotrienes are potent proinflammatory mediators and their concentration has been shown to be high in EBC in asthma and in nasal lavage fluid in SAR. It could be very useful in identifying changes in leukotrienes in EBC in patients with allergic rhinitis. This has the potential to provide information regarding the severity of inflammation, and the need for and response to treatment.

Median concentrations were higher in these non-asthmatic rhinitis subjects compared with healthy controls and increased further during the pollen season. However, careful examination of Fig. 5.3 reveals that the overlap in levels between those with and without rhinitis was considerable. Despite this overlap, a case can be made for treating SAR in subjects with higher levels of leukotrienes, measured in EBC, with leukotriene antagonists.

Leukotrienes were analysed using a specific and sensitive gas chromatography/mass spectrometry (GC/MS) assay. The use of GC/MS reduced the applicability of EBC as this assay is not immediately available to most clinicians. A hand-held portable machine that could measure biomarkers in exhaled breath, such as NO, and in EBC, such as leukotrienes, would be ideal.

Asthma was carefully excluded in these patients with questionnaire and pulmonary function tests, but the leukotrienes measured in EBC were probably of

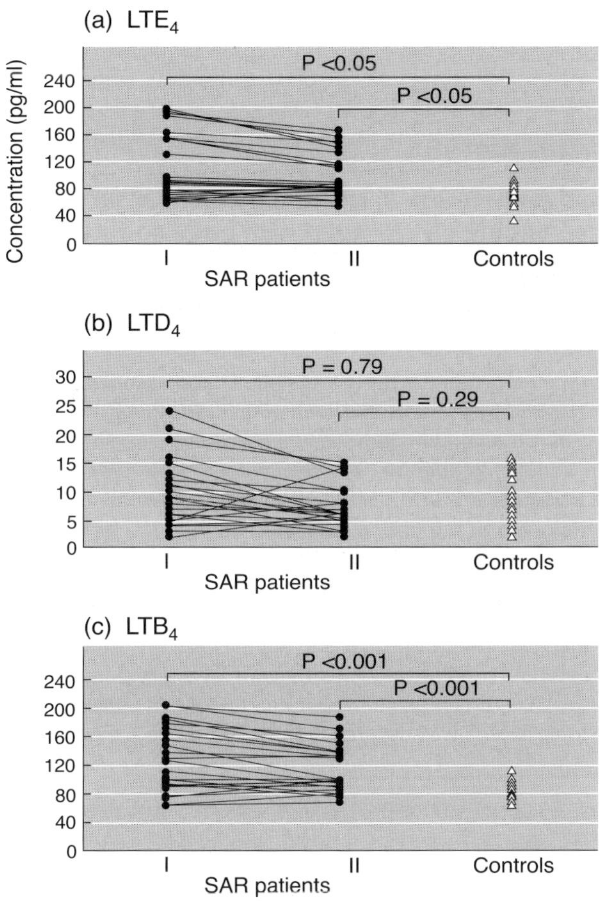

Fig. 5.3 Concentration of leukotrienes in exhaled breath condensate in patients with seasonal allergic rhinitis (I, during pollen season; II, outside the pollen season) and healthy controls. Source: Cap *et al.* (2005).

lower airway origin because a noseclip was used, preventing nasal contamination. This argues strongly for the one airway–one inflammation hypothesis, i.e. the presence of lower airway inflammation in rhinitis subjects with no historical or physiological evidence of asthma.

The relationship of AR and asthma

The concept of asthma and rhinitis being different manifestations of the same disease has been proposed in recent years, giving rise to the term 'united airway disease'. The proposed mechanisms are a common mucosal inflammatory process, bronchial aspiration of nasal contents, and nasal–bronchial reflux. Recent evidence supports this view and extends observations to include otitis media, and further clarifies the extent to which treatment of one disease might improve the other.

Similar allergic inflammation in the middle ear and the upper airway: evidence linking otitis media with effusion to the united airways concept

Nguyen LH, Manoukian JJ, Sobol SE, *et al.* *J Allergy Clin Immunol* 2004; **114**: 1110–15

BACKGROUND. Otitis media with effusion (OME) is a chronic inflammatory disease of the middle ear space characterized by the accumulation of fluid. Previous investigations have suggested that the immunopathological mechanism underlying the development of middle ear effusion in patients with allergy largely involves the effects of Th2 mediators. The investigators set out to determine whether the middle ear compartment may be a component of the united airways in allergic disease by comparing the inflammatory profiles of the middle ear with those of the upper airway. Middle ear effusions, torus tubaris (Eustachian tube mucosa at the nasopharyngeal orifice) and adenoidal tissue biopsies were obtained from 45 patients undergoing simultaneous tympanostomy tube placement for OME and adenoidectomy for adenoid hypertrophy. The cellular and cytokine profiles of each site were investigated by using immunocytochemistry (elastase, CD3, major basic protein) and *in situ* hybridization (IL-4, IL-5 and IFN-γ mRNA). Atopic status was determined for each patient by using skin-prick testing.

INTERPRETATION. Eleven of the 45 patients with OME (24%) were atopic. The middle ear effusions of atopic patients had significantly higher levels of eosinophils, T lymphocytes and IL-4 mRNA-positive cells ($P<0.01$) and significantly lower levels of neutrophils and IFN-γ mRNA-positive cells ($P<0.01$) compared with non-atopic patients. The nasopharyngeal tissue biopsies revealed similar cellular and cytokine profiles. Thus, in atopic patients with OME, the allergic inflammation occurs on both sides of the Eustachian tube, i.e. the middle ear and the nasopharynx.

Comment

OME is defined as chronic inflammation of middle ear mucosa characterized by retention of serous fluid in the middle ear space. Given that the middle ear is an anatomical extension of the airway through the Eustachian tube, it is not surprising that similar allergic mechanisms underlie inflammation in this space. It is known that patients with OME have an increased prevalence of atopic diseases. A Th2-type allergic inflammation with eosinophils and increased expression of IL-4 and IL-5 mRNA has previously been demonstrated in OME. Data from this study provide further confirmation that, in atopic patients, the inflammation in OME is allergic, and that this occurs in the middle ear space and Eustachian tube as well as the nasopharynx. This study supports the concept that the middle ear may be part of the united airway in atopic individuals. These findings have management implications. Treatment of OME is unsatisfactory and many children need surgical intervention. It is conceivable that in atopic patients the treatment of allergic rhinitis with nasal corticosteroids or leukotriene antagonists may improve otitis media. Moreover, other treatment modalities, such as allergen avoidance and specific allergen immunotherapy, may prove to be beneficial.

Asthma-related health care resource use among asthmatic children with and without concomitant allergic rhinitis

Thomas M, Kocevar VS, Zhang Q, Yin DD, Price D. *Pediatrics* 2005; **115**: 129–34

BACKGROUND. Asthmatic children who also have AR seem to have higher morbidity and to use more healthcare resources. This was further investigated to determine the incremental effect of AR on healthcare resource use in children with asthma. The data were from a general practice database in the UK and covered the period 1998–2001. Children aged 6–15 years who had an asthma-related visit to their general practitioner at least once during a defined 12-month period were reviewed.

INTERPRETATION. Of 9522 children with asthma, 1879 (19.7%) had a recorded diagnosis of AR. Compared with children with asthma alone, children with comorbid AR experienced more general practitioner visits (4.4 vs 3.4) and more of them were hospitalized for asthma (1.4 vs 0.5%) during the 12-month follow-up period. In multivariable regression analyses, comorbid AR was an independent predictor of hospitalization for asthma (odds ratio 2.34; 95% confidence interval [CI] 1.41–3.91) and was associated with increases in asthma-related drug costs (mean increase GBP 6.7; 95% CI 6.5–7.0). It was concluded that children with comorbid AR incurred greater prescription drug costs and experienced more general practitioner visits and hospitalizations for asthma than did children with asthma alone.

Comment

Asthma and AR coexist in 25–50% of patients. It has been proposed previously that subjects with coexisting asthma and AR have, in general, more severe disease. This study systematically examined and compared the use of healthcare resources by asthmatic children with and without concomitant AR. As expected, children with both asthma and AR experienced more general practitioner visits and were more often hospitalized despite incurring a higher prescription cost for asthma-related drugs (Fig. 5.4). A similar effect of AR on asthma-related healthcare cost in adults was also reported recently by these authors [**11**].

It is possible that bronchial aspiration of nasal content, with its profile of mediators and cytokines, promotes lower airway inflammation. Further, nasal obstruction leads to mouth breathing, with the loss of warming and humidification of inspired air. This may initiate bronchospasm and result in increased bronchial

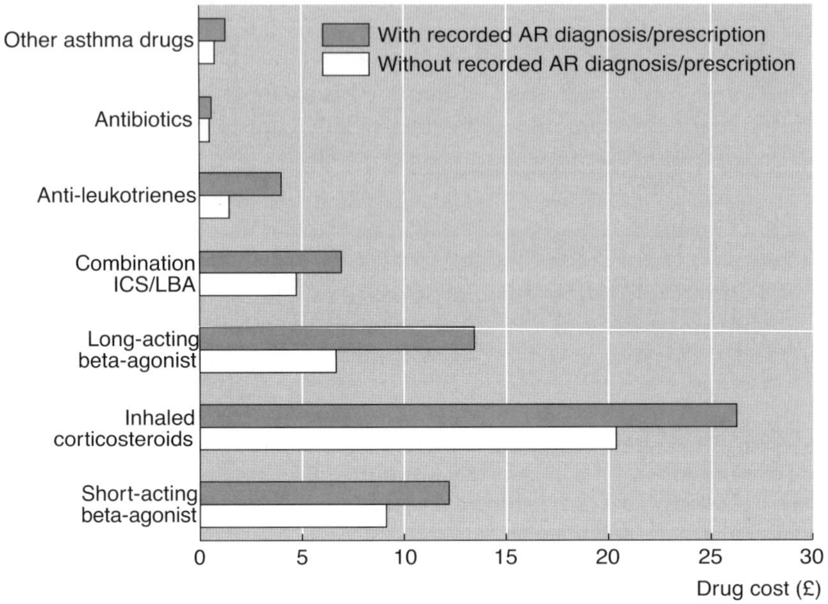

Fig. 5.4 Cost of asthma drug by drug class. Source: Thomas *et al.* (2005).

hyper-responsiveness. These arguments are supported by reports which suggest that treatment of nasal inflammation with topical corticosteroids does improve asthma in these subjects. A unified treatment strategy for asthma and AR, as recommended by the ARIA initiative, might reduce the cost of treating these conditions.

Studies based on general practice data are limited in terms of the details of the recorded information. For example, many patients with mild rhinitis rely on over-the-counter medications and are not diagnosed as having rhinitis. As the authors accept, a 20% diagnosis of AR in those with asthma was probably an under-estimation. The findings of this study may thus be applicable only to asthmatic children with moderate to severe AR.

Effect of immunotherapy on asthma progression, BHR and sputum eosinophils in allergic rhinitis

Polosa R, Li Gotti F, Mangano G, *et al. Allergy* 2004; **59**: 1224–8

BACKGROUND. Subjects with AR have a higher incidence of subsequent development of asthma. Bronchial hyper-responsiveness (BHR) and airway inflammation are frequently associated with allergic rhinitis, and may be important risk factors for the development of asthma. These investigators aimed to assess the

effect of *Parietaria*-specific immunotherapy on rhinitic symptoms, BHR, eosinophilic inflammation and, importantly, on the subsequent development of asthma. Non-asthmatic subjects with seasonal rhinitis were randomly assigned to receive *Parietaria* pollen vaccine ($n = 15$) or matched placebo ($n = 15$). Data on symptoms, medication score, BHR to methacholine and eosinophilia in sputum were collected during the 3-year study period.

INTERPRETATION. By the end of the study, in the placebo group, symptoms and medication scores had increased significantly, by a median (interquartile range) of 121% (15–280) and 263% (0–4400) respectively ($P<0.01$), whereas no significant difference was observed in the group receiving *Parietaria*-specific immunotherapy. No significant changes were detected in sputum eosinophils and BHR to methacholine in either group. After 3 years, two of 14 (14%) in the specific immunotherapy group and seven of 15 (47%) in the placebo group had developed asthma symptoms ($P = 0.056$). In conclusion, *Parietaria*-specific immunotherapy reduces symptom and rescue medication scores without any measurable effect on the BHR to methacholine or sputum eosinophilia. Interestingly, *Parietaria*-specific immunotherapy appears to prevent the progression of allergic rhinitis to asthma, suggesting that specific immunotherapy should be considered earlier in the management of subjects with allergic rhinitis.

Comment

Specific immunotherapy is the only therapy available that has immunomodulatory ability and may influence the natural history of atopic disease. It has been shown that patients with AR without current asthma do carry a risk of subsequent development of asthma, and the presence of BHR may be predictive of this risk [12]. Previous studies have suggested an asthma-preventive role of specific immunotherapy in subjects with AR. However, whether this protective effect is associated with improvement in the underlying BHR is not established. These authors carried out a double-blind study with appropriate assessments. Specific immunotherapy was effective in that significant differences were observed in symptoms and medication score in years 2 and 3. Interestingly, there was no placebo effect and differences in the two groups resulted primarily from increased symptoms and the requirement for medication in the placebo group. Although the asthma-preventive effect was shown in this study despite small numbers of patients, this effect was not related to changes in BHR or sputum eosinophilia. This may be an allergen (*Parietaria*)-specific effect, as reduction in BHR in AR patients treated with specific immunotherapy has been previously shown with mite and grass pollen allergens. Alternatively, the immunomodulatory effect of specific immunotherapy in preventing asthma may not influence bronchial responsiveness. The numbers in this study were too small for a firm conclusion to be made. However, the findings have important public health implications. In this study, nearly 50% of AR patients developed asthma and specific immunotherapy prevented this progression in most of these subjects. In view of this preventive effect, should specific immunotherapy be recommended for all AR subjects, even if their symptoms are well controlled on pharmacotherapy?

Coseasonal sublingual immunotherapy reduces the development of asthma in children with allergic rhinoconjunctivitis

Novembre E, Galli E, Landi F, *et al. J Allergy Clin Immunol* 2004; **114**: 851–7

BACKGROUND. In an open randomized study, these authors sought to determine whether short-term co-seasonal sublingual immunotherapy (SLIT) can reduce the development of asthma in children with hay fever. One hundred and thirteen children aged 5–14 years (mean age 7.7 years) with hay fever limited to grass pollen and no other clinically important allergies were randomized in an open study involving six Italian paediatric allergy centres to receive specific SLIT for 3 years or standard symptomatic therapy. All of the subjects had hay fever symptoms, but at the time of study entry none reported seasonal asthma with more than three episodes per season.

INTERPRETATION. The actively treated children used less medication in the second and third years of therapy, and their symptom scores tended to be lower. From the second year of immunotherapy, subjective evaluation of overall allergy symptoms was favourable in the actively treated children. Development of asthma after 3 years was 3.8 times more frequent (95% confidence limit 1.5–10.0) in the control subjects. Three years of co-seasonal SLIT improves seasonal allergic rhinitis symptoms and reduces the development of seasonal asthma in children with hay fever.

Comment

In recent years several studies have confirmed the efficacy of SLIT in reducing symptoms and medication requirement in patients with seasonal AR. SLIT is safer and easier to use than conventional specific immunotherapy administered by injections. It has been shown previously that subcutaneous specific immunotherapy prevents the development of asthma in those with AR. Whether SLIT has the same preventive effect was the subject of this randomized study. As expected, SLIT was well tolerated and reductions in symptoms and medication scores were observed in the treated group. Importantly, SLIT did prevent the development of asthma after 2–3 years. However, the results of this study should be treated with caution as the study was not double-blind and all assessments (symptoms, asthma diagnosis) were subjective.

Treatment of AR with anti-IgE antibody

AR is an IgE-mediated disease. The binding of inhaled allergens to IgE on the surface of mast cells and basophils triggers the release of pre-formed and newly synthesized mediators, such as histamine, leukotrienes and prostaglandins, initiating the cascade of the inflammatory process and resulting in allergic symptoms. Omalizumab is a humanized monoclonal anti-IgE antibody that binds to IgE in the circulation, rendering it incapable of binding to mast cells and basophils, thus blocking IgE-mediated allergic reaction. It does not interact with cell-bound IgE and therefore does not cause the release of mediators. This approach to the treatment of allergic disease is logically sound. In asthmatic subjects, omalizumab inhibits early- and late-phase reactions following allergen challenge and reduces exacerbation and the steroid requirement. Several studies have confirmed its efficacy in asthma and it is now a licensed treatment for allergic asthma in many countries.

There is a paucity of treatment for patients with severe AR. Moreover, asthma and AR coexist in a significant number of patients. Omalizumab has been shown to be effective in AR induced by birch pollen and ragweed. Recent studies also showed an improvement in rhinitis symptoms and rhinitis-specific quality of life in patients who had coexistent allergic asthma and AR.

Effects of omalizumab, a humanized monoclonal anti-IgE antibody, on nasal reactivity to allergen and local IgE synthesis

Corren J, Diaz-Sanchez D, Saxon A, *et al. Ann Allergy Asthma Immunol* 2004; **93**: 243–8

BACKGROUND. Treatment with omalizumab has been shown to reduce serum free IgE concentrations and to have beneficial effects on allergic airway disease. However, its effect on local IgE synthesis is unknown. The authors investigated whether omalizumab therapy diminishes nasal reactivity to allergen and local IgE production. Nineteen patients with perennial allergic rhinitis were treated with intravenous omalizumab every 2 weeks for 26 weeks in an open-label study. Serum free and total IgE concentrations were measured at baseline and every 2 weeks throughout the study. Nasal challenge to dust mite allergen was performed at baseline and after 12 and 24 weeks of treatment. Nasal lavage fluid obtained before and after each nasal challenge was evaluated for mite-specific antibodies, plaque-forming cells and productive epsilon mRNA.

INTERPRETATION. During treatment, serum free IgE concentrations were decreased by 97–99% and the nasal response to allergen challenge was significantly reduced on days 80 and 164. The post-challenge increase in mite-specific IgE in nasal lavage was also significantly reduced by treatment with omalizumab on day 168. However, IgE plaque-forming cells and productive epsilon mRNA were not significantly affected by omalizumab treatment. Overall, omalizumab treatment markedly reduced serum free IgE and the clinical response to nasal allergen challenge. However, it did not significantly modulate the synthesis of nasal IgE.

Comment

This study was designed to improve our understanding of the mechanisms of anti-IgE treatment in AR. Omalizumab not only reduces free serum IgE but also inhibits the expression of high-affinity receptors on immune effector cells, further reducing IgE-mediated allergic reactivity. Moreover, *in vitro* studies have suggested that omalizumab causes inhibition of allergen-induced IgE synthesis, which is a useful additional effect as IgE itself promotes allergic inflammation and inhibition of IgE synthesis would be a desirable outcome.

This study reported that, following administration of omalizumab, serum free IgE was reduced by 99% of the pre-treatment level, resulting in a diminished nasal response to allergen challenge. However, it failed to show inhibition of local IgE synthesis *in vivo* in nasal mucosa following allergen challenge.

Conclusion

Latvala *et al.*, in their study of young army recruits, suggest that the prevalence of asthma and AR may still be rising, even in the developed world. This is in contrast to recent reports that the prevalence of asthma and allergy may have peaked. Further studies are required to clarify this important issue. The natural history of AR, in terms of spontaneous remission, is another important subject that requires further investigation, because the presumed high remission rate in adults may not be evidence-based.

The new classification proposed by ARIA has yet to be accepted universally by clinicians. Ciprandi *et al.* did confirm that the traditional classification of seasonal and perennial allergic rhinitis is not helpful, as most patients could not be classified into one of these groups. Further, there is now evidence that the new classification is different from the traditional one and characterizes patients better in terms of severity.

Objective monitoring of nasal inflammation with biomarkers can potentially improve the diagnosis, prognosis and treatment of AR. The review by Howarth *et al.* outlines the available methods and their current use. So far, none of these procedures has found general clinical acceptability. However, nasal NO is being investigated actively and may prove to be a useful tool in the management of AR.

Although the association of asthma and rhinitis has been known for some time, in recent years data have accumulated indicating how one disease affects another. Children and adults with asthma and AR tend to have higher asthma-related healthcare needs and drug costs than those with asthma alone. Polosa *et al.* confirmed that specific immunotherapy for AR caused by *Parietaria* prevents the development of asthma in these subjects. Novembre *et al.* suggest that SLIT may have the same beneficial effect. There is also evidence that similar allergic inflammation may occur in the middle ear in atopic subjects. This may have implications for the management of serous otitis media. Thus, in atopic subjects, asthma, AR and even serous otitis media may be considered different manifestations of the same disease. In these patients, treatments with systemic effects, such as leukotriene antagonists, omalizumab and specific immunotherapy, may be used increasingly in the coming years.

References

1. World Allergy Organisation. Combined allergic rhinitis and asthma syndrome. http://www.worldallergy.org/professional/allergy_update/caras/airwayssynopsis.shtml.
2. Leynaert B, Neukirch F, Demoly P, Bousquet J. Epidemiologic evidence for asthma and rhinitis comorbidity. *J Allergy Clin Immunol* 2000; **106**: 201–5.
3. Arshad SH, Kurukulaaratchy R, Fenn M, Waterhouse L, Matthews S. Rhinitis in 10-year-old children and early life risk factors for its development. *Acta Paediatrica* 2002; **91**: 1334–8.
4. Toren K, Olin AC, Hellgren J, Hermansson BA. Rhinitis increase the risk for adult-onset asthma—a Swedish population-based case–control study (MAP-study). *Respir Med* 2002; **96**: 635–41.
5. Boulay ME, Boulet LP. The relationships between atopy, rhinitis and asthma: pathophysiological considerations. *Curr Opin Allergy Clin Immunol* 2003; **3**: 51–5.
6. Taramarcaz P, Gibson PG. The effectiveness of intranasal corticosteroids in combined allergic rhinitis and asthma syndrome. *Clin Exp Allergy* 2004; **34**: 1883–9.
7. Gosepath J, Amedee RG, Mann WJ. Nasal provocation testing as an international standard for evaluation of allergic and non-allergic rhinitis. *Laryngoscope* 2005; **115**: 512–16.
8. Braun-Fahrländer C, Gassner M, Grize L, Takken-Sahli K, Neu U, Stricker T, Varonier HS, Wüthrich B, Sennhauser FH; the Swiss Study on Childhood Allergy and Respiratory Symptoms. No further increase in asthma, hay fever and atopic sensitisation in adolescents living in Switzerland. *Eur Respir J* 2004; **23**: 407–13.
9. Plaschke PP, Janson C, Norrman E, Bjornsson E, Ellbjar S, Jarvholm B. Onset and remission of allergic rhinitis and asthma and the relationship with atopic sensitization and smoking. *Am J Respir Crit Care Med* 2000; **162**: 920–4.
10. Bousquet J, Van Cauwenberge P, Khaltaev N; Aria Workshop Group; World Health Organization. Allergic rhinitis and its impact on asthma. *J Allergy Clin Immunol* 2001; **108**: S147–334.
11. Price D, Zhang Q, Kocevar VS, Yin DD, Thomas M. Effect of a concomitant diagnosis of allergic rhinitis on asthma-related health care use by adults. *Clin Exp Allergy* 2005; **35**: 282–7.
12. Braman SS, Barrows AA, DeCotiis BA, Settipane GA, Corrao WM. Airway hyper-responsiveness in allergic rhinitis; a risk factor for asthma. *Chest* 1987; **91**: 671–4.

6

Systemic allergic reactions

GRAHAM ROBERTS

Introduction

Systemic allergic reactions are a relatively common clinical emergency. In their mildest form, they may just manifest as systemic cutaneous reactions with pruritis, urticaria and angio-oedema. In more severe cases there are cardiorespiratory symptoms such as stridor, wheeze, difficulty in breathing or hypotension. Anaphylaxis has been defined as a 'severe, life-threatening generalized or systemic hypersensitivity reaction' [1]. The prevalence of systemic allergic reactions is unclear because of the lack of a clear, consistent definition and large prospective population studies. Up to 8% of infants and around 2% of older children and adults are thought to have food allergy [2]. The prevalence of severe allergic reactions has been estimated to be 0.5–3 cases per 10 000 people [3] and it is thought that there are likely to be between one and three deaths from anaphylaxis per million people. The commonest causes of systemic allergic reactions are food, drugs, insect stings and latex [4]. The commonest foods involved are peanut, tree nuts, egg, fish, legumes, milk, crustaceans and wheat [5]. In a systemic allergic reaction, there is systemic release of mediators by mast cells and basophils. Without specific treatment, the reaction is likely to progress, with increasingly severe respiratory and cardiovascular problems. In this chapter some of the latest literature concerning systemic allergic reactions will be reviewed and their implications for clinical practice will be discussed.

Anaphylaxis

Clinical features and severity grading of anaphylaxis

Brown SG. *J Allergy Clin Immunol* 2004; **114**: 371–6.

Background. Definitions of anaphylaxis vary considerably, impeding the comparison of different clinical studies. Different definitions of anaphylaxis have been

© Atlas Medical Publishing Ltd

developed as clinical descriptions of severe allergic reactions, different authors emphasizing different symptoms.

Interpretation. The author aimed to develop a simple clinical grading system and definition for anaphylaxis using clinical data. He retrospectively analysed 1149 case records (median age 29 years) with systemic allergic reactions (30% venom allergy, 22% iatrogenic allergy, 18% food allergy) from an emergency department in Australia. A third required treatment with intramuscular adrenaline and three patients died despite treatment. Confusion, collapse, unconsciousness and incontinence were strongly associated with severe reactions where there was cardiorespiratory failure. Diaphoresis, vomiting, presyncope, dyspnoea, stridor, wheeze, chest or throat tightness, nausea, vomiting and abdominal pain defined moderate reactions. Reactions limited to the skin were defined as mild. These grades correlated well with treatment with adrenaline. Older age, insect venom, iatrogenic causes and pre-existing lung disease were independent predictors of severity.

Comment

The author has developed an impressive database of subjects with allergic reactions presenting to the emergency room. The subsequent analysis is, however, dependent on the accuracy of the diagnosis by the emergency room team in the absence of skin-prick testing, serum specific immunoglobulin E (IgE) or provocation challenge. The study highlights key symptoms that should alert families and healthcare workers to the development of a severe allergic reaction. Interestingly, gastrointestinal symptoms seem to highlight the presence of a moderately severe reaction. Looking at the data more closely, nausea, vomiting and diarrhoea are significantly associated with hypotension. These gastrointestinal symptoms are all too often dismissed as not being important; it looks as if it is time to alter this attitude. The author proposed the following definition of anaphylaxis: 'Multiple-organ hypersensitivity characterized by the presence of significant gastrointestinal, respiratory, or cardiovascular involvement (nausea, vomiting, abdominal pain, throat or chest tightness, breathlessness, wheeze, stridor, hypotension, hypoxia, confusion, collapse, loss of consciousness, or incontinence)' which is usually accompanied by 'skin features (erythema, urticaria, or angioedema)'. This definition makes clinical sense but the lack of a gold standard diagnostic test for allergy in this paper means that the data presented cannot be used to substantiate this as a definitive definition of anaphylaxis. A number of consensus statements concerning anaphylaxis have been published recently. The World Allergy Organization has recently defined anaphylaxis as a severe, life-threatening generalized or systemic hypersensitivity reaction |**1**|. A useful paper from a North American multidisciplinary symposium has reviewed the epidemiology, pathophysiology, aetiology, diagnosis and management of anaphylaxis |**6**|. These authors offer a complicated definition of anaphylaxis based on the fulfilment of one of three clinical criteria: skin and respiratory or circulatory involvement; involvement of two systems after exposure to a known allergen; or hypotension after exposure to a known allergen. The American Academy of Allergy, Asthma and Immunology and the American College of Allergy,

Asthma and Immunology have also recently published a practice parameter on anaphylaxis [7]. This document provides a very useful clinical approach to a patient with possible anaphylaxis.

Insect sting hypersensitivity

Insect sting hypersensitivity is an important cause of severe allergic reactions [4]. Bees and wasps are the usual culprits. Immunotherapy is a very effective therapy for bee and wasp allergy. The therapy is not without its risks and many children with systemic reactions to insect stings seem to outgrow the problem with time.

Outcomes of allergy to insect stings in children, with and without venom immunotherapy

Golden DBK, Kagey-Sobotka A, Norman PS, Hamilton RG, Lichtenstein LM. *N Engl J Med* 2004; **351**: 668–74

BACKGROUND. It has been thought that children with insect sting hypersensitivity have a much better prognosis than adults. This has been the basis for the different thresholds for recommending immunotherapy for children and adults with insect sting hypersensitivity. Until now, there has been very little long-term follow-up data to support this policy.

INTERPRETATION. The authors have followed up children who were diagnosed with insect sting hypersensitivity 10–20 years previously. They managed to contact 512 subjects, half the 1033 children diagnosed with insect sting hypersensitivity during this time. A third had received specific venom immunotherapy (mean duration 3.5 years). Forty-three per cent of the subjects had a repeat sting during the follow-up period (mean 18 years). Systemic reactions occurred less frequently in subjects who had received immunotherapy (3 vs 17%; $P = 0.007$). This difference was even more apparent in those with previous moderate to severe reactions (5 vs 32%; $P = 0.007$).

Comment

Although seemingly very effective, specific immunotherapy has potentially severe adverse effects. It is therefore important that it is only used for children who are at risk of further systemic reactions to insect stings and that a clinically important long-term benefit can be demonstrated. This paper contributes useful evidence on both of these points. In the group of children who did not receive immunotherapy, a third of those with a previous moderate or severe systemic reaction (cardio-respiratory symptoms) had another systemic reaction to a further sting. This compares favourably with the adult data that would suggest that over half will go on to develop systemic allergic reactions [8]. Focusing on the children with less severe initial reactions, 13% of those with an initial mild systemic reaction (only cutaneous symptoms) and 7% of those with only an initial large local reaction had a

Table 6.1 Risk of systemic reaction to future stings in untreated patients with insect sting hypersensitivity

Original sting reaction		**Risk of systemic reaction**	
Severity	**Age**	**1–9 years later**	**10–20 years later**
No reaction	Adult	17%	
Large local	All	10%	10%
Cutaneous systemic	Child	10%	5%
Cutaneous systemic	Adult	20%	10%
Anaphylaxis	Child	40%	30%
Anaphylaxis	Adult	60%	40%

Source: Adkinson *et al.* (2003) **[12]**.

systemic reaction during follow-up. None of these systemic reactions was severe. This paper also again emphasizes that children with systemic cutaneous reactions have a relatively low rate of subsequently developing future systemic reactions. A summary of the risk of further reactions is outlined in Table 6.1. The key importance of this paper is the length of the follow-up, which is unrivalled. Even after 18 years of average follow-up, immunotherapy would still seem to be of benefit. In this study only 3% of those who received immunotherapy had a subsequent systemic reaction, 5-fold less than in the non-treated group. Many of these reactions occurred many years after the children had finished receiving immunotherapy. This compares well with previous studies with much shorter follow-up durations **[8,9]**. Since these patients were treated, it has been suggested that immunotherapy should be continued for 5 years or, for the most severely affected subjects, even life **[10]**. The follow-up results might have been even better had the duration of treatment been longer. A note of caution: this is an observational paper with mostly non-random allocation of subjects to immunotherapy or no treatment. We therefore need to be a little circumspect in extrapolating the results to our own patients. However, we are unlikely to see many better data sets with such an impressive length of follow-up. An updated practice parameter on the management of insect sting hypersensitivity has recently been published **[11]**.

Food allergy

Food allergy is a major cause of severe allergic reactions, particularly in children. Eggs and milk are the commonest cause in infants. Most children outgrow this problem by the age of 5 years. With increasing age, allergies to peanuts, tree nuts, fish and shellfish become more prevalent. No cure is currently available for food allergy. Management must therefore be focused on identification of the allergen, avoidance of the allergen and managing any allergic reactions.

Efficacy of a management plan based on severity assessment in longitudinal and case–controlled studies of 747 children with nut allergy: proposal for good practice

Ewan PW, Clark AT. *Clin Exp Allergy* 2005; **35**: 751–6

BACKGROUND. Food allergy is the commonest cause of allergic reactions in children and adults. Many of these are potentially life-threatening cardiorespiratory reactions. Each patient must also have a personalized management plan to deal with any future reactions. A key question in developing these is whether a device for the self-injection of adrenaline (e.g. EpiPen or Anapen) should be prescribed. To address this question, we need to understand the natural history of food allergy and be able to identify who is at risk of having a severe reaction.

INTERPRETATION. A total of 747 children with peanut or tree nut allergy were seen annually by this group for a median of 3.3 years. A self-injectable adrenaline device was given if there was a history of reactions with airway narrowing, milder reactions to low-dose exposure or concomitant asthma. Only 17 of the 395 (4.3%; 95% confidence interval 2.5–6.8%) subjects with a non-life-threatening initial reaction had a cardiorespiratory reaction during the follow-up period. All these reactions involved only mild bronchospasm or stridor and none required therapy with adrenaline.

Comment

There is considerable inconsistency in the prescription of self-injection devices. In recent years we have been prescribing more devices in response to data from a North American group [**13**]. They studied a group of 83 young children with peanut allergy; 61 of them had a non-life threatening initial reaction. A third of this group of 61 children subsequently had a potentially life-threatening cardiorespiratory reaction during the 6-year median follow-up period. These data effectively demand that all children with a reaction to peanut of any severity should have access to a self-injectable adrenaline device. These results contrast with the data from this group of 747 British children allergic to peanuts or tree nuts. There was a difference of more than 7-fold in the rate of subsequent severe reactions, which cannot be explained by the difference in the duration of follow-up. There are two possible explanations for these contrasting results. Firstly, the American study focused on the first reaction while the British one focused on the most severe reaction during the 2-year median period between first reaction and assessment in an allergy clinic. Secondly, only the British patients were all reviewed at yearly intervals, when avoidance education was reinforced. Both papers demonstrate that the severity of previous reactions cannot be used to identify a group of children with nut allergy who are at zero risk of further systemic reactions. However, with a risk of a severe reaction of only around 1% per year, some clinicians may feel that prescribing self-injectable adrenaline is not justified. Arguments for this would be that devices are too inconvenient to carry and are often left at home, the need for training to ensure that they are used correctly, their expense and short shelf-life, and the existence of a rapid-response paramedic service for the rare event of a severe reaction. But the very real risk of a future potentially life-threatening severe reaction has to be kept in mind. The decision about the provision of a self-injectable adrenaline device should be made in conjunction with the family.

Parental use of EpiPen for children with food allergies

Kim JS, Sinacore JM, Pongracic JA. *J Allergy Clin Immunol* 2005; **116**: 164–8

BACKGROUND. Families frequently do not use their self-injectable adrenaline device, even when their child is experiencing a potentially life-threatening cardiorespiratory allergic reaction to a food allergen [14]. Fatal anaphylaxis is rare but well recognized and the early use of intramuscular adrenaline may be life-saving.

INTERPRETATION. The authors investigated whether the under-use of a self-injectable adrenaline EpiPen for allergic reactions to foods might be attributed to parental discomfort with the administration of the device and lack of knowledge of the proper method of administration. A total of 165 parents of a food-allergic child completed the survey. Parents were happier to administer adrenaline if they had previously used it ($P = 0.009$), they had been trained to use the device ($P = 0.005$) and felt empowered ($P<0.0005$). Interestingly, neither a history of previous anaphylaxis nor a high level of knowledge was associated with a high level of comfort in using the self-injectable adrenaline device.

Comment

Many families do not use their self-injectable adrenaline EpiPen device to treat severe allergic reactions. Parents have been found to not know the symptoms of anaphylaxis and to not understand how to use the device [14]. This survey highlights these issues and the authors then seek to understand the reasons behind the problem. Only 83% of parents had received training in the use of the device and only 78% reported carrying it with them always or almost always. Half were uncomfortable with administering an EpiPen to their child, mainly because they were concerned that they would not be able to recognize the symptoms of anaphylaxis. The results emphasize the need for training, preferably with a trainer device. They also highlight the importance of empowerment as this was directly correlated with increased comfort with using adrenaline. Experiencing your child having a severe allergic reaction must be very stressful, and it is therefore not surprising that psychological factors are important in this situation. Fear may impede parents from reacting in the way that they have been taught. As allergists we must help parents to take ownership of the management of their child's allergic reactions to help them feel empowered and comfortable with delivering the correct emergency treatment. This needs to be delivered within a structured multidisciplinary educational strategy [15].

Lupin flour anaphylaxis

Radcliffe M, Scadding G, Brown HM. *Lancet* 2005; **365**: 1360

BACKGROUND. Lupin is a member of the legume family and seems to be the latest novel food allergen. There are, however, isolated reports of lupin flour as an allergen from as far back as 1994 [16]. The new factor is the introduction of lupin flour into large-scale food manufacturing, particularly as a wheat or soya substitute. This has been a particular problem in France. Typical foods that have been found to sometimes contain lupin flour are bread, pastries, pasta, pizza base, pitta bread and yogurt.

INTERPRETATION. The authors describe a 25-year-old women who had an anaphylactic reaction to a restaurant meal requiring multiple doses of intramuscular adrenaline. She was known to have a severe peanut allergy. It was considered that the meal could not have been contaminated with peanut, but the onion ring batter contained lupin flour. A skin-prick test to lupin gave a 14 mm weal (crude 1:100 w/v eluate of lupin) and serum specific IgE was 12.5 kU_A/l (UniCAP test, Pharmacia Diagnostics, Uppsala, Sweden). The patient declined to be challenged.

Comment

The common factor for this and the other cases of lupin allergy in the literature seems to be coexistent legume allergy, in particular to peanut, soya or pea. Peanut-allergic subjects may have a 50% chance of being sensitized to lupin [**17**]. However, we do not know how many of these have clinical allergy to lupin flour. Is this just an example of cross-sensitization without coexistent allergy? We urgently need to know the answer to this question and to determine the prevalence of lupin allergy in the general population. Additionally, we need a better understanding of which products are likely to contain lupin. This would be considerably helped if lupin flour were added to the 12 other potential allergenic ingredients in the new European Union directive on food labelling (see Mills *et al.*, reviewed below). It is frustrating that these problems could have been anticipated prior to the introduction of lupin flour into our food chain. Prior testing of legume-allergic subjects would have highlighted the problem. This would have at least prompted the early introduction of labelling, if not a complete ban on the introduction of this new ingredient into our food chain.

Information provision for allergic consumers—where are we going with food allergen labelling?

Mills ENC, Valovirta E, Madsen C, *et al.* *Allergy* 2004: **59**: 1262–8

BACKGROUND. Food allergy is a relatively common problem. Despite this, we still do not have any specific therapy for the problem. Avoidance of the offending allergen

is therefore the mainstay of the management of food allergy. To achieve this, patients and their families must be appropriately educated and be able to rely on the accurate and informative labelling of food. Unfortunately this has not been in place up until now. Legislation has previously allowed non-declaration of potentially allergic ingredients on the labels (the European 25% rule says that ingredients making up less than 25% of the finished product do not need to be declared) while not outlawing defensive 'may contain labels' on products that should not contain a specific allergen.

Interpretation. The paper presents an overview of the new European Union directive on food labelling. The new European Union food labelling directive abolishes the old 25% rule and now expects manufacturers to declare all the ingredients. Additionally, it cites a list of twelve food allergens (peanuts, tree nuts, soybeans, eggs, milk, fish, crustaceans, celery, mustard, sesame seed, cereals containing gluten, sulphur dioxide and sulphites). The presence of any of these or any product derived from them must be clearly indicated on food products. The paper goes onto discuss the problem of defensive labelling for consumers.

Comment

Food-allergic consumers have been asking for potentially allergenic foods to be declared on the label in a clear, understandable and easy-to-read manner. For the first time the regulators have listened to this request. This new European Union regulation is being added to the national laws in the Member States and consumers should expect to see changes in labelling from early 2006. The introduction of these regulations will represent a considerable challenge to manufacturers. Good record-keeping and communication will be required throughout their global supply chains. This will be complicated by the constant change in constituents, reflecting the availability and price of raw products. The problem of defensive labelling is unfortunately not tackled by this new European Union directive. These labels make the lives of food-allergic consumers even more difficult. Many frustrated patients often ignore the warning, putting themselves at risk of suffering a potentially life-threatening allergic reaction if they are unlucky enough to consume a contaminated product. Many manufacturing facilities are unfortunately not set up to minimize the cross-contamination during the production process. Given this, the introduction of the new directive may increase the amount of defensive labelling. Thus, although the new European Union directive is a good start, a follow-up directive to deal with this defensive labelling is urgently required.

Development of a questionnaire to measure quality of life in families with a child with food allergy

Cohen BL, Noone S, Munoz-Furlong A, Sicherer SH. *J Allergy Clin Immunol* 2004; **114**: 1159–63

Background. No cure is available for food allergy and food-allergic patients and their families are therefore burdened with the need to constantly avoid allergenic food

while worrying about the potential effect of any accidental exposure. Living with food allergy can therefore be expected to impair the quality of life of the sufferer and their family. Until now, this issue has only been explored in food allergy with generic quality of life questionnaires such as the Child Health Questionnaire Parent Form 50 (CHQ-PF50). Disease-specific health-related quality of life questionnaires focus on areas that are most relevant to a specific disease and can therefore be expected to be more sensitive. Until now, there has been no validated health-related quality of life questionnaire for food allergy.

INTERPRETATION. The authors set out to develop and validate a food allergy-specific health-related quality of life questionnaire to measure the parental burden associated with having a child with food allergy: the Food Allergy Quality of Life–Parental Burden (FAQL–PB) questionnaire. A total of 74 items affecting families with children with food allergy were identified. The highest-impact items were used to develop a final short questionnaire. This covers family/social activities, school, meal preparation, health concerns and emotional issues. Good internal validity and reliability was demonstrated. There was good correlation with the parents' expectation of the seriousness of their child's problem and with scores on a generic health-related quality of life questionnaire. The questionnaire was able to discriminate between families with different burdens of disease.

Comment

The authors have used well-established principles to develop a disease-specific health-related quality of life questionnaire to measure the burden of childhood food allergy on parents. They have then validated this instrument in a group of 352 families with a child with food allergy. Of note, these families were mostly affluent and white and there was an over-representation of children with severe allergic reactions. The developmental process that was needed to generate the questionnaire highlighted all the issues that affect families with food allergy. These include purchasing food and preparing meals, family and social activities, such as school, holidays, meals out and child care. Parents may be anxious about reactions and worried that their child may not have a normal upbringing. The one issue with this new questionnaire is its generalizability to other populations. The authors need to demonstrate that it is valid in less affluent families with less severe food allergy. Additionally, care must be taken when applying it to populations outside the USA as these questionnaires do not always work as well, even in other English-speaking countries, because of country-specific questions. With these reservations, the FAQL–PB questionnaire is a useful health-related quality of life end-point for food allergy studies and will be useful when we come to assess the effectiveness of interventions to treat food allergy.

Adverse reactions to allergen immunotherapy

Immunotherapy is a useful therapy. It seems to be particularly effective for bee and wasp hypersensitivity and allergic rhinitis |**18**|. Unfortunately, it is rarely associated with severe allergic reactions. This has severely restricted its use in the UK, although it is still a very popular treatment option in the rest of Europe and the USA.

Twelve-year survey of fatal reactions to allergen injections and skin testing: 1990–2001

Bernstein DI, Wanner M, Borish L, Liss GM; Immunotherapy Committee, American Academy of Allergy, Asthma and Immunology. *J Allergy Clin Immunol* 2004; **113**: 1129–36

BACKGROUND. Specific allergen immunotherapy is a very effective therapy for many forms of allergic disease. Unfortunately, there is a small risk of fatal allergic reactions associated with its use. The risk factors for severe reactions are now well known: dosing errors, coexistent asthma, concomitant use of β-blockers, previous systemic reactions to immunotherapy and administration during peak seasonal allergen exposure. Protocols have been adjusted to allow for these factors.

INTERPRETATION. A postal survey was undertaken to ascertain all the fatal and near-fatal reactions related to immunotherapy from 1990 to 2001 in US and Canadian populations. A quarter of the 2404 allergy practices responded. Forty-one fatal immunotherapy reactions were reported and full details were available for 17 (Table 6.2). Almost all reactions involved patients with asthma; some had poorly controlled disease. Three cases occurred in settings without medical supervision. One case was associated with an 18-fold overdose. Most reactions occurred during the maintenance phase of treatment. Three reactions commenced 30–60 min after an injection. In a third of cases, adrenaline was given more than 5 min after the start of a reaction; it was almost always given subcutaneously. None of the patients experiencing a fatal reaction was receiving β-blockers but one was being treated with an angiotensin-converting enzyme inhibitor. It was estimated that one fatality occurred per 2.5 million injections. One other fatality was confirmed after skin-prick testing with 90 food allergens in a patient with poorly controlled asthma (forced expiratory volume in 1 s less than 50% of predicted).

Comment

In many ways the results of this survey are disappointing, given that it demonstrated a rate of fatalities similar to those in earlier surveys [**19,20**] despite the introduction of national practice parameters [**21**]. Additionally, given the poor response rate to the survey, it is possible that it has underestimated the actual fatality rate. As with previous studies, most fatalities occurred in asthmatic people, and often their asthma was poorly controlled. These findings lend further support to the UK view that perennial asthma should generally be a contraindication to immunotherapy. The results additionally emphasize the necessity that immunotherapy should only be administered in a medically supervised setting. The supervising personnel should be trained to treat the first sign of anaphylaxis immediately with adrenaline. The intramuscular route should be used as we know that intramuscular adrenaline is more effective than subcutaneous adrenaline [**22**].

Additionally, the results demonstrate the need for a 60 min observation period. The reporting of the first known fatal reaction to skin-prick testing is concerning. All previously reported fatal reactions associated with skin testing have been with intradermal testing [19,20]. Although this was only a single case, it suggests that skin-prick testing should be postponed if a patient's asthma is poorly controlled or that serum specific IgE testing should be used.

Latex allergy

The prevalence of latex allergy has increased worldwide over the last few decades with the introduction of universal precautions and the ubiquitous latex glove. The risk factors for allergy are well known. These include previous multiple operations, particularly urological, atopic predisposition or occupational exposure.

Latex allergy in infants younger than 1 year

Kimata H. *Clin Exp Allergy* 2004; **34**: 1910–15

BACKGROUND. The literature on the prevalence of latex allergy in the general population is unclear. The prevalence has been estimated as ranging from zero in children [23] to 6.5% in adult blood donors [24]. Subjects with latex allergy generally fall into one of the well-known high-risk groups. Latex allergy is very unusual in infants.

INTERPRETATION. Nine cases of proven latex allergy in infants are reported. The author reviews the symptoms and risk factors of latex allergy in these infants. None had any congenital abnormalities or had undergone any operations. Six patients had atopic dermatitis and another had atopic asthma. Infants presented with wheezing, angio-oedema, urticaria or anaphylaxis with latex contact. The causative products included bottle teats, pacifiers, nose cleaners, balloons, or enema tubes. All had positive skin-prick test to latex and eight were positive for serum specific IgE for latex. Six patients had a parent with latex allergy.

Comment

The presentation of latex allergy during infancy is very rare, making this an unusual group of patients. The group is characterized by their atopic tendency, as demonstrated by sensitization to food and aeroallergens and their expression of clinical atopic disease. Given the relative rarity of latex allergy, it is surprising that so many of the parents also had evidence of latex allergy. This suggests that there may be strong genetic influences on the development of latex allergy. The authors are unable to give any estimate of the minimum prevalence of latex allergy in Japanese infants as these cases seem to have been referred to them from across Japan. We have recently looked at the prevalence of latex allergy in a large community sample of 7-year-olds in the UK [23]. A total of 1877 subjects were skin-prick tested to latex (ALK-Abello, Horsholm, Denmark). Only four subjects had

Table 6.2 Characteristics of individual fatal reactions to immunotherapy injections in 17 patients from long surveys

Patient number	Onset (minutes)	Initial symptoms	Symptoms	Allergen dose for adverse reactions	Risk factors	Cause of death
1	>30	Pruritis	Lower airway obstruction, shock	Maintenance	Previous systemic reaction	Anaphylactic shock
2	10–20	Lower airway obstruction	Lower airway obstruction, hypotension	Up-dosing	Previous systemic reaction, unstable asthma	Asthma, cardiovascular collapse
3	>30	Lower airway obstruction	Lower airway obstruction, hypotension	Maintenance	Recent exacerbation of asthma	Asthma, arrhythmia, airway oedema
4	Not known	Unwell	Lower airway obstruction	Maintenance	None	Anaphylactic shock
5	Not known	Dyspnoea	Dead on arrival	Up-dosing	Recent asthma exacerbation	No information
6	0–3	Upper airway obstruction	Upper and lower airway obstruction, hypotension	Up-dosing	Switched from unstandardized to standardized extract	Anaphylactic shock
7	3–10	Facial erythema	Lower airway obstruction	Up-dosing	Poor asthma control	Asthma, seizure
8	10–20	Upper airway obstruction	Lower and upper airway obstruction, hypotension	Maintenance	Previous systemic reaction, ACE inhibitor	Anaphylactic shock
9	0–3	Lower airway obstruction, shock	Lower airway obstruction, shock	Maintenance	Poor asthma control, self-administered, peak pollen season	Anaphylactic shock

10	Not known	Upper airway obstruction	Upper airway obstruction, angio-oedema	Maintenance	None	Upper airway oedema
11	0–3	Gastrointestinal	Upper and lower airway obstruction, shock	Maintenance	None	Upper airway oedema
12	Not known	Upper airway obstruction	Upper and lower airway obstruction, hypotension	Up-dosing	Height of pollen season, recent asthma exacerbation	Asthma, anaphylactic shock
13	3–10	Shortness of breath	Upper and lower airway obstruction, hypotension	Maintenance	Recent asthma exacerbation	Asthma, laryngeal oedema
14	0–3	Upper airway obstruction	Upper and lower airway obstruction, hypotension	Maintenance	Poorly control asthma	Upper airway oedema
15	10–20	Lower airway obstruction	Lower airway obstruction, shock, cyanosis	Maintenance	Left clinic within minutes of injection	Asthma, anaphylactic shock
16	3–10	Lower airway obstruction	Lower airway obstruction, shock	Up-dosing	Height of pollen season, previous systemic reaction, unstable asthma	Anaphylactic shock, asthma, cardiac arrhythmia
17	>30	Something in throat	Angio-oedema, hypotension, upper airway obstruction	Up-dosing	None	Anaphylactic shock, pulmonary oedema

ACE, angiotensin-converting enzyme.
Source: Bernstein *et al.* (2004).

positive reactions and none had a history of clinical reaction to latex. This gives a general population prevalence of sensitization and clinical allergy to latex of 0.2% (95% confidence interval 0.1–0.6%) and 0.0% (0–0.2%) respectively. The epidemic of latex allergy in healthcare workers seems to be abating with the realization of the importance of reducing latex exposure. In Germany, powdered latex gloves were banned in 1998. Data have recently been published comparing the annual numbers of reported cases of occupational latex allergy from 1996 to 2002 with the purchase of latex gloves from 1986 to 2002 [25]. In the late 1980s and early 1990s the number of gloves purchased increased over 10-fold. This coincided with a huge increase in occupational latex allergy. From 1998 the number of non-powdered latex gloves purchased exceeded the number of powdered ones. After 1998, the incidence of new cases dropped by 80%. Although this was not a controlled interventional study, the data strongly suggest that latex exposure is a key factor in the development of latex allergy and suggest that controlling latex exposure is an effective intervention. We need to ensure that our patients' exposure to latex is also minimized.

Conclusion

With systemic allergic reactions, allergy is associated with both morbidity and mortality. Our efforts to understand anaphylaxis have been impeded by the lack of a consensus definition of anaphylaxis. Advances have been made in this in the last few years ([1,6,7] and Brown, reviewed above) but it remains to be seen if any of these become universally accepted. Insect hypersensitivity is one of the more important and treatable causes of systemic allergic reactions. The contribution of Golden *et al.* [10] to this area provides long-term outcome data to support our approach to using immunotherapy to manage children with severe insect hypersensitivity. Will the increase in duration of therapy to 5 years further improve the outcome for this patient group? It is still concerning that fatal reactions to immunotherapy continue to be reported despite the implementations of international practice parameters (Bernstein *et al.*, reviewed above). This emphasizes the need to further develop this therapeutic intervention to minimize the risks while maintaining its benefits. An obvious approach would be to use a monoclonal anti-IgE antibody to cover the up-dosing period, when reactions are most frequent. We still lack a curative therapeutic intervention for food allergy, and novel food allergens continue to emerge. This must add to the impaired quality of life associated with food allergy (Cohen *et al.*, reviewed above). Lupin flour is the latest novel food allergen to cause major problems (Radcliffe *et al.*, reviewed above). We must hope that when a novel food is next introduced into our food chain, it is first properly evaluated for allergenicity. Hopefully, lupin will soon be added to the new EU list of food allergens that must be identified on food products (Mills *et al.*, reviewed above). Self-injectable adrenaline is the therapy of choice for a systemic reaction in the community. There is huge variation in their prescription, however. The data from Ewan *et al.* (reviewed above) are likely to add to the discussion.

Although they suggest that the risk of a systemic allergic reaction in a child with previous mild reactions to peanut and tree nuts is lower than previously suggested [13], there is still a very real but small risk of anaphylaxis in this group. Will we be able to identify a low-risk group of nut-allergic patients or do they all need access to self-injectable adrenaline? Even if we provide self-injectable adrenaline, families must be prepared to use them. To facilitate this, we need to effectively engage the family in the management plan (Kim *et al.*, reviewed above). It had looked as though we were winning the battle with latex allergy as the incidence dropped with the stricter environmental controls on latex gloves, but it is concerning that a sizeable group of infants have been identified with latex allergy in Japan (Kimata, reviewed above). Is there a common latex source that they have been exposed to? This might explain why this pattern of latex allergy has not been seen in the rest of the world. There is still much we need to learn about systemic allergic reactions and we desperately need better therapeutic interventions for patients at risk of anaphylaxis.

References

1. Johansson SGO, Bieber T, Dahl R, Friedmann PS, Lanier BQ, Lockey RF, Motala C, Ortega Martell JA, Platts-Mills TA, Ring J, Thien F, Van Cauwenberge P, Williams HC. Revised nomenclature for allergy for global use: Report of the Nomenclature Review Committee of the World Allergy Organization, October 2003. *J Allergy Clin Immunol* 2004; **113**: 832–6.
2. Sicherer SH. Food allergy. *Lancet* 2002; **360**: 701–10.
3. Moneret-Vautrin DA, Morisset M, Flabbee J, Beaudouin E, Kanny G. Epidemiology of life-threatening and lethal anaphylaxis: a review. *Allergy* 2005; **60**: 443–51.
4. Dibs S, Baker M. Anaphylaxis in children: a 5-year experience. *Pediatrics* 1997; **99**: 1–5.
5. Moneret-Vautrin DA, Romano MC, Kanny G, Morisset M, Beaudouin E, Parisot L, Croizier A, Hatahet R. Le Projet d'Accueil Individualisé pour urgence allergique: situation en France métropolitaine et dans les Dom-Tom en 2002. *Presse Med* 2003; **32**: 61–6.
6. Sampson HA, Munoz-Furlong A, Bock SA, Schmitt C, Bass R, Chowdhury BA, Decker WW, Furlong TJ, Galli SJ, Golden DB, Gruchalla RS, Harlor AD Jr, Hepner DL, Howarth M, Kaplan AP, Levy JH, Lewis LM, Lieberman PL, Metcalfe DD, Murphy R, Pollart SM, Pumphrey RS, Rosenwasser LJ, Simons FE, Wood JP, Camargo CA Jr. Symposium on the definition and management of anaphylaxis: summary report. *J Allergy Clin Immunol* 2005; **115**: 584–91.
7. Joint Task Force on Practice Parameters; American Academy of Allergy, Asthma and Immunology; American College of Allergy, Asthma and Immunology; Joint Council of

Allergy, Asthma and Immunology. The diagnosis and management of anaphylaxis: an updated practice parameter. *J Allergy Clin Immunol* 2005; **115**: S483–523.

8. Reisman RE. Natural history of insect sting allergy: relationship of severity of symptoms of initial sting anaphylaxis to re-sting reactions. *J Allergy Clin Immunol* 1992; **90**: 335–9.
9. Valentine MD, Schuberth KC, Kagey-Sobotka A, Graft DF, Kwiterovich KA, Szklo M, Lichtenstein LM. The value of immunotherapy with venom in children with allergy to insect stings. *N Engl J Med* 1990; **323**: 1601–3.
10. Golden DBK. Insect sting allergy and venom immunotherapy: a model and a mystery. *J Allergy Clin Immunol* 2005; **115**: 439–47.
11. Moffitt JE, Golden DB, Reisman RE, Lee R, Nicklas R, Freeman T, deShazo R, Tracy J, Bernstein IL, Blessing-Moore J, Khan DA, Lang DM, Portnoy JM, Schuller DE, Spector SL, Tilles SA. Stinging insect hypersensitivity: a practice parameter update. *J Allergy Clin Immunol* 2004; **114**: 869–86.
12. Yunginger JW. Insect allergy. In: Adkinson NF, Yunginger JW, Busse WW, Bochner BS, Holgate ST, Simons FER (eds). *Middleton's allergy: Principles and practice.* 6th edn. St Louis: Mosby, 2003; pp 1475–86.
13. Vander Leek TK, Liu AH, Stefanski K, Blacker B, Bock SA. The natural history of peanut allergy in young children and its association with serum peanut-specific IgE. *J Pediatr* 2000; **137**: 749–55.
14. Gold MS, Sainsbury R. First aid anaphylaxis management in children who were prescribed an epinephrine autoinjector device (EpiPen). *J Allergy Clin Immunol* 2000; **106**: 171–6.
15. Kapoor S, Roberts G, Bynoe Y, Gaughan M, Habibi P, Lack G. Influence of a multidisciplinary paediatric allergy clinic on parental knowledge and rate of subsequent allergic reactions. *Allergy* 2004; **59**: 185–91.
16. Hefle SL, Lemanske RF, Bush RK. Adverse reaction to lupin fortified pasta. *J Allergy Clin Immunol* 1994; **33**: 256–67.
17. Moneret-Vautrin DA, Guerin D, Danny G, Flabbee J, Morisset M. Cross-allergenicity of peanut and lupin: the risk of lupin allergy in patients allergic to peanuts. *J Allergy Clin Immunol* 1999; **104**: 883–8.
18. Anon. Allergen immunotherapy: therapeutic vaccines for allergic diseases. Geneva: 27–29 January 1997. *Allergy* 1998; **53**(44 Suppl): 1–42.
19. Lockey RF, Nicoara-Kasti GL, Theodoropoulos DS, Bukantz SC. Systemic reactions and fatalities associated with allergen immunotherapy. *Ann Allergy Asthma Immunol* 2001; **87**: 47–55.
20. Lockey RF, Benedict LM, Turkeltaub PC, Bukantz SC. Fatalities from immunotherapy and skin testing. *J Allergy Clin Immunol* 1987; **79**: 660–77.
21. Joint Task Force on Practice Parameters, representing the American Academy of Allergy, Asthma and Immunology, the American College of Allergy, Asthma and Immunology, and the Joint Council of Allergy, Asthma and Immunology. Practice parameters for allergen immunotherapy. *J Allergy Clin Immunol* 1996; **98**: 1001–11.
22. Simons FER, Roberts JR, Gu X, Simons KJ. Epinephrine absorption in children with a history of anaphylaxis. *J Allergy Clin Immunol* 1998; **101**: 33–7.

23. Roberts G, Lack G, Northstone K, Golding J. Prevalence of latex allergy in the community at age 7 years. *Clin Exp Allergy* 2005; **35**: 299–300.

24. Ownby DR, Ownby HE, McCullough J, Shafer AW. The prevalence of anti-latex IgE antibodies in 1000 volunteer blood donors. *J Allergy Clin Immunol* 1996; **97**: 1188–92.

25. Allmers H, Schmengler J, John SM. Decreasing incidence of occupational contact urticaria caused by natural rubber latex allergy in German health care workers. *J Allergy Clin Immunol* 2004; **114**: 347–51.

7

Food allergy

TARANEH DEAN

Introduction

A task force of the European Academy of Allergy and Clinical Immunology [1] has recently suggested that any adverse reactions to food should be called 'food hypersensitivity'. When immunological mechanisms have been demonstrated, the appropriate term is 'food allergy'. Where the role of immunoglobulin E (IgE) is confirmed, it is suggested that the form of allergy should be known as 'IgE-mediated food allergy'. They suggest that other reactions, previously sometimes referred to as 'food intolerance', should be referred to as 'non-allergic food hypersensitivity'. Severe, generalized allergic reactions to food are classified as 'anaphylaxis' [1]. It is important to recognize that food hypersensitivity is not a single disease. An individual with food hypersensitivity could have one of several conditions, such as atopic eczema/dermatitis syndrome, isolated urticaria or asthma. It is also interesting to note that although the diversity of the human diet is enormous, only a few foods account for most cases of food hypersensitivity globally.

The evidence in the area of food hypersensitivity has grown over the last few years and subsequently our knowledge of how to diagnose and manage food hypersensitivity has increased. Perhaps one of the most significant contributions to evidence about food hypersensitivity is our knowledge of the size of the problem. A number of government-funded projects across Europe have recently addressed the issue of the scale of food hypersensitivity. Researchers from many countries have now established the prevalence of food hypersensitivity within their geographical areas and potential risk factors are explored. Diagnosis of food hypersensitivity is not straightforward and the diagnostic work-up usually includes skin-prick tests [2] and/or the measurement of food-specific IgE antibodies [3] and, more recently, the atopy patch test [4]. Food challenges, in particular the double-blind, placebo-controlled food challenge (DBPCFC), remain the current gold standard for the diagnosis of food hypersensitivity [5,6]. Once food hypersensitivity is diagnosed, currently the only effective mode of treatment is avoidance. Individuals with food hypersensitivity need to learn to identify and avoid the implicated food and to know what to do if any is accidentally ingested and they experience symptoms. Apart from the clinical and social burden that accompanies food hypersensitivity, the economic impact of food hypersensitivity and its cost to

© Atlas Medical Publishing Ltd

society is beginning to be recognized [6]. The economic burden affects not only individuals with food hypersensitivity but also their carers and households, the healthcare sector and the food industry.

In this chapter a selection of recent studies addressing some of these issues is critically reviewed.

Prevalence of food hypersensitivity

Prevalence of adverse reactions to food in Germany: a population study

Zuberbier T, Edenharter G, Worm M, *et al.* *Allergy* 2004; **59**: 338–45

BACKGROUND. Because of the lack of existing data, the German Ministry of Health funded a study in Berlin during 1999–2000 to establish the prevalence of food hypersensitivity in Berlin and then project the findings to the whole German adult population using the 1998 national health census data. Using a cross-sectional survey, 13 300 inhabitants of all ages in Berlin were contacted, and 4093 responded. All respondents mentioning any sign of food hypersensitivity were followed up by telephone and, in appropriate cases, invited to attend the allergy clinic for further investigation.

INTERPRETATION. The prevalence of self-reported lifetime food hypersensitivity and that of food hypersensitivity confirmed by DBPCFC in the Berlin population was 34.9 and 3.6%, respectively. Considering only the adult population in Berlin, the point prevalence of food hypersensitivity confirmed by DBPCFC was 3.7% (18–79 years; 95% confidence interval [CI] 3.1–4.4%). Among these, 2.5% were IgE-mediated and 1.1% non-IgE-mediated. On the basis of a statistical comparison with available data of adults from the national health census, the prevalence of food hypersensitivity in the adult population of Germany was calculated to be 2.6% (95% CI 2.1–3.2%). When the researchers explored IgE-mediated versus non-IgE-mediated food allergy, they found that the highest frequency of IgE-mediated allergy was seen in 20- to 39-year-olds. Interestingly, for the non-IgE-mediated food allergy, the highest frequency was noted in the age group of 6 years and older (Figs 7.1 and 7.2).

Comment

This large-scale study gives a fairly accurate assessment of the prevalence of food hypersensitivity among adults in Germany. Although the response rate was only 31%, the sample required to report an expected prevalence rate of 2% was 4000. This study, alongside a number of previous studies, highlights the significant difference (greater than 10-fold in this case) between the rate of self-reported food hypersensitivity and that of objectively assessed food hypersensitivity. The main limitation of this study is the use of prick-to-prick testing to assess rates of

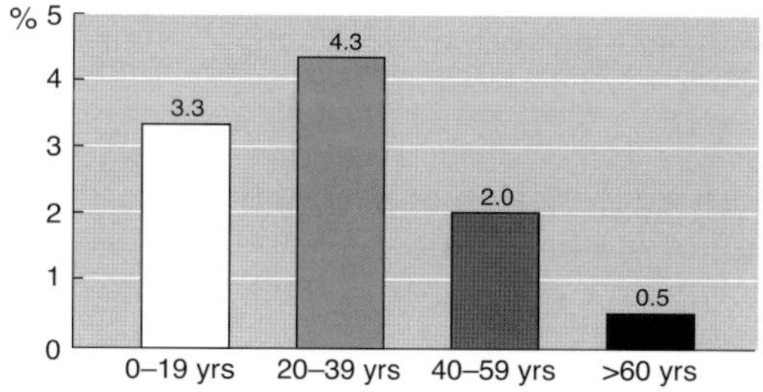

Fig. 7.1 Calculated prevalence of DBPCFC-proven IgE-mediated food allergy according to age. Source: Zuberbier *et al.* (2004).

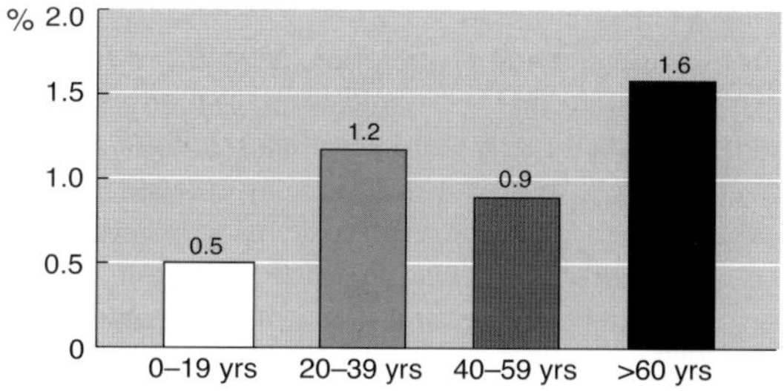

Fig. 7.2 Calculated prevalence of DBPCFC-proven food allergy according to age. Source: Zuberbier *et al.* (2004).

sensitization to foods and the lack of information provided on challenges (e.g. doses used in the challenge, number of adults and children challenged, and reactions experienced during challenges). In this study, 804 respondents (who included both adults and children; no breakdown provided) were given the skin-prick test using the prick-to-prick technique and the authors reported that the most frequent sensitization observed was to pollen-related foods, such as apple and hazelnut. It is impossible to compare the prick-to-prick sensitization data between different studies and populations because this procedure is not standardized. Looking at specific IgE antibodies to foods, they reported that 11.2% had positive specific IgE to at least one of the following food allergens: wheat, milk, egg, soy and fish. This is rather an interesting observation as the corresponding numbers for the prick-to-prick test were 4.7, 0.6, 0.8, 3.3 and 0.5% for wheat, milk, egg, soy and herring respectively. With regard to the final end-point (the DBPCFC), the authors state that, for both IgE- and non-IgE-mediated reactions, the foods that elicited a reaction were mostly pollen-related, such as hazelnut and apple.

The fact that food hypersensitivity was more frequent in Berlin (3.7%) than in the whole German population (2.6%) could suggest that perhaps the study sample was not representative. However, the authors argue that higher rates of allergies are often observed in urban areas compared with the countryside.

Prevalence and main characteristics of schoolchildren diagnosed with food allergies in France

Rance F, Grandmottet X, Grandjean H. *Clin Exp Allergy* 2005; **35**: 167–72

BACKGROUND. This study was another cross-sectional study, and it aimed to establish the prevalence of food hypersensitivity among schoolchildren in France. The research was conducted in schools in Toulouse using a questionnaire, which was distributed to children in their classes. The anonymous questionnaire was distributed to 3500 children and 2716 (77.6%) returned the completed questionnaire. No further investigation was carried out.

INTERPRETATION. Of the questionnaires returned, 2524 (92.9%) reported no food hypersensitivity. Of the 192 questionnaires reporting food hypersensitivity, ten were excluded and 182 were retained as reporting true food hypersensitivity. On the basis of this information the authors concluded that the cumulative and point prevalences were 6.7% (95% CI 5.8–7.6) and 4.7% (95% CI 3.9–5.5) respectively. The point prevalence was 4% for children aged 2–5% years, 6.8% for children aged 6–10 years, and 3.4% for children aged 11–14 years. The main foods reported as causing food hypersensitivity were milk, eggs, kiwi fruit, peanuts, fish, tree nuts and shrimps. The clinical signs of the food hypersensitivity were cutaneous (62.7%), digestive (30.3%) and respiratory (6.9%) signs, and anaphylactic shock (4.9%).

Comment

This study is one of the first population-based studies that has specifically aimed to establish the prevalence of food hypersensitivity among children. However, the results need to be treated with caution. To begin with, the results are based solely on parental report and, as discussed earlier, there is a significant difference between perceptions of food hypersensitivity and objectively assessed food hypersensitivity. Fewer than a third of the respondents had their food hypersensitivity diagnosed using food challenges. The anonymous aspect of data collection did not allow the researchers to investigate the degree of non-response bias. The age range covered was 2–14 years, and when cumulative prevalence is calculated the estimate will be subject to significant recall bias. This is particularly important considering that the point prevalence was lowest among the older children. The authors hope to confirm the reported food hypersensitivity in future using food challenges.

Prevalence of sensitization to food allergens, reported adverse reactions to foods, food avoidance, and food hypersensitivity among teenagers

Pereira B, Venter C, Grundy J, Clayton CB, Arshad SH, Dean T. *J Allergy Clin Immunol* 2005; **116**: 884–92

BACKGROUND. This population-based cross-sectional study, funded by a UK government agency, aimed to establish the rate of sensitization to food allergens, reported food hypersensitivity, food avoidance and objectively assessed food hypersensitivity in 11- and 15-year-olds living on the Isle of Wight, UK. The researchers approached the teenagers via their schools, and a questionnaire completed by the parents and children formed the basis of capturing data to determine the prevalence of current reported food hypersensitivity and rates of food avoidance. This information was available on 775 individuals aged 11 years and 757 aged 15 years. All consenting teenagers (699 aged 11 years and 649 aged 15 years) were given the skin-prick test using a predefined panel of standardized food allergens. Children with a positive skin-prick test who had never knowingly eaten a large amount of the food and those who reported a previous reaction to a certain food (regardless of the skin-prick test data) were invited for food challenges. In order to account for both the immediate and delayed reactions, 1-day or 1-week challenges were performed depending on the clinical history. Initially, open food challenges were conducted and only those with a positive reaction were asked to undergo a DBPCFC.

INTERPRETATION. The prevalence of reported food hypersensitivity among the 11- and 15-year-olds was 11.6 and 12.4% respectively. A total of 122 (15.7%) 11-year-olds and 142 (18.7%) 15-year-olds were avoiding some food or food ingredients. The rates of sensitization to the food allergens were 5.1 and 4.9% for the 11- and 15-year-olds respectively. The individual rate of food sensitization to the predefined panel of allergens is shown in Fig. 7.3.

Atopic children were significantly more likely to report a problem with any food in both the 11-year-old cohort (odds ratio [OR] 2.33; 95% CI 1.41–3.83; $P = 0.001$) and the 15-year-old cohort (OR 1.9; 95% CI 1.17–3.11; $P = 0.009$). The researchers observed significant differences between the rates of sensitization in boys and girls, boys having significantly higher rates of sensitization. The prevalence of food hypersensitivity, confirmed by open food challenges and a positive skin-prick test plus a convincing history of adverse reactions, was 2.3% for both the 11-year-olds and the 15-year-olds.

Comment

This study aimed specifically to look at population-based food hypersensitivity among teenagers. These are an important group as most severe allergic reactions and deaths caused by food hypersensitivity appear to be in the teenage population [7]. Most studies attempting to address population rates of sensitization to foods have been conducted in adult populations. The study by Zuberbier *et al.* described in this section included both adults and children but only prick-to-prick tests were

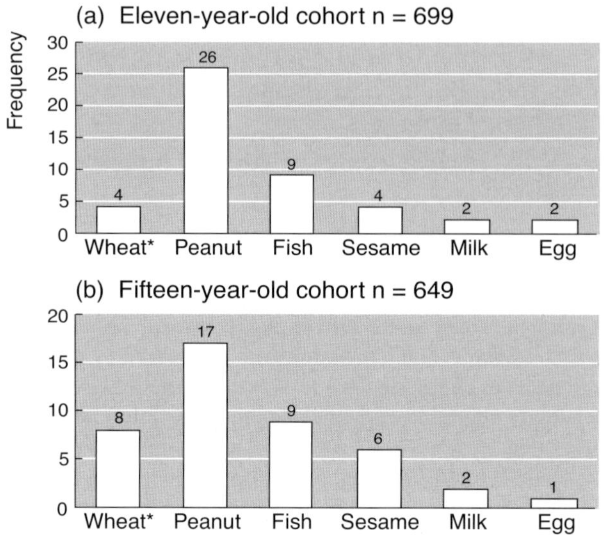

Fig. 7.3 Frequency of sensitization to the predefined food panel. Source: Pereira *et al.* (2005).

carried out and data on children are not presented separately; consequently, a direct comparison cannot be made. What is interesting, though, is the difference between the foods to which the populations in the two studies were sensitized. In the study by Zuberbier *et al.* the main food allergens were pollen-related foods, such as apple and hazelnut, whilst in the study by Pereira *et al.* peanuts and fish were the most frequent allergen to which the teenagers were sensitized.

This study showed that although perception of food hypersensitivity is common among teenagers (up to 12%), true food hypersensitivity could only be confirmed in 18–19% of this group who perceived that they had food hypersensitivity despite attempts to mimic the history in terms of the dose needed and the duration of exposure.

Diagnosis of food hypersensitivity

The relationship of allergen-specific IgE levels and oral food challenge outcome

Perry TT, Matsui EC, Conover-Walker MK, Wood RA. *J Allergy Clin Immunol* 2005; **114**: 144–9

BACKGROUND. Diagnosis of food hypersensitivity is a clinical challenge and the only current definitive test is the DBPCFC. Although the DBPCFC is the current gold standard, it is difficult to perform and is very time-consuming. Hence, researchers are continually evaluating new tests and assessing the value of the available serum tests. This study assessed the value of food-specific IgE levels in predicting the likelihood that patients with presumed milk, egg, peanut, soy or wheat allergy have acquired oral tolerance or might have been given an incorrect diagnosis because of a false-positive test result. The study retrospectively reviewed the outcome of 604 open food challenges in 391 children and investigated this in relation to the food-specific IgE levels measured before the challenge.

INTERPRETATION. Challenge pass rates (i.e. percentages of those who passed the challenge without having a positive reaction), median ages and specific IgE levels at the time of challenge are presented in Table 7.1. Among those who had a positive food challenge test result, urticaria or another skin manifestation occurred in 77%, gastrointestinal symptoms occurred in 43%, upper respiratory symptoms in 24% and lower respiratory symptoms in 26%; 60% of reactions involved two or more systems. Specific IgE levels were higher among patients who had a positive food challenge test result ($P \leq 0.03$ for each food). A cut-off level of 2 kUA/l (kilounits of antibody per litre)

Table 7.1 Pass rate, median age and median food-specific IgE results for 391 children who underwent 604 challenges

	Median age (years)*	Passed	Median IgE level: all*	Median IgE level: fail*	Median IgE level: pass*	*P*-value†
All challenges (*n* = 604)	5.3	57%	–	–	–	–
Milk (*n* = 166)	5.3	45%	1.34	2.0	0.9	<0.001
Egg (*n* = 138)	5.6	57%	0.94	1.2	0.7	0.024
Peanut (*n* = 173)	5.6	59%	1.13	1.9	0.5	<0.001
Wheat (*n* = 46)	4.2	67%	8.63	19.6	4.6	0.011
Soy (*n* = 81)	4.4	72%	3.88	9.3	3.2	0.030

* Median age and food-specific IgE results are based on data at the time of the challenge.
† *P*-value for the comparison of median IgE results between those who passed and failed challenges.
Source: Perry *et al.* (2005).

(for milk, egg and peanut) indicated a 50% likelihood of the challenge having a positive result. From these data the authors concluded that concentrations of allergen-specific IgEs to milk, egg and peanut serve as useful predictors of challenge outcome and should be considered when selecting patients for oral challenges to these foods.

Comment

In 1997, Sampson and colleagues published their study showing positive predictive values of 90% for specific IgEs to milk and eggs and 95% for specific IgE to peanuts [3,8]. These thresholds are most useful in deciding when a patient's specific IgE is so high that a challenge is unnecessary. This study has approached the same question from the opposite perspective. Here the researchers looked at the prediction of a negative challenge result at lower IgE levels. This is particularly useful for patients who may have outgrown their allergy or who have had false-positive test results. Although their data for milk, eggs and peanuts suggested a cut-off of 2 kUA/l for wheat and soy, the data were less clear. Despite the authors' interesting findings, one needs to consider that selection bias could have influenced their findings. Their study population consisted of children referred to a tertiary care facility, many of whom had multiple food allergies. In addition, because open food challenges were used the data are subject to reporting bias as well as observer bias.

The diagnostic accuracy of the atopy patch test in diagnosing hypersensitivity to cow's milk and hen's egg in unselected children with and without atopic dermatitis

Osterballe M, Andersen KE, Bindslev-Jensen C. *J Am Acad Dermatol* 2004; **51**: 556–62

BACKGROUND. Over the last 5 years some studies [9,10] have suggested that the atopy patch test (APT) may be a useful test in children with atopic dermatitis who have suspected food hypersensitivity and may even obviate the need for oral challenges. An alternative test to oral challenges with high sensitivity and specificity would be helpful in the diagnosis of food hypersensitivity. This study examined the clinical relevance of APT in diagnosing hypersensitivity to cow's milk or hen's egg compared with the skin-prick test, histamine release and specific IgE in an unselected group of children. The lifetime prevalence of atopic dermatitis was recorded by the Danish questionnaire developed from the UK Working Party's questionnaire for atopic dermatitis. Moreover, the severity of atopic dermatitis was scored according to the SCORAD (SCORing Atopic Dermatitis) index. The skin-prick test was performed with fresh cow's milk and hen's egg using the prick-to-prick technique. The atopy patch test was performed by placing one drop (20 μl) of fresh whole egg and fresh cow's milk (3.5% fat) on filter paper and applying it to uninvolved skin of the back using an 8 mm aluminium cup on adhesive tape. The application site was checked after 20 min and scored finally after 72 h. Immediate reactions (20 min) were defined as inconclusive; if such a reaction occurred further testing was stopped.

Table 7.2 Hen's egg: the diagnostic value (%) of the atopy patch test, skin-prick test, histamine release and specific IgE compared with the outcome of oral challenge and case history of possible hypersensitivity to hen's egg

	Atopy patch test	Skin-prick test	Histamine release	Specific IgE
Sensitivity	40	88	71	75
Specificity	99	99	96	89
Positive predictive value	39	59	22	10
Negative predictive value	99	99	99	99

Source: Osterballe *et al.* (2004).

The outcome of the atopy patch test was scored as follows: + indicated a weak positive reaction (erythema and slight infiltration); ++ indicated a strong positive reaction (erythema, infiltration and papules); +++ indicated a very strong reaction (erythema, infiltration, papules and vesicles). A positive outcome of the atopy patch test was defined as a score of + or greater, with infiltration as the major criterion.

INTERPRETATION. In this study 455 children were examined for atopic dermatitis and food hypersensitivity. Atopic dermatitis was confirmed in 74 (16.3%) children. Of these children, ten were suspected to have food hypersensitivity and this was confirmed in five of them (6.8%). Among those without atopic dermatitis ($n = 381$, 83.7%), twelve were suspected to have food hypersensitivity, which was subsequently confirmed in six (1.6%). The frequency of food hypersensitivity confirmed by oral challenges was 1.6% to hen's egg and 0.6 to cow's milk. No hypersensitivity to cow's milk or hen's egg was predicted by the atopy patch test alone. The performance characteristics of the different diagnostic tests are shown in Tables 7.2 and 7.3.

Comment

The information from this study has contradicted the earlier findings by Roehr *et al.* |**10**|, who reported that a combination of the atopy patch test and specific IgE could predict clinical reactivity with more than 95% certainty, and in fact a positive

Table 7.3 Cow's milk: the diagnostic value (%) of the atopy patch test, skin-prick test, histamine release and specific IgE compared with the outcome of oral challenge and case history of possible hypersensitivity to cow's milk

	Atopy patch test	Skin-prick test	Histamine release	Specific IgE
Sensitivity	0	67	67	50
Specificity	99	100	94	98
Positive predictive value	0	45	6	14
Negative predictive value	99	99	99	99

Source: Osterballe *et al.* (2004).

predictive value of 100% was reported for the atopy patch test when the specific IgE was above 17.5 kU/l. However, the study by Roehr *et al.* was conducted in a selected group of children with atopic dermatitis. In this select population it is likely that the prevalence of food hypersensitivity is quite high and the positive predictive value is a measure that is sensitive to prevalence. It is therefore not surprising that in an unselected group of children such as the cohort in this paper the positive predictive value was 39% for hen's egg. From the evidence generated from the study under review, the atopy patch test cannot be recommended in the diagnosis of food hypersensitivity in children.

Operational issues on food challenges

The DBPFC is considered to be the gold standard in the diagnosis of food hypersensitivity; i.e. it is regarded as the most specific and sensitive test to diagnose food hypersensitivity. Having said this, there are no standardized methods for carrying out the DBPCFC. Procedures vary widely, challenge materials differ and results of different studies cannot be compared easily. The next three studies reviewed in this chapter have addressed some interesting areas with regard to the operation of food challenges.

Development and validation of challenge materials for double-blind, placebo-controlled food challenges in children

Vlieg-Boerstra BJ, Bijleveld CMA, van der Heide S, *et al.* *J Allergy Clin Immunol* 2004; **113**: 341–6

BACKGROUND. The challenge materials used at different centres vary considerably. Some centres use freeze-dried foods, some use concentrated foods masked in other foods or capsules, and some use freshly prepared foods. This study aimed to develop and validate a number of recipes for DBPCFCs in children. Common allergenic foods, cow's milk, egg, soy, peanut, hazelnut and wheat were used where possible in their usual edible form. For each allergenic food an active recipe and a placebo test recipe was developed. All recipes met a series of criteria which included acceptable taste, optimal matrix ingredients, allowance of a challenge dose high enough to elicit allergic reactions, and good matching of sensory properties of placebo and active test food recipes. A group of volunteers and a panel of professional tasters participated in the validation study. Validation was conducted on the basis of sensory tests for difference by using the triangle test and the paired comparison test. Recipes were considered to be validated if no statistically significant differences were found.

INTERPRETATION. Seventeen recipes were validated. All validated recipes are available in the journal's online repository. These include recipes for milk, egg, soy, peanut, hazelnut and wheat. For all recipes, except for peanut and hazelnut, the maximum doses masked were 1.75 g of food protein. However, for peanut and hazelnut only 0.35 g of the protein could be masked.

Comment

For a DBPCFC to work effectively it is essential to blind the challenge food. Yet the blinding of challenge materials is rarely tested formally. This study used fresh foods in their recipes; these are readily available and the recipes can be replicated in future studies.

In this rigorously executed study, only 17 of the 27 recipes developed were validated and ten were identified correctly as placebo or active by the professional panel of testers. The volunteer panel could not decode any of the 27 recipes. It could be argued that if healthy volunteers cannot decode the challenge material, it is likely that the patient with suspected food hypersensitivity cannot either. However, many individuals with food hypersensitivity have highly sensitive tasting ability, particularly to the food implicated in their hypersensitivity, and therefore good masking will be essential. Many previous studies have reported using challenge doses that have been much higher than those used in the present study. This raises the question of the degree of blindness of the DBPCFCs reported in the literature.

Sensory testing of recipes masking peanut or hazelnut for double-blind placebo-controlled food challenges

Ronteltap A, van Schaik J, Wensing M, Rynia FJ, Knulst AC, de Vries JHM. *Allergy* 2004; **59**: 457–60

BACKGROUND. This study used the method of paired comparisons and tested the suitability of peanut and hazelnut recipes. Two recipes, each with three concentrations of peanut or hazelnut, were used. The recipe for peanut consisted of mashed potatoes with 2.7, 8.9 or 26.8 mg of peanut flour (equivalent to 0.7, 2.3 and 6.8 mg of peanut protein in a 15 g portion of the recipe). The recipe for hazelnut consisted of oatmeal porridge, and a 15 g portion of the food contained 11.6, 39 or 117 mg of hazelnut protein. Recipes were offered together with a placebo and were evaluated on sensory features by 81 volunteers.

INTERPRETATION. The volunteers did not discriminate between foods with any of the three doses of peanuts and the placebo. However, they clearly discriminated between the foods with hazelnut and their placebos.

Comment

Unlike the study by Vlieg-Boerstra *et al.* described earlier, this study used healthy volunteers as opposed to professional testers and it is not clear whether the findings would be the same with skilled testers. Nevertheless, the sensory testing approach (using the paired comparison method) put forward by this group can easily be used by clinicians for DBPCFCs.

Risk of oral food challenges

Perry TT, Matsui EC, Conover-Walker MK, Wood RA. *J Allergy Clin Immunol* 2004; **114**: 1164–8

BACKGROUND. Oral food challenges pose significant risks to patients and can result in symptoms ranging from mild cutaneous to systemic and potentially life-threatening reactions. This study addressed the risk and severity of reactions associated with oral food challenges in a group of highly atopic patients undergoing open oral food challenges to milk, egg, peanut, soy and/or wheat at a specialist centre. The study was conducted by retrospectively reviewing the notes of 253 patients who had positive food challenge results during a 7-year period.

INTERPRETATION. Of the 253 patients with a positive food challenge result, 197 had a cutaneous reaction, 108 gastrointestinal, 66 oral, 67 lower respiratory and 62 upper respiratory reactions. Patients with a positive peanut challenge result were more likely to have oral (($P \leq 0.01$) and upper respiratory symptoms ($P \leq 0.01$) compared with patients with a positive challenge result for other foods. All patients with a positive wheat challenge had skin symptoms (($P = 0.03$). There were no statistically significant trends for lower respiratory or gastrointestinal symptoms for any of the foods. Of the reactions observed, 39% were mild, 33% were moderate and 28% were severe. Antihistamines were the most common treatment; 77% of those with a positive challenge received antihistamines. Eleven per cent received epinephrine, 6% received steroids and 4% received albuterol.

Comment

Many families and patients with suspected food hypersensitivity are reluctant to undergo food challenges because of the risk of adverse reactions. It is important for clinicians performing these challenges to be able to quantify and communicate these potential risks to the patient. The most life-threatening symptoms of an allergic reaction to food are cardiovascular and respiratory reactions. It was therefore reassuring that this retrospective review of over 200 positive challenges did not find evidence of any cardiovascular symptoms and only 26% of patients presented with lower respiratory symptoms. From a practical point of view, one of the interesting findings of this study was that cumulative exposure did not increase the reaction severity. In conclusion, the results of this study may allow clinicians and patients to make more informed decisions about the risks and benefits of food challenges. The study showed that food challenges can be performed safely and that symptoms of reactions experienced during challenges are reversible with prompt treatment and termination of the challenge at the earliest dose eliciting symptoms.

Prediction of tolerance to food allergens

Determination of food specific IgE levels over time can predict the development of tolerance in cow's milk and hen's egg allergy

Shek LPC, Soderstorm L, Ahlstedt S, Beyer K, Sampson HA. *J Allergy Clin Immunol* 2004; **114**: 387–91

BACKGROUND. Many young children with food hypersensitivity outgrow it and develop tolerance within the first 3–5 years of life [11]. By and large, milk and egg are the most common allergens for children under 3 years of age. Although we know that there is a high likelihood that many will outgrow their allergy, there are no robust indices that can predict when and in whom this occurs. This study attempted to address this systematically by prospectively following a group of children with milk and egg allergy (*n* = 88 and 49, respectively). Children were divided into two groups: those with at least two positive DBPCFCs, representing those who remained allergic, and those with an initial positive DBPCFC followed by a negative one, representing those who had become tolerant. Challenges were performed yearly for up to 10 years or until a final clinical decision could be made to establish the child as being either tolerant or having persistent allergy. Serum samples were obtained at the time of challenges and were stored. These samples were analysed retrospectively for specific IgE (sIgE) to cow's milk and hen's egg. Logistic regression was used to evaluate the relationship between tolerance and sIgE levels over a period of time. The logistic model was applied separately for egg and milk.

INTERPRETATION. Twenty-eight (32%) children had become tolerant to hen's egg and 16 (33%) had become tolerant to milk. The sIgE at the first challenge (i.e. at diagnosis) was significantly less in the 'tolerant' group than in the 'persistent' group for egg allergy, and a similar trend was seen for milk allergy (P<0.001 and P = 0.06 respectively). When the logistic model was applied the researchers found that for both egg and milk there was a significant relationship between the decrease in sIgE levels and the probability of developing tolerance (P = 0.0014 and P = 0.0175 respectively). For egg there was an influence of the time between the first and last challenge (P = 0.06), but this was not the case for milk. Stratification into two age groups—those below 4 years of age and those above 4 years of age at the time of the first challenge—had an effect: the younger age group were more likely to develop clinical tolerance in relation to the rate of decrease in serum IgE. Using the logistic model, the researchers developed estimates for the probability of a child becoming tolerant to milk and egg, based on serum IgE levels and time (Fig. 7.4).

Comment

One of the main strengths of this study was that the cases of milk and egg allergy were defined appropriately and all the initial diagnoses were based on the DBPCFC,

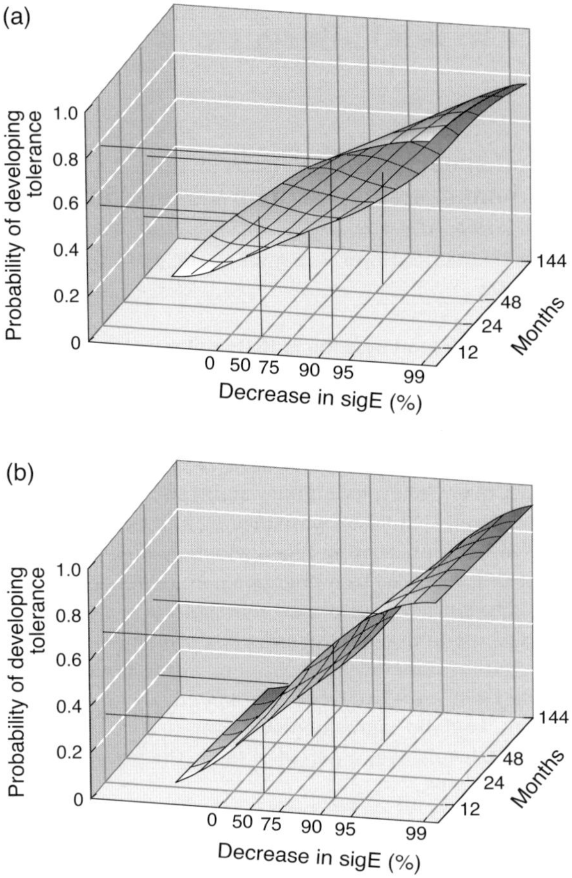

Fig. 7.4 The relationship between developing tolerance and the relative change in specific IgE antibody concentration and time for (a) hen's egg and age below 4 years and (b) cow's milk and age below 4 years at challenge. Source: Shek *et al.* (2004).

which eliminates the problem of uncertain diagnosis. In addition, the investigators included the interval between challenges in their statistical model, which allowed them to standardize their estimates to a 12-month period. The proposed model is very useful in identifying those in whom tolerance is likely to develop, and in practice it can be used to time challenges in allergic patients. Having said this, it is important to realize that these researchers investigated the predictive role of IgE in patients with IgE-mediated milk and egg allergy. A significant proportion of patients with milk allergy have non-IgE-mediated reactions and this model will be inappropriate for them. In addition, many of the children in this study had atopic dermatitis and thus constituted a population in which IgE levels are greater than in patients without atopic dermatitis. Additional studies will be needed to see if the model can be applied to patients without atopic dermatitis. This, however, may be logistically difficult to do as most infants with cow's milk and hen's egg allergy have atopic dermatitis.

Cow's milk-specific immunoglobulin E levels as predictors of clinical reactivity in the follow-up of the cow's milk allergy infants

Garcia-Ara MC, Boyano-Martinez MT, Diaz-Pena JM, Martin-Munoz MF, Martin-Esteban M. *Clin Exp Allergy* 2004; **34**: 866–70

BACKGROUND. This study addressed a similar area, and confirms the importance of finding appropriate methods that avoid unnecessary food challenges, which are costly and impose a greater burden on the patient in terms of time and convenience. In this study, 66 infants (age range 1–11 months, 31 males) with cow's milk allergy were followed up prospectively and periodic assessment was carried out every 6 months until they were 2 years old and then annually until tolerance was achieved or until the last follow-up in which tolerance had not been achieved. The follow-period ranged from 9 to 99 months (mean of 32.9 months). At each follow-up assessment, the skin-prick test was performed and sIgE to cow's milk and its protein was measured. In addition, the patients underwent open challenges to verify whether tolerance had been achieved.

INTERPRETATION. During the study time, 45 of 66 infants (68%) became tolerant. The mean age of the group who developed tolerance was 24.7 months. Those with persistent cow's milk allergy had a mean age of 61.7 months at the last follow-up. Fifteen patients had developed tolerance by their first follow-up assessment (age range 13–18 months) and a further ten had developed tolerance by their second assessment (age range 19–24 months). Eighteen had developed tolerance at the third assessment (age range 25–36 months) and two additional patients had outgrown their cow's milk allergy at the fourth assessment. The remaining patients ($n = 21$) did not develop tolerance in the remaining follow-up period. The medians of sIgE to milk and its proteins among the tolerant group were significantly lower for both the initial assessment and the final follow-up compared with medians in those with persistent cow's milk allergy. The sIgE level, which was a predictor of clinical reactivity (i.e. positive predictive value was ≥90%), was directly associated with the age of infants. The authors calculated that for cow's milk the cut-off value of sIgE that provided a 90% positive predictive value was 1.5 kU/l in the age range 13–18 months, 6 kU/l in the age range 19–24 months and 14 kU/l in the third year of life. The same calculations were carried out to establish the cut-off values for individual milk proteins.

Comment

There are a number of issues which need to be taken into consideration with this paper. The main point relates to the diagnostic criteria used to define cow's milk allergy. The children in the study had a clinical history of cow's milk allergy which was confirmed by the skin-prick test, sIgE measurement and open challenge with cow's milk. Challenges were not carried out in eight children on account of severe symptoms. Unlike the study by Shek *et al.*, this study did not involve any of the children undergoing double-blind placebo-controlled challenges. The other issue is that at follow-up assessment food challenges were not conducted if the parents reported that the child had had a clinical reaction within the last 3 months due to accidental exposure. In fact, nine children did not undergo challenges at any of the follow-up assessments. However, the researchers argue that in most cases the reactions experienced during these accidental exposures were immediate cutaneous symptoms. The researchers report that they carried out the skin-prick test at diagnosis and at the follow-ups; however, it is disappointing that these data are not presented. The skin-prick test data could have shed light on the allergic status of the children. One needs to be aware of these shortcomings in taking this study into account. In addition, it is important to appreciate changes in predictive values with changes prevalent of the condition, and the results can be applied to other populations in which the prevalence of milk allergy is different from that found in Spain.

Prediction of the development of tolerance to milk in children with cow's milk hypersensitivity

Vanto T, Helppila S, Juntunen-Backman K, *et al. J Pedatr* 2004; **144**: 218–22

BACKGROUND. This article is the third study published in 2004 that has addressed predictive indicators of tolerance to milk in cow's milk hypersensitivity. The children who participated in this Finnish study were participating in a clinical trial of infant feeding in which they were randomized to receive either a soy-based or a whey-based, extensively hydrolysed formula as a supplement to breast-feeding when needed. A total of 162 children with cow's milk hypersensitivity diagnosed before 12 months of age were followed up to 4 years of age. It is important to note that, unlike the children in the previous studies in this section, the children in this study included those with both immediate (*n* = 95) and delayed (*n* = 67) reactions to milk. Among the immediate reactors, 66% had an IgE-mediated reaction while among the delayed reactors only 31% had an IgE-mediated reaction. Cow's milk hypersensitivity was diagnosed by means of DBPCFC, except in four infants with a history of anaphylactic reactions, who also had a positive skin-prick test result and elevated sIgE to cow's milk. The challenges were designed such that both immediate and delayed reactions were detected. Children were reviewed at 2, 3 and 4 years of age, when sIgE measurements, skin-prick tests and DBPCFCs were carried out.

INTERPRETATION. Forty-four per cent of the children had developed tolerance by 2 years of age, 69% by 3 years of age and 77% by 4 years of age. The development of tolerance did not differ between the groups who were supplemented with soy- or whey-based, extensively hydrolysed infant formulae. Children with delayed reactions developed tolerance faster than those with immediate reactions by 2, 3 and 4 years of age (64, 92 and 96% respectively vs 31, 53 and 63%). A wheal size of less than 5 mm in the skin-prick test correctly identified 83% of 124 infants who developed tolerance by 4 years of age, and a wheal size of at least 5 mm in the skin-prick test correctly identified 71% of 39 infants with persistent cow's milk hypersensitivity. Milk sIgE below 2 kU/l correctly identified 82% of infants who developed tolerance and sIgE of at least 2 kU/l correctly identified 71% of infants with persistent cow's milk hypersensitivity.

Comment

This study confirms earlier studies [**11,12**], which reported that those with IgE-mediated, often immediate reactions were shown to have more persistent cow's milk hypersensitivity than those with non-IgE-mediated, often delayed reactions. The researchers reported that the predictive value of the skin-prick test response to cow's milk was similar to that of milk-specific IgE and that combining the two did not improve the predictive value. This study adds to the consistency of the evidence reported in the previous two studies discussed here, which show that sIgE and the skin-prick test are useful prognostic indicators of the development of tolerance to cow's milk.

Conclusion

This chapter has concentrated on key published findings in the area of food hypersensitivity over the last 12–18 months. There is no remaining doubt that the frequency of perception of food hypersensitivity far exceeds the frequency of objectively assessed food hypersensitivity. All three studies in this chapter that focused on this area reported large discrepancies between perceived and proven food hypersensitivity. The reason for this high rate of perception of food hypersensitivity is not known at present. One could postulate that this might be due to an increased awareness of food hypersensitivity accentuated by the popular media coverage. Clearly, this area needs to be explored further as the false perception could have an impact on the individual's life and it could be resource-intensive in terms of diagnostic procedures, consultation time, etc.

These three studies also highlight the differences between three European countries in terms of the foods implicated in food hypersensitivity.

In terms of objective outcome measures, the DBPCFC remains the gold standard in the diagnosis of food hypersensitivity. What is extremely promising and clinically relevant is the generation of predicting models that could allow clinicians to predict the development of tolerance using sIgE measurements. A better understanding of the predictive information that can be obtained from the results of sIgE measurements and skin-prick tests and how these can be used in clinical settings are excellent opportunities for patients and clinicians and can aid the clinical decision-making processes.

References

1. Johansson SG, Bieber T, Dahl R, Friedmann PS, Lanier BQ, Lockey RF, Motala C, Ortega Martell JA, Platts-Mills TA, Ring J, Thien F, Van Cauwenberge P, Williams HC. Revised nomenclature for allergy for global use: report of the Nomenclature Review Committee of the World Allergy Organization, October 2003. *J Allergy Clin Immunol* 2004; **113**: 832–6.
2. Dreborg S, Frew A (eds). Position paper: allergen standardization and skin tests. *Allergy* 1993; **47**(Suppl 14): 48–82.
3. Sampson HA. Utility of food-specific IgE concentrations in predicting symptomatic food allergy. *J Allergy Clin Immunol* 2001; **107**: 891–6.
4. Roehr C, Reibel S, Ziegert M, Sommerfeld C, Wahn U, Niggeman B. Atopy patch test together with level of specific IgE reduces the need for oral food challenges in children with atopic dermatitis. *J Allergy Clin Immunol* 2001; **107**: 548–53.
5. Sicherer SH. Food allergy: when and how to perform oral food challenges. *Pediatr Allergy Immunol* 1999; **10**: 226–34.
6. Miles S, Fordham R, Mills C, Valovirta E, Mugford M. A framework for measuring costs to society of IgE-mediated food allergy. *Allergy* 2005; **60**: 996–1003.
7. Pumphrey RS. Lessons for management of anaphylaxis from a study of fatal reactions. *Clin Exp Allergy* 2000; **30**: 1144–50.
8. Sampson HA, Ho DG. Relationship between food-specific IgE concentrations and the risk of positive food challenges in children and adolescents. *J Allergy Clin Immunol* 1997; **100**: 444–51.
9. Stromberg L. Diagnostic accuracy of the atopy patch test and the skin-prick test for the diagnosis of food allergy in young children with atopic eczema/dermatitis syndrome. *Acta Paediatr* 2002; **91**: 1044–9.
10. Roehr CC, Reibel S, Ziegert M, Sommerfeld C, Wahn U, Niggemann B. Atopy patch tests, together with determination of specific IgE levels, reduce the need for oral food challenges in children with atopic dermatitis. *J Allergy Clin Immunol* 2001; **107**: 548–53.
11. Host A, Halken S, Jacobson HP, Christensen AE, Herskind AM, Plesner K. Clinical course of cow's milk protein allergy/intolerance and atopic disease in childhood. *Pediatr Allergy Immunol* 2003; **13**(Suppl 15): 23–8.
12. James JM, Sampson HA. Immunologic changes associated with the development of tolerance in children with cow milk allergy. *J Pediatr* 1992; **121**: 371–7.

8

Drug allergy

JOHN MUCKLOW

Introduction

The large majority of adverse reactions to medicines are dose-related, predictable from knowledge of the responsible agent's pharmacology, and largely avoidable. Allergic reactions are usually unpredictable, and account for no more than about 10% of adverse reactions. In the experience of the individual prescriber, they are uncommon and seldom severe.

This chapter presents a selection of recent publications on drug allergy and illustrates the variety of approaches to the investigation, prevention and management of this problem.

Allergic reactions to medicines are classified according to the nature of the immunological mechanism involved, insofar as this is understood, based on the Gell and Coombs system [1]. Table 8.1 illustrates the categories and likely mechanisms, describes the clinical manifestations of each, and gives some examples of medicines that behave in this way [2]. It will be obvious from Table 8.1 that penicillins can result in all types of reaction that involve immunological mechanisms, including immunoglobulin (Ig) E-mediated hypersensitivity, IgG-mediated haemolysis, antigen-antibody complex-mediated serum sickness, T-cell-mediated contact dermatitis and antibody-mediated cytolysis [3]. However, individuals who have experienced an allergic reaction to a penicillin, and who react following re-exposure, tend to react in a stereotypical way.

The risk of penicillin allergy following re-exposure

Suspected drug allergy is not easy to investigate. In the UK, few centres have the necessary facilities and expertise, the evidence base of the available diagnostic tests is not robust, and their interpretation is not straightforward [4]. This has led many clinicians increasingly to rely on the patient's recollection of previous response to individual medicines when anticipating the likely tolerability of future exposure. There is controversy about the need to perform skin testing. It is acknowledged that no more than 10–20% of patients with a history of penicillin allergy react positively to skin tests, and the likelihood of a positive reaction diminishes with time after the

© Atlas Medical Publishing Ltd

Table 8.1 Classification of allergic reactions to medicines

Reaction type	Mechanism	Clinical characteristics	Examples
Type 1 (immediate)	IgE antibodies fixed to mast cells, which release chemical mediators (e.g. histamine, leukotrienes) after exposure to circulating antigen	Urticaria, angio-oedema, wheezing, hypotension, nausea, vomiting, abdominal pain, diarrhoea	Beta-lactams and other antibiotics, insulin, enzymes, antisera, monoclonal antibodies, protamine, heparin
Type 2 (cytotoxic)	IgG, IgM, IgA antibodies to cell-bound antigens (drug or metabolite) borne by erythrocytes, leucocytes and platelets	Haemolytic anaemia	Beta-lactams, quinidine, methyldopa
		Granulocytopenia,	Phenothiazines, thiouracils, sulphonamides, anticonvulsants
		Thrombocytopenia	Quinine, quinidine, paracetamol, sulphonamides, gold, propylthiouracil
Type 3 (immune complex)	Circulating immune complexes and complement activation 1–3 weeks after exposure	Fever, urticaria, arthralgia, lymphadenopathy	Beta-lactams, sulphonamides, phenytoin, streptomycin
Type 4 (delayed)	T cell mediated 8–120 h after subsequent exposure	Skin erythema, blistering, pruritus	Penicillin, local anaesthetics, antihistamines, neomycin, preservatives, excipients (e.g. parabens, lanolin)
Morbilliform	T cell mediated 4–10 days after start of exposure (may occur up to 2 weeks after therapy ceases)	Maculopapular exanthema, becoming confluent, pruritus, low-grade fever (may progress to erythroderma and exfoliation	Penicillins, sulphonamides, phenytoin, NSAIDs
Erythema multiforme	T cell mediated 1–2 weeks after exposure	Distinctive cutaneous target lesions, spreading from hands and feet	Beta-lactams, sulphonamides, NSAIDs, phenytoin, phenothiazines, barbiturates, imidazoles, quinolones, allopurinol
Stevens–Johnson syndrome		Erythema multiforme + bullous lesions affecting skin and mucous membranes, constitutional symptoms and high fever	

Table 8.1 *Continued*

Reaction type	Mechanism characteristics	Clinical	Examples
Toxic epidermal necrolysis		Stevens–Johnson syndrome + skin detachment	
Anaphylactoid	Direct release of chemical mediators from mast cells and basophils	Pruritus, urticaria, angio-oedema, bronchospasm, hypotension	Opioids, aspirin, radiocontrast agents

Source: Volcheck *et al.* (2004) [2].

initial event. However, the risk of an allergic reaction to penicillin following re-exposure is greater if the skin test is positive (about 50%) than if it is negative (3–4%). If skin tests can be performed reliably and safely, these figures would seem to support their wider use. Investigators in the USA have shown that skin tests can be performed safely in selected patients. In one large series, having excluded those with reactions suggesting hepatitis, nephritis, exfoliative dermatitis, Stevens–Johnson syndrome or toxic epidermal necrolysis, only 0.12% of patients had a systemic reaction following skin testing, although the incidence was higher among those whose skin test was positive (2.3%) [5].

Represcription of penicillin after allergic-like events

Apter AJ, Kinman JL, Bilker WB, *et al. J Allergy Clin Immunol* 2004; **113**: 764–70

BACKGROUND. It is said that whereas the overall frequency of allergic reactions to beta-lactam antibiotics is 2% per course [6], the frequency of reactions after re-exposure increases to 60%. These data are estimates obtained from studies in small series of hospital inpatients and may not reflect the true incidence of reactions in outpatients, for whom the majority of antibiotic courses are prescribed. In this retrospective cohort study (relating to patients treated between 1987 and 2001), the authors used data obtained from the UK General Practice Research Database (GPRD), which includes primary care medical records as well as prescriptions from 687 general practitioner practices throughout England and Wales, providing healthcare to 6% of the population.

INTERPRETATION. At least one prescription for penicillin was given to 3 375 162 patients. Of 6212 (0.18%) patients who experienced an event suggesting an allergic (hypersensitivity) reaction within 30 days of the initial prescription, 48.5% were given a second prescription subsequently (after at least 60 days), compared with 59.8% of those who did not experience such an event (risk ratio 0.81; 95% confidence interval [CI] 0.79–0.83). Of 2 017 957 patients who took two or more prescriptions for penicillin (the reference cohort), 3014 (0.15%) experienced a hypersensitivity-like event after the first prescription, and 57 (1.89%) had another event after the second prescription (Fig. 8.1). The unadjusted odds ratio of a hypersensitivity-like event after the second prescription for those who experienced such an event after the first prescription, compared with those who had no initial event, was 11.2 (95% CI 8.6–14.6). Adjustment for a prior history of similar events reduced the odds ratio to 9.9 (95% CI 9.8–10.0). However, the absolute difference in the incidence of events was small (1.72%) (Table 8.2).

Comment

This was a comprehensive study encompassing a huge amount of data. Although the authors admit that they might have overlooked events relating to more trivial adverse reactions, it is unlikely that any serious events went unrecorded and thereby escaped their attention.

Perhaps the most striking observation was that almost half of the patients experiencing an allergic-like event after a prescription of penicillin were given a further dose. The most common event recorded (75%) was urticaria, but the database included reports of erythema multiforme, angio-oedema, laryngospasm, anaphylaxis and toxic epidermal necrolysis. Although three-quarters of the prescriptions were for amoxicillin, the nature of the events recorded indicate that the majority of reactions were IgE-mediated, rather than the late pseudo-allergic

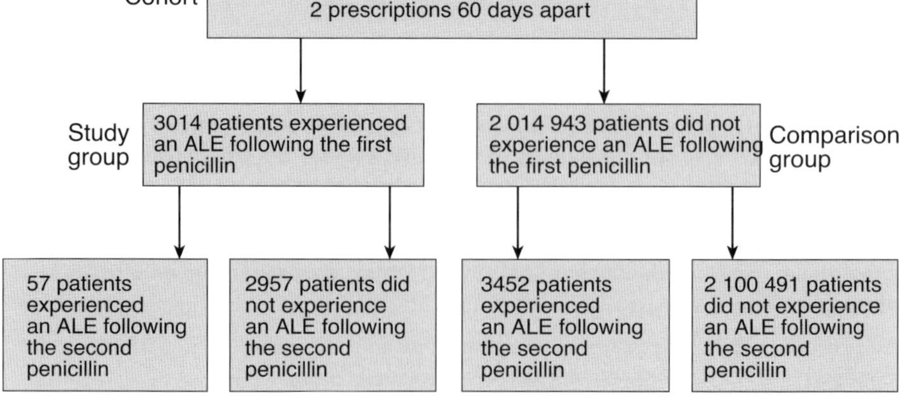

Fig. 8.1 Schematic representation of the study protocol. Source: Apter *et al.* (2004).

Table 8.2 Description of the allergic-like event following the first and second penicillin prescriptions

Event type	First penicillin *n* (%)	Second penicillin *n* (%)
Anaphylaxis	16 (0.53)	32 (0.91)
Angio-oedema	106 (3.52)	131 (3.73)
Laryngospasm	19 (0.63)	18 (0.51)
Urticaria	2275 (75.48)	2589 (73.78)
Erythema multiforme	237 (7.86)	220 (6.27)
Toxic epidermal necrolysis	6 (0.2)	11 (0.31)
Dermatitis due to an ingested drug	11 (0.36)	11 (0.31)
Adverse drug reaction to an ingested drug	344 (11.41)	497 (14.16)
Total	3014	3509

Source: Apter *et al.* (2004).

reaction characteristic of exposure to amoxicillin. It is surprising, though reassuring, that only 1 in 53 patients who had an event after the first prescription experienced another one after the second. This suggests that immediate hypersensitivity occurs less frequently among outpatients exposed to repeated doses of penicillin than was previously thought. Moreover, the overall incidence of anaphylaxis (8–16 per million prescriptions) was also much less frequent than previously reported estimates of 100–500 per million prescriptions [6].

The role of skin testing in delayed reactions to penicillins

The use of skin tests as an aid to diagnosis in patients with suspected allergy to penicillin is usually considered in the context of IgE-mediated reactions. It is not customary to use this approach in the investigation of patients with non-immediate allergic reactions, such as maculopapular erythema and urticaria of late onset, as these reactions involve T cell mediated events. Published studies show that about half of all patients who have experienced maculopapular or erythematous reactions to aminopenicillins manifest delayed hypersensitivity in response to patch testing or intradermal tests where reading is delayed [5].

Skin test evaluation in non-immediate allergic reactions to penicillins

Torres M-J, Sánchez-Sabaté E, Álvarez J, *et al.* *Allergy* 2004; **59**: 219–24

BACKGROUND. This study compared the diagnostic value of intradermal tests and patch tests in 20 patients with non-immediate reactions to penicillin (none had IgE

antibodies to benzylpenicillin or amoxicillin detectable using a commercial RAST [radioallergosorbent test] method), using 30 patients tolerant to penicillin as controls. Intradermal tests assessed reactivity to injection of major and minor determinants of benzylpenicillin, amoxicillin and ampicillin. Patch testing involved the same hapten solutions used for intradermal testing, either embedded in a patch disk or mixed with petrolatum.

Interpretation. Among the 20 patients investigated, six had experienced desquamative exanthema, three maculopapular erythema and eleven urticaria (with or without angio-oedema) occurring at least 4 h after drug administration. The clinical characteristics of the patients are shown in Table 8.3. The mean interval between the clinical event and the skin test was 8 years (range 1 month to 30 years). There were no reactions to any drug in the control patients. No patient reacted to intradermal injection of the major or minor determinants of benzylpenicillin. Reactions to intradermal injection of ampicillin and amoxicillin occurred in all 20 patients, and comprised indurated erythema (varying in size between 7 × 6 mm and 10 × 16 mm). In four patients, these were accompanied by small vesicles (three cases) or a bulla (one case). All changes appeared between 24 and 96 h after injection (Table 8.4). Eighteen of the 20 patients reacted positively (and similarly) to both patch tests. Biopsies of the abnormal skin

Table 8.3 Clinical characteristics of the patients included in the study

						Interval
ID	**Age**	**Sex**	**Drug**	**Reaction**	**Drug reaction (h)**	**Reaction study (years)**
1	30	M	Ampicillin	DE	48	30
2	47	F	Amoxicillin	DE	6	7
3	72	F	Amoxicillin	MPE	48	20
4	64	M	Ampicillin	DE	168	15
5	69	F	Benzylpenicillin	Urticaria	8	6
6	67	M	Amoxicillin	DE	48	0.08
7	58	F	Amoxicillin	Urticaria	21	5
8	49	F	Benzylpenicillin	Urticaria	12	10
9	57	F	Amoxicillin	MPE	8	0.08
10	43	F	Ampicillin	Urticaria	4	15
11	41	F	Ampicillin	Urticaria	24	2
12	43	M	Amoxicillin	Urticaria	48	3
13	42	F	Amoxicillin	Urti/Angio	32	0.08
14	37	M	Amoxicillin	DE	144	0.5
15	50	F	Amoxicillin	Urticaria	24	0.5
16	60	F	Ampicillin	Urticaria	48	3
17	40	F	Ampicillin	Urticaria	4	3
18	52	F	Benzylpenicillin	Urti/angio	48	20
19	62	M	Benzylpenicillin	MPE	12	10
20	53	F	Amoxicillin	DE	24	10

DE, desquamative exanthema; MPE, maculopapular erythema; Urti/angio, urticaria and angio-oedema.
Source: Torres *et al.* (2004).

Table 8.4 Results of intradermal and patch testing and the optimal times in the study patients

	Intradermal tests		Patch tests			
			Saline		Petrolatum	
Patient	**Amoxicillin**	**Ampicillin**	**Amoxicillin**	**Ampicillin**	**Amoxicillin**	**Ampicillin**
1	8 × 9 (48 h)	10 × 9 (48 h)	+ 48 h	+ 48 h	+ 48 h	+ 48 h
2	10 × 16 (24 h)	9 × 16 (24 h)	+++ 48 h	+++ 48 h	+++ 48 h	+++ 48 h
3	7 × 6 (48 h)	8 × 7 (48 h)	+ 48 h	+ 48 h	+ 48 h	+ 48 h
4	10 × 12 (48 h)	9 × 7 (48 h)	++ 48 h	++ 48 h	++ 48 h	++ 48 h
5	8 × 7 (48 h)	10 × 12 (48 h)	++ 48 h	++ 48 h	++ 48 h	++ 48 h
6	7 × 6 (48 h)	8 × 9 (48 h)	+ 48 h	+ 48 h	+ 48 h	+ 48 h
7	10 × 12 (48 h)	10 × 14 (48 h)	++ 48 h	++ 48 h	++ 48 h	++ 48 h
8	8 × 9 (48 h)	7 × 6 (48 h)	++ 48 h	++ 48 h	++ 48 h	++ 48 h
9	10 × 15 (48 h)	10 × 16 (48 h)	+++ 48 h	+++ 48 h	+++ 48 h	+++ 48 h
10	7 × 7 (24 h)	8 × 9 (24 h)	–	–	–	–
11	7 × 6 (48 h)	10 × 12 (48 h)	+ 48 h	+ 48 h	+ 48 h	+ 48 h
12	8 × 12 (96 h)	10 × 12 (96 h)	++ 240 h	++ 240 h	++ 240 h	++ 240 h
13	8 × 10 (48 h)	12 × 14 (48 h)	++ 48 h	++ 48 h	++ 48 h	++ 48 h
14	7 × 8 (48 h)	8 × 9 (48 h)	++ 48 h	++ 48 h	++ 48 h	++ 48 h
15	9 × 13 (96 h)	8 × 14 (96 h)	++ 96 h	++ 96 h	++ 96 h	++ 96 h
16	9 × 10 (48 h)	9 × 14 (48 h)	++ 48 h	++ 48 h	++ 48 h	++ 48 h
17	7 × 8 (24 h)	9 × 9 (24 h)	–	–	–	–
18	14 × 15 (48 h)	10 × 13 (48 h)	++ 48 h	++ 48 h	++ 48 h	++ 48 h
19	9 × 10 (48 h)	9 × 11 (48 h)	++ 96 h	++ 96 h	++ 96 h	++ 96 h
20	11 × 15 (48 h)	10 × 13 (48 h)	++ 48 h	++ 48 h	++ 48 h	++ 48 h

Tests were undertaken with amoxicillin (AX) and ampicillin (AM) at the following doses: intradermal and patch testing diluted in saline at 20 mg/ml and patch testing in petrolatum at 50% w/w.
Source: Torres *et al.* (2004).

consistently revealed a mononuclear cell infiltrate consisting largely of lymphocytes (perivascular CD4 cells and intradermal CD8 cells). The authors concluded that intradermal testing gave more consistent responses than patch testing, and that a single reading after 48 h appeared optimal.

Comment

Intradermal injections are commonly used in addition to prick tests when carrying out skin tests in patients who have experienced immediate reactions to penicillins, but the response is generally apparent within an hour. In this study, no response was apparent for at least 24 (and usually 48) h and no patient had IgE antibodies to penicillins in the blood. This diagnostic method would seem to offer a useful approach in patients who have experienced symptoms consistent with a non-immediate reaction to penicillin, in whom the role of the penicillin cannot be clearly identified because of concurrent infection or treatment with other drugs.

Cross-reactivity with other beta-lactams and related drugs

Approximately 10–15% of patients report a history of allergy to penicillin. Of these, a proportion (estimates vary, some being as high as 15%) will also react to cephalosporins, owing to their shared beta-lactam ring [5]. Whereas the beta-lactam ring of penicillin is conjugated to a five-sided thiazolidine ring, that of cephalosporins is conjugated to a six-sided sulphur-containing ring, and that of carbapenems is attached to a five-sided ring containing carbon or oxygen in place of the sulphur in penicillin. The cross-reactivity rate among patients treated with first-generation cephalosporins was relatively high, partly because these compounds also shared a side chain with benzylpenicillin, and partly because they contained trace amounts of penicillin. The risk of an IgE-mediated reaction to a third-generation cephalosporin in a patient with a history of penicillin allergy is thought to be no higher than the equivalent risk of a reaction to an unrelated antibiotic. However, enduring concern about cross-reactivity has led to the recommendation that all patients who give a history of penicillin allergy should undergo penicillin skin testing before being treated with a cephalosporin. The value of such precaution is questionable: the likelihood of a reaction to cephalosporin in a patient with a history of allergy to penicillin cannot be predicted reliably by penicillin skin tests [7,8].

Safety of cephalosporin administration to patients with histories of penicillin allergy

Daulat S, Solensky R. *J Allergy Clin Immunol* 2004; **113**: 1220–2

Background. This retrospective cohort study attempted to identify the incidence of adverse reactions to cephalosporin treatment among patients giving a history of a

non-specific or trivial reaction to penicillin with no features suggestive of immediate hypersensitivity, and who had not undergone a skin test.

INTERPRETATION. The authors identified 23 270 hospital inpatients who had been given treatment (usually parenteral) with a cephalosporin (42% first generation, 21% second generation, 37% third or fourth generation). Of these, 606 reported a history of penicillin allergy (not judged to have been severe) before starting treatment. In all, 16 patients (0.07%) experienced an adverse reaction to cephalosporin treatment, but only one (0.17%) of those who had reported a history of penicillin allergy experienced an adverse reaction (a worsening of her underlying eczema). This incidence is much lower than the previously reported cross-reactivity rates of 8–12% in patients reporting allergy to penicillin who are not skin-tested before treatment with a cephalosporin.

Comment

The outcome of the study is reassuring. The likelihood of an allergic reaction after cephalosporin treatment, in a patient who claims to be allergic to penicillin but whose history includes no features suggestive of severity, is very small. Yet many prescribers accept patients' assertions that they are allergic to penicillin without question, routinely denying them treatment with any beta-lactam. This may lead to the individual patient being treated with an antimicrobial agent that is either less effective against the organism in question or more expensive (or both). It may also mean that a more recently marketed antimicrobial agent is chosen, accelerating its wider use and hastening the development of microbial resistance to its effects. The findings of this study appear to support the use of cephalosporins in such patients, provided the risk of a reaction has been carefully assessed, and call into question the need to engage in time-consuming and expensive skin tests.

Is it safe to use carbapenems in patients with a history of allergy to penicillin?

Sodhi M, Axtell, SS, Callahan J, Shekar R. *J Antimicrob Chemother* 2004; **54**: 1155–7

BACKGROUND. Carbapenems, such as imepenem/cilastatin and meropenem, have a chemical structure similar to penicillins, and the manufacturers of these drugs warn that hypersensitivity reactions, some of which have been serious, have occurred in patients with a history of beta-lactam hypersensitivity. Estimates of the incidence of cross-reactivity, determined by skin tests, have been as high as 47%, compared with an estimated incidence of carbapenem-associated hypersensitivity in the general population of 1–3%. This study involved a retrospective review of patients treated with carbapenems in two hospitals over a 2-year period.

INTERPRETATION. The study identified 266 patients who were given at least 1 day's treatment with either imepenim/cilastatin or meropenem. Of these, 163 (61%) reported allergy to penicillin. A total of 19 patients (7.1%) experienced a hypersensitivity reaction that appeared after an average interval of 3.6–5.5 days. In 14 of these, the reaction

Table 8.5 Comparisons of patients with reported penicillin allergy and without penicillin allergy

	Patients with penicillin allergy (*n* = 163)	**Patients without penicillin allergy (*n* = 103)**
Mean age, years (range)	70.6 (32–91)	74 (39–91)
Sex, male/female (% male)	69/94 (42)	65/38 (63)
Classification of reported reaction	%	%
Rash	34.9	0
Facial swelling and/or anaphylaxis	6.1	0
Unknown	54	0
Other	4.9	0
Other antibiotic allergies		
Cephalosporins	4.3	4.9
Sulpha drugs	22	10.7
Fluoroquinolones	10.4	1.9
Macrolides	5.5	1.9
Allergic reaction to carbapenem	9.2	3.9
Maculopapular rash	6.7	2.9
Drug fever and rash	0.6	1
Facial oedema	0.6	0
Pruritus	0.6	0

Source: Sodhi *et al.* (2004).

took the form of a maculopapular rash, sometimes with additional features such as fever, pruritus or facial oedema. The incidence of reactions among those who reported allergy to penicillin (15; 9.2%) appeared higher than among those who did not (4; 3.9%), but the difference was not statistically significant ($P = 0.164$) (Table 8.5). No serious reactions were encountered, even in the patient who reported previous anaphylaxis after penicillin, and all reactions subsided shortly after the carbapenem was discontinued.

Comment

The results of this study suggest that the incidence of cross-reactivity between penicillins and carbapenems is considerably lower than previous estimates. The authors reflected on the higher incidence of reactions among those who reported allergies to other antibiotics as well as penicillin, and the likelihood that many of the patients who reported penicillin allergy were not truly allergic. Retrospective studies such as this must be interpreted with some caution owing to their dependence on the quality of documentation found in the medical records, and the authors acknowledge that a prospective study would have allowed more accurate and complete assessment of both the patient's previous reactions and the response to the carbapenem. One feature of this study, unusual in a retrospective review, was the observation that when clinical features suggestive of a reaction occurred in these patients, many of whom were being treated with more than one antimicrobial agent, only one drug was discontinued at a time, increasing the precision with which the causative agent was identified.

Apparent allergy to more than one antibiotic

Multiple antibiotic allergy syndrome

Macy E. *Immunol Allergy N Am* 2004; **24**: 533–43

BACKGROUND. Patients (and many doctors) frequently use the term 'allergy' when referring to any adverse drug reaction, even one that has no features of an IgE-mediated response. However, IgE-mediated allergy explains only about 10% of all adverse reactions to antibiotics. Patients who have experienced unexplained symptoms during treatment with two or more antibiotics are often said to have 'multiple antibiotic allergy'; using this definition, the description can be applied to one patient in every 22. Yet if one applies the strict definition, which requires documented evidence (positive skin test or detection of specific IgE) of reactivity to two unrelated antibiotics, the syndrome is rare. Setting semantic issues aside, this review addressed the more interesting question of whether a patient who experiences a documented allergy to one antibiotic is more likely to experience an allergic reaction to another, unrelated to the first.

INTERPRETATION. The review found that the investigation of multiple antibiotic allergies was complicated by several confounding factors. First, well-validated widely used tests for clinically significant IgE directed against antibiotics other than penicillins do not exist. Second, reactions are more common in HIV-infected patients and those with chronic urticaria, cystic fibrosis, or a concurrent viral infection. Third, reactions are more likely to occur after parenteral than oral administration. Fourth, a patient's readiness to report a suspected adverse reaction to a drug is influenced by the individual's psychological make-up. The review found no convincing evidence that patients with histories of multiple antibiotic allergies produce IgE directed against unrelated antibiotics. Penicillin skin tests can be useful in selected individuals but do not predict reactivity to drugs other than penicillins. Management should focus on careful documentation of the clinical history, which allows the development of a patient-specific plan stating which antibiotics should be used preferentially and which should be avoided (Table 8.6). In difficult cases, such as cystic fibrosis or HIV infection, it may be appropriate to consider the use of pre-medication, oral tolerance testing or desensitization.

Comment

This is an extremely sensible approach to a complex and poorly understood problem. It is very important to adopt a rigorous approach to patients who claim to be allergic to multiple antibiotics, who can become so obsessed with the risk of

Table 8.6 Essential elements of an effective multiple antibiotic allergy consultation

Collect the following data for each antibiotic associated with an adverse reaction:

- type of infection last used for
- prior exposures without reaction
- prior exposures with reaction
- dose with last reaction
- route of administration with last reaction
- number of doses taken before onset of last reaction
- number of doses taken after onset of last reaction
- type of adverse reaction
- duration of adverse reaction symptoms
- treatment given for adverse reaction symptoms
- permanent sequelae
- diagnostic tests obtained

Collect the following data for each antibiotic tolerated:

- type of infection last used for
- dose with last exposure
- route of administration with last exposure
- prior exposures without reaction

Other important historical factors

- list all other drugs associated with adverse reactions and dates of last exposure
- document the existence, if any, of the following risk factors: chronic urticaria, dermographism, NSAID intolerance, liver disease, renal dysfunction, immune deficiency, HIV, cystic fibrosis

Elements of an effective treatment plan

- antibiotic OK to use if clinically indicated
- antibiotic should be avoided
- antibiotic can be used with pre-treatment (provide pre-treatment plan)
- antibiotic can be used if a test dose tolerated (provide test dose plan)
- antibiotic can only be used with prior desensitization (provide desensitization plan)

NSAID, non-steroidal anti-inflammatory drug.
Source: Macy (2004).

future exposure that they are willing to deny themselves effective, or even life-saving treatment. The sooner the nettle is grasped the better, before the endorsement of any assumptions by ill-informed health professionals, which can make the patient's conviction difficult to shake. The careful differentiation of symptoms consistent with allergy from those that represent intolerance is the first step, followed if necessary by further objective tests, arriving eventually at a practical management plan in which the patient can have confidence.

The value of drug provocation tests

Although skin tests for investigation of penicillin allergy are widely recommended and carried out, there is less agreement on the value of skin tests to other drugs, and in particular on the advisability of drug provocation tests. There are no guidelines in the USA on the advisability or conduct of such tests. In the UK, the current consensus is that they should be undertaken only when other investigations have been exhausted and benefit and risk have been carefully weighed, and should be avoided in patients who have experienced anaphylaxis unless there is no suitable alternative form of treatment [4]. The European Academy of Allergology and Clinical Immunology, however, recommends the use of drug provocation tests to confirm drug hypersensitivity reactions.

Drug provocation tests in patients with a history suggesting an immediate drug hypersensitivity reaction

Messaad D, Sahla H, Benahmed S, Godard P, Bousquet, Demoly P. *Ann Intern Med* 2004; **140**: 1001–6

BACKGROUND. This French study describes an energetic approach to drug provocation tests in patients whose history suggested a previous reaction. The authors investigated 898 consecutive patients (including 126 children) with suspected immediate drug allergy over a 5-year period, excluding only those who had experienced severe skin reactions, or those with positive skin tests to beta-lactams, as well as those with non-compatible clinical histories (Fig. 8.2). They administered increasing doses of the suspected causal drug by ingestion or injection (whichever route had been used before) every 30 min until the usual daily dosage had been given or symptoms suggestive of a reaction occurred.

INTERPRETATION. The study involved 1372 provocation tests, using various drugs including beta-lactams (30.3%), aspirin (14.5%), non-steroidal anti-inflammatory drugs (11.7%), paracetamol (8.9%), macrolides (7.4%) and quinolones (2.4%). Of these tests, 241 (17.6%) proved positive, and tended to reproduce the same symptoms that patients had experienced previously. The reactions included anaphylactic shock (13; 5.4%), anaphylaxis without shock (17; 7.0%), laryngeal oedema (10; 4.1%), bronchospasm (19; 7.9%), urticaria (160; 66.4%), and maculopapular eruption (22; 9.1%) (Table 8.7).

Comment

The authors expressed the view that relying on the history to prove or exclude drug hypersensitivity was not possible, and felt that the routine use of drug provocation tests in such patients was justified by their results. They obtained written informed consent to perform the test, but were not required to seek ethical approval for the study because there was no alternative test for drug allergy and patients needed to take the drugs in question. Given the range of alternative drugs available, readers might reasonably question the necessity of such tests in respect of aspirin and paracetamol, and perhaps macrolides and quinolones. They monitored the patients very carefully, inserted intravenous cannulas in advance into patients who had previously experienced anaphylaxis, and ensured that full resuscitation facilities were available. However, one cannot escape the concern that deliberate exposure of patients to the risks of anaphylaxis, laryngeal oedema and bronchospasm as a

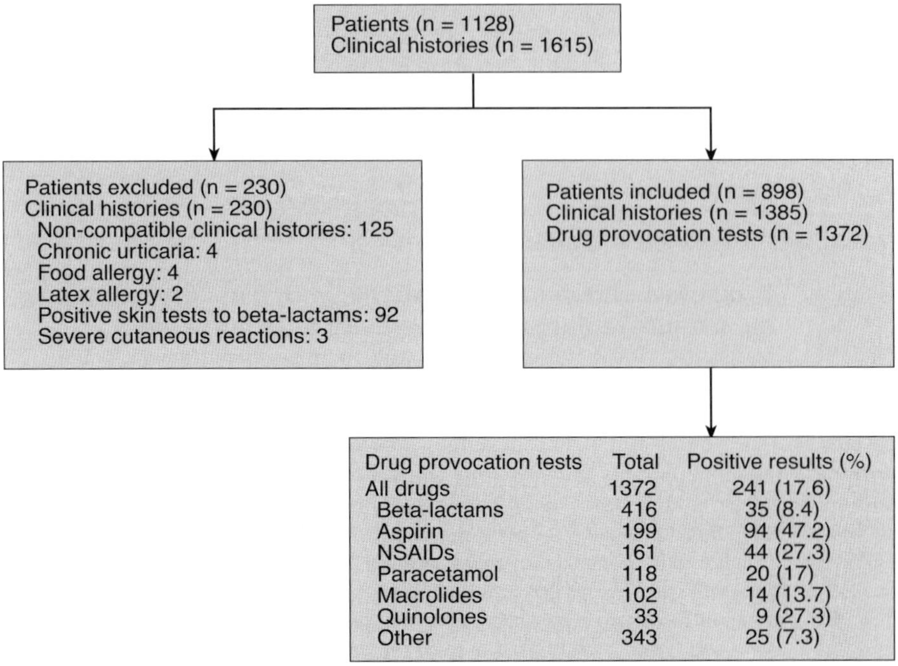

Drug provocation tests	Total	Positive results (%)
All drugs	1372	241 (17.6)
Beta-lactams	416	35 (8.4)
Aspirin	199	94 (47.2)
NSAIDs	161	44 (27.3)
Paracetamol	118	20 (17)
Macrolides	102	14 (13.7)
Quinolones	33	9 (27.3)
Other	343	25 (7.3)

Fig. 8.2 Flow chart of study patients and results of drug provocation tests.
Source: Messaad *et al.* (2004).

matter of course is likely to result eventually in serious mishap, unless one is blessed with sustained good luck in large measure. It would be interesting to learn the experiences of patients who presented with a history consistent with serious reactions such as these, when exposed subsequently to the same drugs in the confident knowledge that their provocation test was negative. The risks of this procedure can be justified only by establishing its validity and reliability beyond doubt.

Reactions to lidocaine

Hypersensitivity to lidocaine is very rare. Reported reactions among patients in whom lidocaine has been used as a local anaesthetic agent are most commonly vasovagal attacks, anxiety or hyperventilation. Events that do involve an allergic mechanism are most commonly reactions to a preservative used to prevent deterioration in a multi-use vial, such as methylparaben or, in formulations that include adrenaline (epinephrine), the anti-oxidant sodium metabisulphite |**9,10**|. However,

Table 8.7 Characteristics of patients with positive drug provocation test results

Patient characteristic	Patients	Positive drug provocation test results (%)
Sex		
Female	945	15.4
Male	427	22.2
Age (years)		
≤18	144	15.9
18–65	986	17.7
>65	242	17.8
Drug class		
Beta-lactam	416	8.4
Aspirin	199	47.2
NSAIDs	161	27.3
Paracetamol	118	17.0
Macrolides	102	13.7
Quinolones	33	27.3
Other (local anaesthetics, vaccines, narcotics, corticosteroids)	343	7.3
Symptoms		
Anaphylactic shock	64	32.8
Anaphylaxis without shock	57	29.8
Laryngeal oedema	90	27.8
Bronchospasm	94	20.2
Urticaria	718	17.8
Maculopapular eruption	300	10.3
Other (faintness, conjunctivitis, fever, itching)	49	0
Interval between last dose of drug and onset of symptoms (h)		
≤1	448	24.8
1–8	184	24.5
8–12	556	12.2
12–24	184	9.2

NSAI, non-steroidal anti-inflammatory drug.
Source: Messaad *et al.* (2004).

the rarity of lidocaine allergy is not widely known and many patients who claim to be either allergic or intolerant are either obliged to undergo a procedure without local anaesthesia, or subjected unnecessarily to general anaesthesia. Skin testing has been advocated as a guide to predicting future reactions, but is poorly reproducible and frequently results in a false-positive result.

Evaluation of re-challenge in patients with suspected lidocaine allergy

Amsler E, Flahault A, Mathelier-Fusade P, Aractingi S. *Dermatology* 2004; **208**: 109–11

BACKGROUND. The authors of this study sent questionnaires to members of the French Society of Dermatology, seeking information about their experience with lidocaine and for details of any adverse reactions (Table 8.8).

INTERPRETATION. There was a 38.5% response to the questionnaire. Of 597 respondents, 391 (65.5%) had encountered patients claiming to be either allergic to or intolerant of lidocaine. Where allergy to lidocaine was suspected, 186 (36.5%) had carried out formal skin testing (no details were provided on the outcome of skin testing or subsequent exposure in these patients), whereas 199 (39.5%) had simply re-injected lidocaine as a discrete procedure. Among patients who had been re-challenged rather than skin-tested, only 11 (5.5%) had experienced an adverse reaction, none of which was severe, and in only one of these was the mechanism subsequently shown to involve hypersensitivity; the others were either vasovagal (nine) or psychogenic (one).

Table 8.8 Lidocaine hypersensitivity questionnaire

1. How many lidocaine injections have you done during the past week?
    <5 5–10 10–20 >20 other
2. Have you already encountered an adverse reaction to lidocaine injected during the last few years?
    Yes No
3. Did any patients tell you they were 'allergic' or intolerant to lidocaine?
    Yes No
4. When you suspect an allergy to lidocaine, do you carry out skin testing?
    Yes No
5. When you last gave lidocaine to a patient with lidocaine intolerance, did you note the occurrence of an adverse reaction afterwards?
    Yes No
6. If a reaction occurred, what was its nature?
    Urticaria
    Deep urticaria or angio-oedema
    Dyspnoea with laryngeal oedema
    Bronchospasm
    Vasovagal syncope
    Anaphylactoid reaction
    Other, be precise if possible

Source: Amsler *et al.* (2004).

Comment

Questionnaire studies tell us nothing about those who did not respond. However a 38.5% response is quite creditable, and in this case produced a respectable amount of data. Moreover, this is a topic that tends to arouse interest, and one would have expected those who had thought at all seriously about the problem to accept an invitation to share their experiences. The results support the use of re-challenge rather than formal skin testing as a means of assessing the likely safety of lidocaine use. The authors recommend that this be done as a discrete procedure, in circumstances where facilities for treatment of any reaction are available, in advance of any intended use of the drug as a local anaesthetic.

Immediate reactions to aspirin and related drugs

Aspirin can result in symptoms suggestive of IgE-mediated drug allergy. However, because it has never proved possible to identify specific IgE antibodies directed against the relevant drug hapten, immediate reactions to aspirin are usually referred to as anaphylactoid or pseudo-allergic. With the exception of patients with aspirin-exacerbated respiratory disease (see below), and those with chronic idiopathic urticaria, who may experience flares when challenged with aspirin, such reactions are rare. However, all non-steroidal anti-inflammatory drugs (NSAIDs) that inhibit cyclooxygenase (COX)-1 can cause hypersensitivity, in the form of urticaria, angio-oedema and anaphylaxis, and specific IgE antibodies to individual NSAIDs have been demonstrated in a few instances [11]. Controversy therefore surrounds the issue of whether these reactions should be referred to as allergic or anaphylactoid.

Prehospital use of aspirin rarely is associated with adverse events

Quan D, LoVecchio F, Clark B, Gallagher JV. *Prehosp Disast Med* 2004; **19**: 362–5

BACKGROUND. Although immediate reactions to aspirin in the general population are uncommon, the increasing frequency with which it is being given to reduce the incidence of myocardial infarction in patients with acute chest pain by paramedical teams in the community has led to concern about reactions to its use in this setting. This study examined 25 600 encounters with pre-hospital personnel during a 6-month period in Phoenix, Arizona, which involved 2399 patients with potential acute coronary syndrome. It sought evidence of adverse events such as urticaria, angio-oedema and bronchoconstriction during the first 24 h after administration of aspirin.

INTERPRETATION. The study excluded patients who had been taking prophylactic aspirin before the event or had taken a dose before the emergency team arrived, or reported intolerance to aspirin. This left 892 individuals who were given aspirin by pre-hospital personnel (Table 8.9). Of the 229 whose chest pain was subsequently judged to

Table 8.9 Patients with presumed coronary syndromes

	Participating facilities	**Other facilities**	**Total**
No aspirin	183	626	809
Refused or 'allergy' to aspirin	53	60	113
Patient-administered aspirin	123	462	585
Pre-hospital administration of aspirin	228	664	892
Presumed coronary syndrome	587	1812	2399

Source: Quan *et al.* (2004).

Table 8.10 Amalgamated results from the participating hospitals

	Total
Unavailable charts	10
Emergency department discharge or 6 h post-emergency medical service encounter	0/106
24 h post-emergency medical service encounter	0/113
Adverse events reported	0/219

Source: Quan *et al.* (2004).

be of cardiac origin, 219 had records that were subsequently available for scrutiny. No adverse reactions to aspirin were apparent from the medical records (Table 8.10).

Comment

The investigators relied totally upon a retrospective examination of medical records and did not discuss the outcome of any treatment event with the patients themselves. The data comprised clinical observations by pre-hospital personnel during the journey to hospital and by nursing and ancillary staff in the hospital itself. Nevertheless, the study findings suggest that the pre-hospital administration of aspirin to patients with acute coronary syndrome is unlikely to result in an acute adverse reaction, provided careful enquiry is made about intolerance before the drug is given.

Systematic review of prevalence of aspirin induced asthma and its implications for clinical practice

Jenkins C, Costello J, Hodge L. *BMJ* 2004; **328**: 434–7

BACKGROUND. There is a widely held view that aspirin and NSAIDs should not be prescribed for patients with asthma lest they trigger an acute attack. In fact, a minority of patients with asthma react in this way. The true prevalence of sensitivity is difficult to assess, chiefly because most studies have sampled patients referred to

hospital, who tend to have more severe asthma; those who react adversely to aspirin and NSAIDs are over-represented in this population. Apart from rare cases of hypersensitivity pneumonitis, most patients with asthma who are sensitive to aspirin and NSAIDs have associated rhinitis, nasal polyps and chronic sinusitis. Their underlying problem is not aspirin sensitivity but aspirin-exacerbated respiratory disease, a pseudo-allergic condition seen almost exclusively in adults, usually between 20 and 40 years of age, and more commonly in women. The condition starts typically after a viral upper respiratory tract infection with persisting rhinitis progressing to pansinusitis, with the later appearance of nasal polyps. Most of these patients will never develop aspirin sensitivity, but in the 30–40% who do sensitivity always develops after the appearance of upper respiratory symptoms. Reactions take the form of acute bronchospasm (which can be severe), sometimes associated with cutaneous, gastrointestinal and vascular effects |12|. Sensitive patients who require treatment with aspirin or NSAIDs can be desensitized, which not only permits continued treatment with these agents but also reduces upper airway mucosal congestion, nasal polyp formation, and the need for systemic steroids.

This meta-analysis examined 66 papers reporting the prevalence of aspirin-induced asthma, of which 21 fulfilled the authors' criteria for inclusion. Some of these studies had examined patients with a history of aspirin-induced asthma; others had not.

INTERPRETATION. The pooled incidence of aspirin-induced asthma was 21% (95% CI 14%–29%), regardless of whether the patients had a history of aspirin-induced asthma or markers for an increased risk. Estimates of prevalence that relied on history alone were much lower than those incorporating a provocation test. Among patients who had reacted positively to a provocation test, about half reacted to doses of aspirin no greater than 80 mg. The estimated prevalence among children was much lower—around 5% (95% CI 0%–14%). The authors recommended formal provocation testing with facilities for resuscitation in all patients aged less than 40 years with asthma requiring either aspirin or an NSAID, in whom the history neither supported nor excluded aspirin-induced asthma.

Comment

This high value for prevalence was surprising, and contrary to the experience of most clinicians treating patients with asthma on an everyday basis. The authors acknowledged that their review was limited by the retrospective nature of the analysis and the heterogeneity of the patient population. They had been unable to acquire information on the clinical status of all the patients, the challenge tests had lacked uniformity, and some studies included very few patients. Considering these limitations, the blanket recommendation seems somewhat excessive. When challenged in correspondence a few months later |**13–15**| on the grounds of both clinical relevance and practicality, the authors agreed that a routine provocation test would be difficult to arrange in practice and that clear advice about the risks would have to suffice if testing was impracticable. They emphasized that their analysis should not be taken to imply that all patients with asthma should avoid aspirin and NSAIDs. They also acknowledged that most of the studies in their analysis had involved patients referred to tertiary hospital outpatient clinics, and almost certainly represented a group of patients with more severe asthma than those who never present to hospital. They agreed that more studies were required to determine the prevalence and severity of aspirin-sensitive asthma in the total asthma population. One cannot escape the feeling that this should have been one of the chief conclusions of the meta-analysis itself.

Adverse reactions to selective cyclo-oxygenase-2 inhibitors

Sánchez-Borges M, Capriles-Hulett A, Caballero-Fonseca F. *Am J Ther* 2004; **11**: 494–500

BACKGROUND. The cross-sensitivity between aspirin and NSAIDs in patients who manifest pseudo-allergic reactions to aspirin affecting the respiratory tract occurs because NSAIDs, like aspirin, inhibit COX-1, so that arachidonic acid metabolism is diverted towards the 5-lipoxygenase pathway, with resulting increased production of cysteinyl leukotrienes, which mediate the appearance of symptoms such as rhinitis and asthma. Selective inhibitors of COX-2 were developed primarily to reduce the incidence of adverse events affecting the gastrointestinal tract, but the possibility that these agents might be less likely to result in other varieties of adverse reaction dependent on COX-1 inhibition has attracted interest. This review examined the evidence for their greater safety in this respect.

INTERPRETATION. The review found that studies of patients with aspirin-exacerbated respiratory disease had revealed no evidence of cross-reactivity with either rofecoxib or celecoxib, but no studies could be found that had examined the safety of other coxibs (valdecoxib, parecoxib, etoricoxib) in such patients. In patients manifesting cutaneous reactions, such as urticaria and angio-oedema, to NSAIDs, the available literature yielded information on 1101 patients who had been challenged with rofecoxib, 18 (1.6%) of whom had experienced urticaria or angio-oedema. By contrast, among 133 patients challenged with celecoxib, 15 (11.2%) had reacted in this way. The authors themselves had challenged 28 patients with valdecoxib, and only one (3.5%) had developed urticaria. No studies had examined the effects of parecoxib or etoricoxib in such patients. The mechanism by which these particular skin reactions occur is unknown. The review makes mention of the fact that celecoxib, valdecoxib and parecoxib all contain a sulphonamide residue (Fig. 8.3) and the European Medicines Evaluation Agency has warned that, owing to this molecular characteristic, these drugs may carry a serious risk of more severe hypersensitivity reactions, such as erythema multiforme, Stevens–Johnson syndrome, exfoliative dermatitis and toxic epidermal necrolysis, which involve a T cell mediated response. One case of valdecoxib-induced epidermal necrolysis has been reported.

Comment

It is clear that the use of COX-2 inhibitors is not without risk. Whereas they are safe to use in patients who manifest respiratory symptoms in response to aspirin and NSAIDs, they can cause urticaria or angio-oedema and can provoke more severe T cell mediated allergic skin reactions. More research is needed to determine the

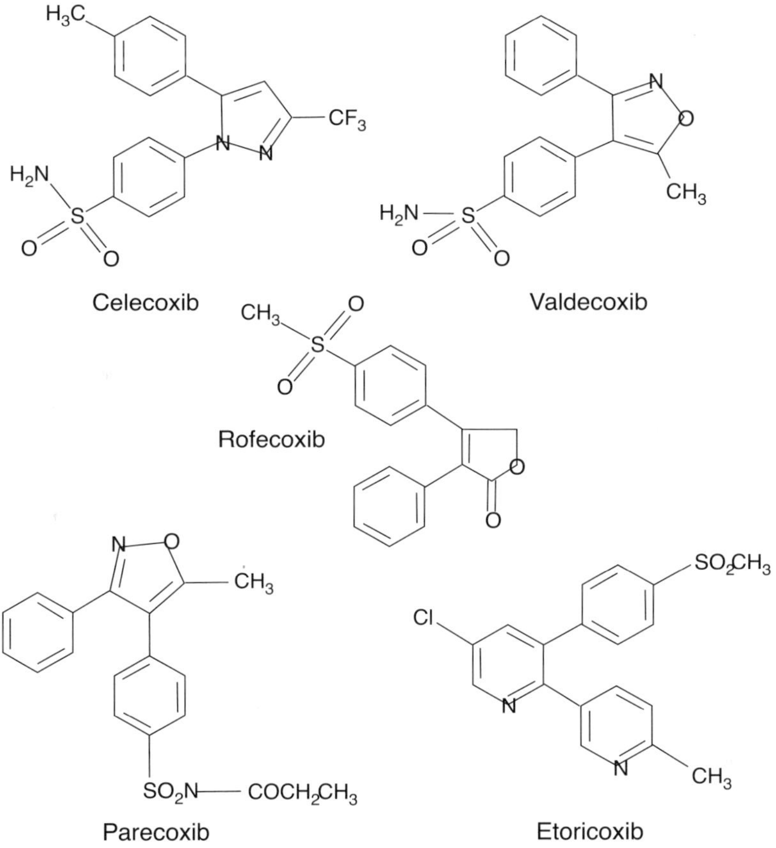

Fig. 8.3 Chemical structure of coxibs. Source: Sánchez–Borges *et al.* (2004).

mechanisms of these reactions more precisely and to identify what predisposes some patients to react in this way. However, the withdrawal of rofecoxib, following the realization that its use is associated with an increased incidence of cardiovascular events, has led to uncertainty over the future of other drugs in this category, particularly those with even greater selectivity than rofecoxib for COX-2 (e.g. etoricoxib).

Conclusion

The potential seriousness of a reaction is sufficient to deter most clinicians from deliberately administering a second course of penicillin to a patient who recalls experiencing symptoms consistent with an IgE-mediated reaction on a previous occasion. It is likely that most re-exposures in such patients are inadvertent—they occur because either the patient or the clinician (or both) overlooked the previous event, which may have occurred many years earlier. Where there is uncertainty about the nature of an adverse reaction to penicillin, a skin-prick test is a prudent move. Skin tests are said to be safe when carried out in suitable conditions by experienced investigators, and a negative skin test substantially reduces the likelihood of a reaction to re-exposure. However, whereas these are widely used in the USA, the necessary reagents are not universally available and few centres in the UK have the necessary specialist expertise to allow their confident interpretation.

The problem facing the individual patient is that an accurate estimate of absolute risk is difficult to obtain. Published studies vary widely in the completeness of their data and the denominator they use when calculating the risk. Apter and colleagues found that, having had one allergic reaction to penicillin, an individual is ten times more likely to react a second time following re-exposure, although the NNH (number needed to harm) is still only one in 53. This is substantially smaller than previous estimates, smaller than the published risk of an adverse reaction in those with a negative skin-prick test, and similar to the risk of a systemic reaction to skin testing itself in those who test positive |**5**|.

An additional difficulty is that many patients who recall reacting adversely to penicillin do not report symptoms suggesting an IgE-mediated reaction. The history is frequently vague and non-specific. Some investigators argue that the history alone affords an acceptable guide to the risk of re-exposure, while others quote studies showing that positive skin tests can occur even in those with non-specific histories |**5**|.

The easier solution to this dilemma is to avoid penicillins in all patients who have reacted adversely, and prefer another antimicrobial agent. Where effective alternatives exist, it is difficult to argue that this is unsound. Where there is uncertainty about the effectiveness of alternative agents, the clinician presented with a patient who may be allergic to penicillin must balance the perceived risk of a serious allergic reaction against the seriousness of the infection (and the likely outcome if penicillin is avoided and a less effective antimicrobial is preferred).

If the risk of a reaction following re-exposure to penicillin is small, the risk of one occurring after treatment with a third-generation cephalosporin or a carbapenem would appear even smaller, and caveats based on estimates of cross-reactivity among different beta-lactams should probably be consigned to the archives, as they do not apply to these modern agents. Of greater concern is the patient who reports allergies to multiple antimicrobials, and the careful and rigorous approach advocated by Macy in the review article discussed in this chapter is endorsed.

Drug provocation tests are inherently risky. There is no clear international consensus on their value or on the advisability of their use. It seems sensible to adopt a similar approach to that recommended when considering whether to use penicillin (where penicillin is the preferred treatment) in a patient who gives a history of a previous adverse reaction, and consider the use of such challenges only where:

- treatment with a specific drug is considered necessary;
- alternative forms of treatment are demonstrably inferior; and
- benefit and risk have been carefully weighed.

For example, a test dose of lidocaine in patients with symptoms consistent with allergy following previous exposure helps to anticipate the likelihood of complications occurring in association with a surgical procedure itself. A supervised test dose of aspirin in a patient with asthma in whom regular treatment with aspirin is justified but in whom there is uncertainty about the possibility of aspirin-exacerbated respiratory disease will allow appropriate treatment to be administered promptly in the event of a severe asthma attack. However, provocation tests should not be performed merely out of curiosity where the need for future treatment with a specific drug has not been established and acceptable alternatives are available.

It seems one can be confident that an acute dose of aspirin can be given safely to non-asthmatic patients who report no previous intolerance, and that COX-2 inhibitors can be given to patients with a history of pseudo-allergic reactions to aspirin and/or NSAIDs affecting the respiratory tract, provided they give no history of severe, T cell mediated allergic reactions.

References

1. Coombs RRA, Gell PGH. Classification of allergic reactions responsible for clinical hypersensitivity and disease. In: Gell PGH, Coombs RRA, Lachmann PJ (eds). *Clinical Aspects of Immunology.* Oxford: Blackwell Scientific Publications, 1975; p 761.
2. Volcheck GW. Clinical evaluation and management of drug hypersensitivity. *Immunol Allergy Clin N Am* 2004; **24**: 357–71.
3. Hernandez–Trujillo VP, Lieberman PL, Chowdhury BA. Drug allergens, haptens and anaphylatoxins. *Clin Allergy Immunol* 2004; **18**: 387–419.
4. Royal College of Physicians of London. Ch 8. Common diseases associated with allergy. In: *Allergy: the unmet need—a blueprint for better patient care.* London: Royal College of Physicians 2003; pp 41–51.
5. Thethi AK, Van Dellen RG. Dilemmas and controversies in penicillin allergy. *Immunol Allergy Clin N Am* 2004; **24**: 445–61.
6. Greenberger PA. Drug allergy, part B: allergic reactions to individual drugs: low molecular weight. In: Grammer LC, Greenberger PA (eds). *Patterson's Allergic Diseases.* 6th edn. Philadelphia: Lippincott, Williams & Wilkins, 2002; pp 335–59.
7. Macy E, Burchette R. Oral antibiotic adverse reactions after penicillin skin testing: multi-year follow-up. *Allergy* 2002; **57**: 1151–8.

8. Madaan A, Li T-C. Cephalosporin allergy. *Immunol Allergy Clin N Am* 2004; **24**: 463–76.
9. Eggelston ST, Walsh LW. Understanding allergic reactions to local anesthetics. *Ann Pharmacother* 1996; **30**: 851–7.
10. Wildsmith JAW, Mason A, McKinnon RP, Rae SM. Alleged allergy to local anaesthetic drugs. *Br Dent J* 1998; **184**: 507–10.
11. Stevenson DD. Aspirin and NSAID sensitivity. *Immunol Allergy Clin N Am* 2004; **24**: 491–505.
12. Simon RA. Adverse respiratory reactions to aspirin and non-steroidal anti-inflammatory drugs. *Curr Allergy Asthma Rep* 2004; **4**: 17–24.
13. Sivanandan I, Robinson SM. Aspirin induced asthma. *BMJ* 2004; **328**: 1076.
14. Southward RD. Aspirin induced asthma. *BMJ* 2004; **328**: 1076.
15. Jenkins C, Costello J, Hodge L. Aspirin induced asthma. *BMJ* 2004; **328**: 1076–7.

9

Immunodeficiency

RICHARD BARETTO, SARAH GODDARD, AARNOUD HUISSON, MAMIDIPUDI T KRISHNA

Introduction

Primary immunodeficiencies occur with a frequency approaching that of cystic fibrosis (1:2500 live births) [1]. However, because they are perceived to be very rare and usually present with common infections, they are under-diagnosed. Often the diagnosis is not considered until substantial end-organ damage has occurred, by which time definitive treatment is only partially successful in preventing further infections [2].

While defects of any part of the immune system may result in recurrent infections, abnormalities of antibody production are by far the commonest. Indeed, the first immunodeficiency diagnosed and treated was X-linked agammaglobulinaemia [3]. But the majority of cases of antibody deficiency are not X-linked, and these have historically been grouped together under the catch-all name of 'common variable immunodeficiency' (CVID). It has always been recognized that this diagnosis comprises a number of distinct syndromes that are distinguishable by their clinical and laboratory characteristics. Susceptibility to CVID has been associated with certain human leukocyte antigen (HLA) alleles, and it is also apparent that CVID is inherited in some families. However, the underlying genetic defects have been very slow to emerge.

The molecular basis of a number of primary immunodeficiency phenotypes has now been elucidated, including some directly associated with hypogammaglobulinaemia. It appears that what we currently call CVID probably comprises dozens of distinct genetic abnormalities (as well as a large proportion of non-inherited acquired syndromes). However, recently described defects in genes encoding molecules that are involved primarily in innate immunity have been found also to give rise to clinical phenotypes of antibody deficiency. This demonstrates the importance of the innate immune system in directing the actions of its adaptive counterpart [4,5].

The mainstay of treatment for patients with antibody deficiency is replacement therapy with normal human immunoglobulin (Ig). For several decades, immunoglobulin was conventionally administered by the intramuscular route. In the 1980s

© Atlas Medical Publishing Ltd

intravenous preparations were developed, allowing much higher doses to be administered, with a concomitant rise in serum immunoglobulin trough levels and better clinical outcome. In recent years subcutaneous therapy has become available, enabling trough levels comparable to those achieved with the intravenous route with the convenience of a subcutaneous route; this has permitted more patients to receive treatment in the home, minimizing disruption to their daily lives.

In this chapter we will discuss disorders that form part of the differential diagnosis of CVID. We will also review some recent advances in the pathogenesis of this disease and some literature regarding important aspects of immunoglobulin replacement therapy.

CVID—a diagnosis of exclusion?

ICOS deficiency in patients with common variable immunodeficiency

Salzer U, Maul-Pavicic A, Cunningham-Rundles C, *et al. Clin Immunol* 2004; **113**: 234–40

BACKGROUND. CVID is the most frequent primary immunodeficiency in man that requires medical intervention. Most cases are sporadic, but about 10% are familial, with a predominance of autosomal dominant over autosomal recessive inheritance. It has recently been shown that homozygous loss of the inducible costimulator (ICOS) on activated T cells may result in an adult form of CVID with autosomal recessive inheritance. ICOS belongs to the family of costimulatory T-cell molecules such as CD28 and CTLA-4. ICOS is expressed on activated T cells, particularly those in germinal centres, and co-induces the secretion of a number of cytokines. The interaction of ICOS with its ligand (ICOS-L) is important for normal T–B cell cooperation, promoting the terminal differentiation of B cells into memory cells and plasma cells. The aim of this study was to determine the frequency of defects in ICOS and ICOS-L in a cohort of 194 patients with CVID from Europe and North America.

INTERPRETATION. All 194 CVID patients had a typical clinical history and were diagnosed according to the European Society for Immunodeficiencies (ESID) criteria. One hundred and eighty-one of these cases were sporadic, with a negative family history, and 13 originated from nine families with autosomal recessive CVID, of whom five contained consanguineous unions. In the sporadic CVID patients, the sequence of the five exons and exon–intron boundaries in ICOS revealed no mutations and there was no significant difference in the frequency of four single-nucleotide polymorphisms and one T repeat in patients with CVID compared with a healthy control population. Five patients from two of the nine families with autosomal recessive CVID had a large deletion in ICOS involving exons 2 and 3. This deletion was the same as that reported in the index cases. All the patients with this deletion in ICOS were genotyped at the ICOS locus using polymorphic markers. This analysis showed that all the patients with the ICOS deletion were homozygous for the same allele detected by one of the polymorphic markers. This strongly suggests a common founder for the mutations in all the four families with ICOS deficiency. The remaining seven families with autosomal recessive CVID were screened for mutations in ICOS-L. No loss-of-function mutations were identified in this gene in these seven families.

Comment

ICOS deficiency is the first single-gene defect identified to cause the CVID phenotype and demonstrates how basic mechanistic defects translate into clinical phenotype. The authors have calculated the frequency (the authors state 'prevalence', but this is not accurate) of ICOS deficiency in patients with CVID to be about 5% (that is, nine cases out of 194 CVID families). However, all the families that included individuals with the deletion in ICOS originated from the same region, connected by the Danube River, and genotyping confirmed the likelihood that this mutation was derived from a common founder. The authors suggest that mutations in ICOS should be sought in patients with a recessive pattern of inheritance of CVID. The data from this study and the original work suggest that, unless the patient has origins from the geographical area associated with the Danube, the likelihood of finding this deletion in ICOS is small. However, the possibility remains of novel mutations in this gene causing the CVID phenotype.

Prevalence of SAP gene defects in male patients diagnosed with common variable immunodeficiency

Eastwood D, Gilmour KC, Nistala K, *et al. Clin Exp Immunol* 2004; **137**: 584–8

BACKGROUND. The molecular basis of CVID is unknown and the diagnosis requires the exclusion of other diseases known to cause primary antibody deficiency syndromes, such as X-linked lymphoproliferative disease (XLP). XLP is a rare primary immunodeficiency disease in which severe immunodysregulatory phenomena occur, typically after exposure to Epstein–Barr virus (EBV). The defective gene in XLP is *SAP* (SLAM associated protein, where SLAM is signalling lymphocyte activation molecule), a small SH2 domain containing protein involved in signal transduction events downstream of the SLAM family of receptors. These receptors are known to regulate T and NK cell function. There are three major clinical phenotypes associated with XLP: fulminant infectious mononucleosis, development of lymphoma, and dysgammaglobulinaemia. The last presentation has clinical and immunological similarities with CVID and a number of patients labelled as having CVID have subsequently been found to have mutations in *SAP*. No large-scale analysis has been performed to determine the true prevalence of SAP defects in males with CVID. Therefore, this study screened 60 patients with CVID and hypogammaglobulinaemia to assess the prevalence of XLP.

INTERPRETATION. According to the ESID criteria for the diagnosis of CVID, 35 of the 60 patients were classified as probable and three as possible CVID. The remaining 22 were labelled as having hypogammaglobulinaemia, since immunoglobulin replacement therapy precluded the assessment of antibody responses. Peripheral blood mononuclear cells (PBMCs) from all 60 patients were shown to express SAP by an immunoblot analysis. However, six patients expressed low levels of SAP compared with normal controls. Furthermore, normal expression does not exclude a diagnosis of XLP, as some patients may be able to express a stable SAP protein. Genetic analysis was therefore performed on these six patients with 26 others, including those with a relevant family history or a history of EBV infection. One patient (UPN56) was found to have a substitution in exon 1 of SAP, which was predicted to affect exon splicing. This patient expressed low levels of SAP in PBMCs, as determined by a semi-quantitative method comparing the level of SAP with that in normal controls and with β-actin (Fig. 9.1).

Comment

The single patient out of the 60 screened had a positive family history consistent with XLP, with a brother dying in early childhood of probably fulminant infectious mononucleosis. Reports of other patients initially diagnosed with CVID who were subsequently found to have XLP have identified individuals in whom there was either a family history of affected males or the onset of symptoms after EBV infection. The authors sensibly point out that, given the complexity and limited availability of the assays required to make the diagnosis of XLP and the low prevalence of this disorder in an unselected cohort of CVID patients, this diagnosis

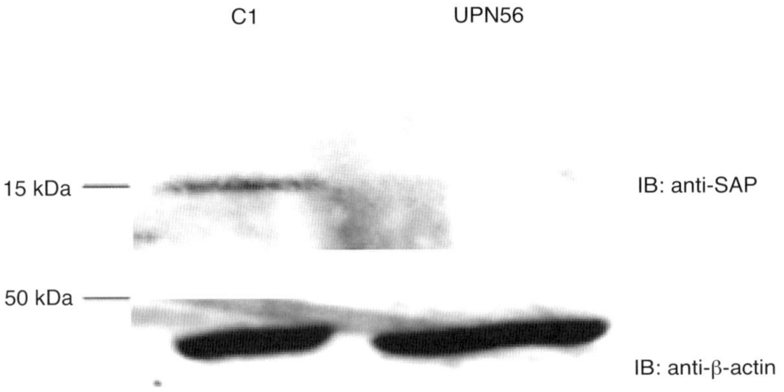

Fig. 9.1 Quantitative analysis of SAP protein expression from a control (C1) and the patient designated UPN56 shows markedly decreased SAP expression in the patient. Equal loading of protein by analysis of β-actin expression is seen in the lower panel. Source: Eastwood *et al.* (2004).

should be sought only in individuals with other clinical features, such as a positive family history and/or a history of EBV-related onset of symptoms.

Primary immunodeficiency to pneumococcal infection due to a defect in toll-like receptor signaling

Currie AJ, Davidson DJ, Reid GS, *et al.* *J Pediatr* 2004; **144**: 512–18

BACKGROUND. The toll-like receptor (TLR) family consists of ten receptors that seem to be critically important in the control of the innate immune system. Recently, two defects in TLR signalling – deficiency of interleukin receptor-associated kinase 4 (IRAK-4) and deficiency of nuclear factor κB (NFκB) essential modulator (NEMO) – have been identified. Patients with the former deficiency suffered with recurrent pyogenic infections as well as with fungal and opportunistic infections, the latter having a phenotype of anhidrotic ectodermal dysplasia with increased susceptibility to pneumococcal infections. This is a report on a 3-year-old boy with recurrent bacteraemia in whom no classical immunodeficiency was found. He was therefore investigated for a possible defect in the TLR signalling pathway.

INTERPRETATION. This boy first presented at 9 months of age with *Staphylococcus aureus* cervical adenitis requiring intensive antimicrobial chemotherapy. At that time, immunological investigations revealed normal blood count and differential leucocyte count, immunoglobulins, complement activity and lymphocyte subset enumeration. Chronic granulomatous disease was excluded using an appropriate test. The patient had an older brother who had died aged 5 years with pneumococcal meningitis. He also had two other brothers who were in good health. At 18 months he suffered an upper respiratory tract infection due to *Streptococcus pneumoniae*. Subsequently, he suffered an episode of bacteraemia and then septic arthritis, both caused by *S. pneumoniae*. Since the last episode he has been started on penicillin prophylaxis and has had no further bacterial infections. All three isolates of *S. pneumoniae* were type 19F. The patient was vaccinated with pneumococcal 7-valent conjugated vaccine and normal levels of antibodies against all covered strains were demonstrable. The patient's mononuclear cells, macrophages and dendritic cells produced significantly lower levels of interleukin (IL)-6 (Fig. 9.2), tumour necrosis factor α, IL-12 and IL-18 when challenged with a range of TLR agonists. IL-1β, IL-18 and lipopolysaccharide signalling also seemed to be impaired, but signalling via CD154, which also uses some components of the TLR pathway, was intact. The TLR signalling pathway was examined in more detail, and a defect in IRAK-4 or NEMO was excluded.

Comment

This is an interesting case report of a boy experiencing recurrent invasive pneumococcal infections before his second birthday who was deficient in TLR-mediated cytokine production with intact IRAK-4 and NEMO function. The fact that this patient had a brother who died of pneumococcal meningitis supports his having an inherited primary immunodeficiency. Furthermore, his phenotype is similar to that of patients with hypomorphic mutations in NEMO and loss-of-

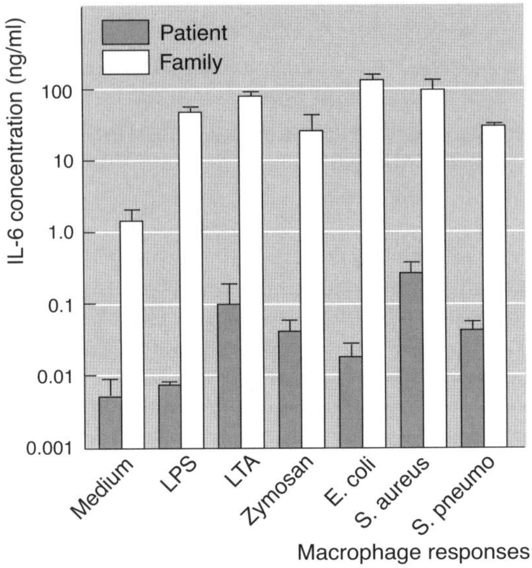

Fig. 9.2 IL-6 production by macrophages from a boy with recurrent bacteraemia and his immediate family after activation with various microbial stimuli. Data shown are mean ± SEM ($n = 3$). The response to *S. pneumoniae* is shown, compared with that of an unrelated healthy adult. Source: Currie *et al.* (2004).

function mutations in IRAK-4, although these disorders have characteristics of primary antibody deficiency. The authors state that the data suggest that, in the presence of protective humoral and phagocytic responses, TLR-mediated recognition of *S. pneumoniae* is a non-redundant innate host defence mechanism.

There are some points that have not been mentioned in this paper which are of importance when considering patients with recurrent pneumococcal infections. Firstly, the presence of a normal functioning spleen has not been commented on. Although this would not cause a defect in TLR signalling, it is part of the differential diagnosis. Secondly, although the discussion states that the patient 'had recurrent pneumococcal infection despite the presence of sufficient antibodies against *S. pneumoniae*', it seems from the case history that he was vaccinated after his last infection; furthermore, there is no record of any pneumococcal-specific antibody levels being measured prior to this or of any failure to respond to the unconjugated vaccine. If he had not responded to the unconjugated vaccine, specific antibody deficiency is a possibility. Alternatively, this may be simply the normal physiological response to polysaccharide antigen since this child's infections occurred before he was 2 years of age and he has remained well since then, albeit with prophylactic penicillin and the conjugate vaccine. Again, however, neither of these conditions would result in impaired TLR signalling.

These points aside, this case report illustrates that defects in TLR signalling should form part of the differential diagnosis of patients with an antibody deficiency phenotype, especially because patients with hypomorphic mutations can have low immunoglobulins. This is possibly due to the use of the TLR signalling pathway by CD154.

Interleukin receptor-associated kinase 4 deficiency associated with bacterial infections and failure to sustain antibody responses

Day N, Tangsinmankong N, Ochs H, *et al.* *J Pediatr* 2004; **144**: 524–6

BACKGROUND. Recently, three patients have been described with IRAK-4 deficiency. IRAK-4 is a critical component of the TLR pathway of the innate immune system. These patients have in common a history of frequent bacterial infections. One of these patients is a young girl, the subject of the report, who continued to have recurring bacterial and fungal infections requiring intravenous immunoglobulin (IVIG) therapy. The authors monitored this patient's response to vaccination with polysaccharide and protein antigens.

INTERPRETATION. The case is of a girl who was born of an incestuous relationship. She was initially hospitalized at 5 weeks of age for buccal cellulitis associated with severe thrush and *Staphylococcus aureus* bacteraemia. She continued to have severe infections, such as pneumonia, septicaemia and septic arthritis, with Gram-positive, Gram-negative, fungal and opportunistic pathogens. These necessitated multiple hospital admissions for intravenous antimicrobial therapy. This patient's PBMCs failed to produce IL-6 in response to a number of TLR ligands, but produced normal amounts of IL-6 when stimulated with pokeweed mitogen. Western and northern blot analysis showed that the patient did not express the protein and the mRNA respectively of IRAK-4. As an infant, before IVIG replacement therapy was begun, the patient was fully immunized with diphtheria and tetanus toxoids. Eighteen months after the fourth immunization, antibodies to these vaccines were undetectable and so she was given a fifth immunization at 3.2 years. One month later antibody levels to diphtheria and tetanus toxoids were borderline and normal respectively. However, six months later antibody levels were significantly lower to both antigens. Table 9.1 shows the patient's antibody response to pneumococcal polysaccharide antigens given at four time-points, again prior to IVIG. There was a suboptimal rise in antibody titre to four of the twelve polysaccharide antigens, but, like the T-dependent antibody responses, these were short-lived.

Comment

This patient with IRAK-4 deficiency suffered from recurrent bacterial infections associated with suboptimal, short-lived antibody responses to both T-dependent and -independent antigens. In contrast, the other two patients reported to have IRAK-4 deficiency gradually improved and both have recently been well. The reason for variable clinical expression of IRAK-4 deficiency is not clear, but such

Table 9.1 Immunological response to pneumococcal polysaccharide vaccine (ng antibody/ml)

Serotype	Before 1st vaccination	* 1 month after 1st vaccination	13 months after 1st vaccination	Before 2nd vaccination* (17 months after 1st vaccination)	6 weeks after 2nd vaccination	5 months after 2nd vaccination	Before 3rd vaccination* (6 months after 2nd vaccination)	1 month after 3rd vaccination	6 months after 3rd vaccination
1	0	0	213	172	311	241	386	402	108
3	0	304	100	50	272	42	103	189	0
4	233	230	338	51	1716	174	139	266	59
6A	4	12	168	81	365	186	316	332	11
7F	0	14	129	97	196	99	251	195	20
8	103	638	521	137	286	233	311	604	47
9N	66	188	68	18	93	194	198	158	84
12F	4	726	173	0	296	60	203	397	10
14	49	100	337	313	642	144	345	281	75
18C	0	0	63	0	152	81	189	211	185
19F	0	0	43	56	43	173	163	244	0
23F	0	647	187	124	484	114	153	223	396

*The 23-valent pneumococcal polysaccharide vaccine was given at 1.6, 3.3 and 3.8 years of age.
Source: Day *et al.* (2004).

genotype–phenotype anomalies are commonly found in primary immunodeficiencies. The severe phenotype observed in this patient could be due to other homozygous gene defects as she is the product of an incestuous union. Conventionally, IRAK-4 and TLRs are considered part of the innate immune system, yet defects in their genes often affect adaptive immunity. This study clearly illustrates how loss-of-function mutations of IRAK-4 can affect antibody production, and although they have not caused pan-hypogammaglobulinaemia they can cause a phenotype similar to that of specific antibody deficiency.

Pathogenesis of CVID

Common variable immunodeficiency is associated with defective functions of dendritic cells

Bayry J, Lacroix-Desmazes S, Kazatchkine MD, *et al. Blood* 2004; **104**: 2441–3

BACKGROUND. CVID is characterized by defects in both antibody production and T-cell function. Therefore, this study investigated the function of dendritic cells (DCs) in CVID to see whether defects in this initiator cell of adaptive immunity could be associated with this disease. The differentiation, maturation and function of monocyte-derived DCs from CVID patients were compared with those of DCs from normal controls and control patients with other primary antibody deficiencies. These DC characteristics were assessed by the expression of CD1a, CD83, CD80, CD40, HLA-DR and CD11c, the ability to induce T-cell proliferation in an allogeneic mixed lymphocyte reaction and the production of cytokine IL-12.

INTERPRETATION. The monocyte-derived DCs from patients with CVID expressed significantly lower levels of CD1a, CD83, CD80, HLA-DR, CD11c and CD40 than normal and disease-matched controls. The DCs from patients with CVID also demonstrated a reduced ability to trigger T-cell proliferation in a mixed lymphocyte reaction, upregulate costimulatory molecules and produce IL-12 in response to CD40L stimulation compared with both control groups. The authors conclude that the defective DC function observed in this study may be responsible for the dysregulation of T-cell and B-cell function observed in patients with CVID.

Comment

This well-designed study shows a significant difference in differentiation, maturation and function in monocyte-derived DCs from patients with CVID and a carefully chosen control group. This consisted of not only normal controls but also patients with other forms of antibody deficiency, such as X-linked agammaglobulinaemia and hyper-IgM syndrome. By including patients recently diagnosed with CVID who were yet to receive replacement immunoglobulin therapy, the authors were able to demonstrate that the observed defects in the DCs were not secondary to therapy.

CVID is a heterogeneous disease, most patients exhibiting reduced serum Ig levels with varying degrees of T-cell dysfunction that manifest *in vivo* as granulomatous disease, autoimmunity and malignancy. The group of CVID patients in this study with T-cell dysfunction-related complications had defective DC function compared with the controls, supporting the hypothesis that defective DC function may be responsible for the myriad defects in immunity observed in patients with CVID.

The use of *in vitro* monocyte-derived DCs is a standard procedure for studying human DCs and remains the only readily available means of examining this cell population. This study showed a significant difference between these cells from CVID patients and those from controls. However, whether these findings can be extrapolated to *in vivo* DCs will require further studies. That all the CVID patients had similar defects in these cells despite the varying clinical presentation suggests that differences in function more subtle than those investigated may be responsible for the different phenotypes.

Exogenous leptin restores in vitro T cell proliferation and cytokine synthesis in patients with common variable immunodeficiency syndrome

Goldberg AC, Eliaschewitz FG, Montor WR, *et al. Clin Immunol* 2005; **114**: 147–53

Background. Leptin is an essential hormone affecting lipid and carbohydrate metabolism and has immune-stimulatory and probably anti-apoptotic effects. Furthermore, the thymic atrophy and suppression of T-cell function associated with acute starvation and low leptin levels can be reversed by the administration of exogenous leptin. T-cell dysfunction is likely to play a role in the pathogenesis of CVID, and many patients with CVID are lymphopenic. The role of leptin in T-cell function in 38 patients with CVID was investigated by assessing the effect of exogenous leptin on T-cell proliferation, apoptosis and cytokine production compared with normal controls.

Interpretation. The mean serum leptin level in 38 patients with CVID was significantly lower than that in normal controls (although there was considerable overlap), but it is not stated whether this correlated with lymphocyte count. (Fig 9.3). On stimulation with phytohaemagglutinin, PBMCs from CVID patients demonstrated reduced proliferation, IL-2 and IL-4 production, and excess apoptosis compared with normal controls. The addition of leptin *in vitro* at least partially reversed the impaired IL-4 secretion and inhibited the excess apoptosis in these cells. The small increases seen in the stimulation index and IL-2 production lost significance on multivariate analysis with sex, age and body mass index as additional independent variables. Addition of leptin to cells from healthy donors had no effect on any of these measures.

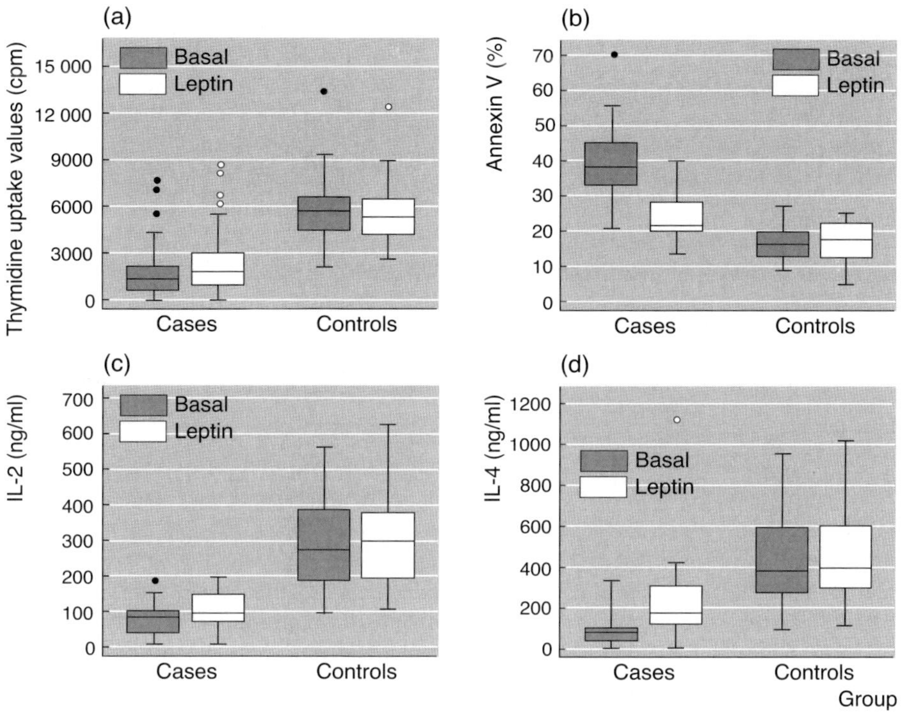

Fig. 9.3 Box plot presentation of results from CVID and control PBMCs (10^6 cells), cultured for 48 h with 2.5 ng/ml phytohaemagglutinin (PHA) in the presence or absence (basal) of 50 ng/ml leptin. (a) Proliferation measured by thymidine uptake; values are in counts per minute. (b) Percentage of apoptosis measured by annexin-V binding using flow cytometry. (c) IL-2 production in ng/ml. (d) IL-4 production in ng/ml, measured by ELISA (enzyme-linked immunosorbent assay). All analyses for the CVID group of patients were significant at $P < 0.001$ compared with controls. Source: Goldberg *et al.* (2005).

Comment

The findings of this study suggest that a low leptin level may be a contributory factor in the pathogenesis of CVID in some patients. The fact that exogenous leptin did not improve T-cell function in all patients suggests that this defect may not be present in all presentations of this heterogeneous disease. Furthermore, addition of leptin did not correct the defective proliferation and cytokine production of PBMCs from patients with CVID, suggesting the involvement of other factors. The precise mechanism of action of leptin is uncertain because, although it is established that monocytes express leptin receptors, the expression of the receptors on T cells is the subject of some controversy. It is possible that the observed effect of leptin on T cells may be mediated via monocytes.

The low leptin levels seen in some patients may assist in understanding the disease progression of a subgroup of CVID patients who lose weight rapidly, and further studies on the effects of leptin in larger numbers of CVID patients may result in a novel leptin-based therapeutic strategy. Given the uncertainty of the mode of action of leptin on lymphocytes, it may be that it acts on lymphoid microenvironments *in vivo* rather than on lymphocytes directly, and thus *in vivo* administration may be more effective. Unfortunately, there is no adequate animal model of CVID to test such a hypothesis.

Abnormal interleukin-7 function in common variable immunodeficiency

Holm AM, Aukrust P, Damas JK, Muller F, Halvorsen B, Froland SS. *Blood* 2005; **105**: 2887–90

BACKGROUND. IL-7 is involved in lymphocyte homeostasis. Elevated levels of IL-7 occur in lymphopenia, and loss of function mutations in the genes encoding the IL-7 receptor α chain cause an autosomal recessive severe combined immunodeficiency (SCID). In view of the T-cell dysfunction associated with CVID, the role of IL-7 in CVID was studied. Plasma levels of IL-7 were determined in 72 patients with CVID compared with 23 healthy controls. T-cell populations, apoptosis, expression of the CC chemokine receptor 7 (CCR7) and production of interferon γ (IFN-γ) and transforming growth factor β (TGF-β) were correlated with the plasma level of IL-7.

INTERPRETATION. A subgroup of 13/72 CVID patients had particularly high levels of IL-7 compared with other CVID patients and normal controls. These patients had significantly higher $CD8^+$ counts than the remaining patients, and although there was no difference in the proportions of $CD45RA^+$ T cells the $IL\text{-}7^{high}$ CVID patients had a significant predominance of $CCR7^-$ effector memory T cells. The proportion of apoptotic cells correlated inversely to IL-7 levels in patients with CVID. Some of the $IL\text{-}7^{high}$ CVID patients had an impaired response to IL-7, as assessed by *in vitro* proliferation and production of IFN-γ and TGF-β.

Comment

The authors describe a subgroup of patients with CVID with high plasma levels of IL-7 associated with elevated numbers of $CD8^+$ T cells and increased proportions of terminally differentiated effector memory T cells that did not show signs of increased proliferation, but appeared to have reduced apoptosis. This suggests that a protective effect of IL-7 may be responsible for the increased percentage of $IL\text{-}7^{high}$ CVID patients who experienced autoimmune phenomena. In addition, these $IL\text{-}7^{high}$ CVID patients also had a high prevalence of bronchiectasis compared with other CVID groups, suggesting that dysregulated IL-7 production may also contribute to the increased susceptibility to infections experienced by patients with CVID. The immunodeficiency may be secondary to abnormal signalling (similar to some forms of SCID) or impaired feedback to IL-7-producing stromal cells due to a primary T-cell defect such as low TGF-β production, as was observed in the CVID patient group. As IL-7 is also involved in DC function, dysregulation may affect T-cell stimulation, resulting in the abnormal T- and B-cell immune responses typical of patients with CVID. This study provides some interesting data regarding possible pathogenic mechanisms of CVID.

The loss of IgM memory B cells correlates with clinical disease in common variable immunodeficiency

Carsetti R, Rosado MM, Donnanno S, *et al. J Allergy Clin Immunol* 2005; **115**: 412–17

BACKGROUND. CVID is characterized by recurrent lower respiratory tract infections caused by encapsulated bacteria, which may cause structural lung damage. However, there exists a group of patients who do not suffer from bacterial pneumonia despite profound hypogammaglobulinaemia. It has been shown previously that IgM memory B cells and natural antibodies play an important role in the defence against encapsulated bacteria. The paradox of patients with hypogammaglobulinaemia and no infections was addressed to see if this clinical finding could be explained by the presence of IgM memory B cells and anti-pneumococcal polysaccharide (anti-PnPS) IgM. The frequency of memory IgM B cells and anti-PnPS IgM antibodies was determined in 54 patients with CVID compared with 27 age-matched controls. The response to vaccination with the 23-valent PnPS vaccine was also assessed.

INTERPRETATION. The 54 CVID patients were divided into three groups. Group 1 consisted of 26 patients with recurrent pneumonia and computed tomographic (CT) findings in the lungs consistent with lung damage. Group 2 included 22 patients with no clinical history of pneumonia or chronic bronchitis and a normal CT scan, and group 3 contained six patients with recurrent pneumonia also with a normal CT scan. (Fig. 9.4). The percentage of total B cells, as assessed by $CD22^+$ and $CD27^-$ staining, was comparable in all groups, including the normal controls. However, the frequency of memory B cells ($CD22^+$ and $CD27^+$) was markedly reduced in group 1 compared not only with the normal controls but also with patients in group 2 (P <0.0001). Switched memory B cells ($CD22^+$, $CD27^+$, IgM^- and IgD^-) were significantly reduced both in group 1 and in group 2 compared with normal controls; however, group 2 patients did not suffer from lower respiratory tract infections. In contrast, IgM memory cells ($CD22^+$, $CD27^+$, IgM^{bright} and IgD^{dull}) were significantly reduced only in patients of group 1 compared with normal controls and group 2 (P <0.0001). In fact, patients in group 2 had higher levels of IgM memory cells than normal healthy controls. The concentration of anti-PnPS IgM was remarkably lower in group 1 than in group 2 (P <0.0003). However, the value for both groups was significantly lower than that for the healthy controls (P <0.0001). There was also a significant correlation between the level of IgM antiPnPS against serotypes 1, 4 and 14 and the frequency of the IgM memory B cells. Based on the presence of IgM memory cells and anti-PnPS IgM antibodies, the six patients in group 3 comprised four patients similar to group 1 and two resembling group 2. In response to vaccination with PnPS vaccine, only patients in group 2 succeeded in making an adequate response.

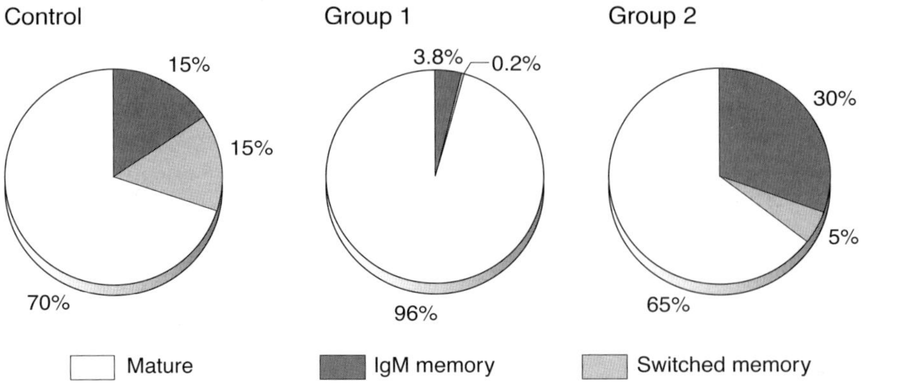

Fig. 9.4 Distribution of B-cell subsets in control subjects and patients with CVID shown as a pie graph. (*White*) Mature B cells; (*black*) IgM memory B cells; (*grey*) switched memory B cells. Source: Carsetti *et al.* (2005).

Comment

This study suggests that anti-PnPS IgM antibodies are protective against lower respiratory tract infections in patients with CVID and that these antibodies are associated with memory IgM B cells. Indeed, there was a significant correlation between the observed defect in IgM memory B cells and bacterial infection of the lower respiratory tract ($P<0.0001$), but not with other clinical complications, such as splenomegaly and autoimmunity. However, the authors correctly note that as there was not an absolute correlation between patients of groups 1 and 2 and that there was an absence of protective cells and antibodies respectively, other parameters are required to predict the risk of pneumonia in these patients. Furthermore, the vast majority of patients with X-linked hyper-IgM syndrome experience bacterial lower respiratory tract infections and have IgM memory B cells, implying that other factors are involved. Despite having IgM and memory IgM B cells, these patients may be unable to produce anti-PnPS immunoglobulin M (IgM) antibodies.

This study also neatly explains why patients with CVID, who are mostly pan-hypogammaglobulinaemic, suffer mainly with infections due to encapsulated organisms. Indeed, switched memory B cells were reduced in both group 1 and group 2, excluding a relevant protective function of this subset against encapsulated bacterial infections and supporting the author's hypothesis of the crucial role of the T-cell-independent antibody response of memory B cells.

Patients with CVID are treated with replacement immunoglobulin. Even when this therapy is instituted early during the course of the disease, these patients can still develop chronic lung disease and bronchiectasis. This may be in part due to the fact that the replacement immunoglobulin contains only IgG and not the IgM which seems to be critical for protection against lower respiratory bacterial infections. Measurement of these cells and antibodies in patients in CVID may allow the identification of patients at risk of recurrent lower respiratory infections and the institution of more aggressive therapeutic strategies.

Treatment with replacement immunoglobulin

Children and adults with primary antibody deficiencies gain quality of life by subcutaneous IgG self-infusions at home

Gardulf A, Nicolay U, Asensio O, *et al.* *J Allergy Clin Immunol* 2004; **114**: 936–42

BACKGROUND. Lifelong immunoglobulin replacement constitutes the mainstay therapy for a large number of paediatric and adult patients with primary antibody deficiencies (PAD). Little is known about the effect of the type of replacement administered on the patient's health-related quality of life (HRQOL) and treatment satisfaction. The authors investigated the effects on HRQOL and treatment satisfaction of switching from hospital-based IVIG to home-based subcutaneous immunoglobulin (SCIG) in a group of 15 paediatric and 22 adult patients. Questionnaires were completed at baseline (when still on IVIG) and at 6 and 10 months into SCIG therapy. The questionnaires comprised the Child Health Questionnaire-Parental Form 50 (children), the Short Form 36 (adults), a quality of life index and a questionnaire related to therapy preferences.

INTERPRETATION. Home-based SCIG therapy significantly improved several important aspects of HRQOL in both the children and the adults surveyed. In particular, children reported better health and improved school/social functioning on home-based SCIG and their parents experienced reduced emotional stress and limitations on personal time and family activities. Adults reported improved mental health and social functioning. Treatment satisfaction scores, as assessed by the quality of life index, also improved on home-based SCIG in both patient groups.

Comment

As data regarding self-reported outcomes in HRQOL and treatment satisfaction due to PAD and its replacement therapy are rare in adults and lacking in children and their families, this well-designed study provides important information about the impact that home-based SCIG has on both paediatric and adult patients. All the improvements in HRQOL and treatment satisfaction gained statistical significance despite the relatively small numbers, and any potential study-specific effects were controlled by including ten patients already established on SCIG in the home.

The authors proposed that some of the improvements in HRQOL and treatment satisfaction could have been due to the relatively stable serum IgG levels attained with weekly SCIG. This stabilization of IgG trough levels may eliminate the increased fatigue and decreased well-being in the week prior to their 3- or 4-weekly IVIG and the unphysiologically high serum IgG levels after IVIG that are suspected of triggering systemic side effects, such as the headache experienced by both patient groups.

The authors also rightly emphasize the effect of therapy in the home environment. For both adults and children, home therapy resulted in a reduced sense of being sick or disabled, and greater independence with less disruption of daily activities such as work, school, leisure and travel. Furthermore, home-based treatment resulted in reduced visits to hospital for children with PAD, with a decreased risk of acquiring infections. This not only contributed to improved health in the children with PAD, but may also have reduced parents' anxiety that their child may become ill with an infection.

Given the positive effects that SCIG itself and treatment in the home may have on HRQOL and treatment satisfaction, the authors concede that it is not possible to be sure which factor is responsible for the improvements observed. They report that the lack of improvement in HRQOL and treatment satisfaction observed in the control patients already established on home-based SCIG supports the argument that the changes can be attributed to the switch from hospital to home-based therapy. The reasoning behind this deduction seems far from clear.

Nevertheless, this study, along with others evaluating SCIG administration and demonstrating its safety, normalized serum IgG levels, protection against infection, patient preference for home therapy and ease of infusion, strongly supports the use of SCIG as an alternative to the intravenous route in adults and children with PAD.

Increased risk of adverse events when changing intravenous immunoglobulin preparations

Ameratunga R, Sinclair J, Kolbe J. *Clin Exp Immunol* 2004; **136**: 111–13

BACKGROUND. IVIG replacement therapy has been a significant advance in the management of patients with primary immunodeficiency, especially those with antibody deficiency. When high-quality IVIG preparations became available in the 1980s the restoration of physiological levels of IgG in the blood was realized. This was associated with a significant reduction in the mortality and morbidity experienced by patients with primary immunodeficiency. With the advent of new technologies comes the opportunity of improving on existing IVIG preparations, with a view to decreasing the chance of viral transmission and minimizing infusion reactions. This study examined the frequency of adverse effects associated with the introduction of a new IVIG preparation. Forty-nine patients receiving Intragam® were changed to Intragam® P without the knowledge of either the clinician or the patient. Intragam had been manufactured by Cohn fractionation of pooled human plasma followed by storage at pH 4.25 in 10% maltose. By contrast, Intragam P is prepared by delipidation of pooled plasma followed by an ion exchange chromatography step to eliminate immunoglobulin aggregates. It is then pasteurized for 10 h at 60°C for viral inactivation before storage at pH 4.25 in 10% maltose.

INTERPRETATION. The 49 patients were receiving IVIG for primary antibody deficiency. The initial preparation, Intragam, had an excellent safety record with no cases of hepatitis C transmission and very occasional serious adverse reaction. Any minor reaction responded well to pre-medication with paracetamol and antihistamines. Following the introduction of Intragam P, 7/49 patients spontaneously reported adverse reactions. All these patients had previously tolerated Intragam without any problem. The reactions included serum sickness, myalgia, fever, neuropathy, vomiting and angio-oedema. Following adjustments to the infusion regime, such as the use of pre-medication and reduction in the infusion rate, all patients were subsequently able to tolerate Intragam P. Given that the clinicians and patients were both unaware of the introduction of the new preparation, it is unlikely that there was biased perception and reporting of side effects. Furthermore, these adverse effects were not batch-related incidents.

Comment

This simple yet highly informative paper succinctly highlights the salient points regarding changing IVIG preparations. In this study, patients were changed from a well-tolerated established preparation to a new formulation from the same company containing fewer aggregates. It was hypothesized that this would result in less immune complex formation than the older preparation, resulting in fewer adverse effects. On the contrary, adverse reactions occurred upon switching to the newer preparation. The patient who suffered a serum-sickness-like reaction was managed with the concomitant administration of the old Intragam preparation, which alleviated the adverse effects of Intragam P. A possible explanation given is the solubilization of immune complexes by the Intragam.

The authors make some recommendations regarding the changing of IVIG preparations. Firstly, patients on home therapy should be given the first few infusions of a new preparation in hospital. The new preparation should be infused at a slower rate than the old preparation, which may allow the clearance of any immune complexes before the activation of effector pathways, and initially patients may benefit from pre-medication with antihistamines and paracetamol. Any changes made to the manufacturing process for replacement immunoglobulin should be communicated to the prescribing physician so that the necessary precautions can be taken. Finally, the authors stress the importance of effective pre- and post-marketing surveillance in the introduction of new IVIG products.

Although this paper is primarily concerned with IVIG, these findings are also relevant to subcutaneous preparations.

Conclusion

CVID is the commonest primary immunodeficiency that requires medical attention, and is an extremely heterogeneous disorder with protean manifestations, probably reflecting different aetiologies. In recent years a number of new primary immunodeficiencies have been identified which form part of the differential diagnosis. These include the defects reviewed in this chapter, but also the recently discovered causes of hyper-IgM syndrome, such as defects in activation-induced cytidine deaminase and uracil-N glycosylase [6]. Thus, CVID should now be considered a diagnosis of exclusion, and indeed a very recent publication has identified mutations in TACI (tumour necrosis factor receptor superfamily, member 13B) as causing CVID [7]. The decision that confronts clinicians faced with established and newly diagnosed patients with CVID is which patients should be screened for possible gene defects. Eastwood and colleagues' approach is most pragmatic; given the rarity of these diseases compared with CVID, screening for alternative diagnoses should be reserved for those patients with other features. In addition, most of the tests are not routinely available at present, rendering the task logistically difficult but not insurmountable. However, as more patients are identified with these defects the respective phenotypes will become apparent, directing future screening programmes. Identification of genetic causes for diseases also has implications for patients and their families.

Until relatively recently, CVID was considered a disorder of B cells. It rapidly became obvious that many patients exhibit T-cell abnormalities. Research into the pathogenesis of CVID has now travelled further upstream in the immune response and focuses on dendritic cells, the initiators of the immune response. Defects in TLR signalling that may mimic CVID certainly support the hypothesis that at least a proportion of CVID may be due to defects in the innate immune system. These experiments suggest interesting theories about CVID, but, given the heterogeneity of the disease, more useful information will be gleaned from so-called experiments of nature.

Replacement immunoglobulin has revolutionized the management of patients with primary antibody deficiency. In particular, IVIG allows high doses to be administered, with all the associated benefits. The advent of SCIG, with its ease of administration, permits more patients to receive therapy at home, which is compatible with a normal life and results in more physiological immunoglobulin levels. Thus, SCIG may replace IVIG as the first choice in patients. Overall, the last 18 months have seen a number of excellent studies that will ultimately improve the diagnosis, management and outlook for patients with antibody deficiency.

References

1. Chapel H, Geha R, Rosen F; IUIS PID (Primary Immunodeficiencies) Classification committee. Primary immunodeficiency diseases: an update. *Clin Exp Immunol* 2003; **132:** 9–15.

2. Seymour B, Miles J, Haeney M. Primary antibody deficiency and diagnostic delay. *J Clin Pathol* 2005; **58:** 546–7.

3. Bruton OC. A decade with agammaglobulinemia. *J Pediatr* 1962; **60**: 672–6.

4. Picard C, Puel A, Bonnet M, Ku CL, Bustamante J, Yang K, Soudais C, Dupuis S, Feinberg J, Fieschi C, Elbim C, Hitchcock R, Lammas D, Davies G, Al-Ghonaium A, Al-Rayes H, Al-Jumaah S, Al-Hajjar S, Al-Mohsen IZ, Frayha HH, Rucker R, Hawn TR, Aderem A, Tufenkeji H, Haraguchi S, Day NK, Good RA, Gougerot-Pocidalo MA, Ozinsky A, Casanova JL. Pyogenic bacterial infections in humans with IRAK-4 deficiency. *Science* 2003; **299**: 2076–9.

5. Doffinger R, Smahi A, Bessia C, Geissmann F, Feinberg J, Durandy A, Bodemer C, Kenwrick S, Dupuis-Girod S, Blanche S, Wood P, Rabia SH, Headon DJ, Overbeek PA, Le Deist F, Holland SM, Belani K, Kumararatne DS, Fischer A, Shapiro R, Conley ME, Reimund E, Kalhoff H, Abinun M, Munnich A, Israel A, Courtois G, Casanova JL. X-linked anhidrotic ectodermal dysplasia with immunodeficiency is caused by impaired NF-kappaB signaling. *Nat Genet* 2001; **27**: 277–85.

6. Durandy A, Revy P, Imai K, Fischer A. Hyper-immunoglobulin M syndromes caused by intrinsic B-lymphocyte defects. *Immunol Rev* 2005; **203**: 67–79.

7. Salzer U, Chapel HM, Webster AD, Pan-Hammarstrom Q, Schmitt-Graeff A, Schlesier M, Peter HH, Rockstroh JK, Schneider P, Schaffer AA, Hammarstrom L, Grimbacher B. Mutations in TNFRSF13B encoding TACI are associated with common variable immunodeficiency in humans. *Nat Genet* 2005; **37**: 820–8.

Part III

Treatment modalities for allergic diseases

10

Environment control

HASAN ARSHAD

Introduction

Asthma and allergic diseases are common in both children and adults. Their development depends on an interaction between genetic and environmental risk factors. Genetic manipulation in multifactorial diseases such as asthma is not feasible in the foreseeable future. However, theoretically, environmental exposures can be controlled in an attempt to stem the rising prevalence of these diseases (primary prevention). Environmental exposures may also influence the frequency of symptoms and the requirement for medication in those with established disease. Thus, avoidance of allergens and irritants should lead to better control of the disease, improved quality of life and reduced medication usage (secondary prevention).

Most allergic disorders have their origins in early life and environmental factors seem to have their maximum impact at this crucial period |**1**|. The proposed factors, both promoting and protecting allergy, include diet (such as antioxidants, omega-3 fatty acids), infections (viral or bacterial), allergens (foods, house dust mite [HDM], pollens, animals, moulds), pollutants (cigarette smoke, nitrogen dioxide [NO_2], ozone, etc.) and endotoxins.

Avoidance of exposure to food and aeroallergens in early life has been investigated in a number of studies. Breast-feeding protects against wheeze and possibly atopic dermatitis in childhood |**2,3**|, but its long-term preventive effect on asthma remains controversial |**4**|. Maternal dietary restriction during pregnancy, to protect the fetus against exposure to allergenic foods, has not been shown to have a protective effect |**5**|. However, similar avoidance during lactation might be of some benefit in children at high risk |**5**|. The use of hydrolysed formula, instead of cows' milk, has shown some protective effect against cows' milk allergy and atopic dermatitis |**6**|. Convincing evidence to support a preventive effect of avoidance of HDM allergen has not been forthcoming |**7**|. The benefit of omega-3 polyunsaturated fatty acids during pregnancy and lactation on the development of wheeze and atopy was minor in the first 18 months of follow-up in a randomized controlled trial |**8**|. There is some evidence that probiotics might be useful in preventing atopic dermatitis |**9**|. Exposure to environmental tobacco smoke is a recognized risk factor for the development of asthma. Randomized controlled trials

© Atlas Medical Publishing Ltd

(RCTs) are not possible, of course, but the evidence from observational studies is convincing [10,11]. The effect of outdoor pollutants in the development of asthma and allergy is not clear. However, the large number of potential risk factors and our inability to accurately predict the development of asthma and allergy has led to conflicting data from recent prevention studies [12].

Secondary prevention aims to achieve better control of disease parameters and improve the prognosis while reducing complications and the consequences of uncontrolled diseases. Apart from pharmacotherapy and immunotherapy, environment control should be an integral part of the management plan. Reduction in allergen exposure can indeed reduce asthma symptoms, the need for medication, and airway hyper-responsiveness. Avoidance of irritants, such as cigarette smoke, pollutants and strong perfumes, improves symptoms and quality of life. Occupational asthma and dermatitis is another area where the value of avoidance is well established. Measures to avoid exposure to HDM, specifically the use of impermeable mattress covers, are generally considered effective in reducing the level of mite allergens and improving asthma control [13]. However, two well-designed, randomized controlled studies failed to show any effect of allergen-impermeable bed covers in asthma and allergic rhinitis [14,15]. Thus, environment control methods should be improved and further research is needed to evaluate their efficacy and cost-effectiveness.

Environment control in primary prevention

Breast-feeding and allergy

The protective effect of breast-feeding on asthma and allergy has been debated for more than 60 years without any hope of a consensus. A major problem is the lack of RCTs. However, breast-feeding has a number of other benefits and should be recommended irrespective of any effect on asthma or allergy. This is why randomized trials are not considered ethical. Thus, we have to rely on observational studies, which have produced conflicting results. Mothers who do or do not breast-feed differ in several environmental exposures, including socio-economic class, smoking and area of living, which influence indoor and outdoor exposure to pollutants. Despite statistical adjustment for these confounding factors, the evidence is never as robust as it would be with an RCT. Two systemic reviews on this subject reached the conclusion that exclusive breast-feeding does seem to have some protective effect against the development of allergy [3,16].

Breast-feeding reduces the risk of asthma during the first 4 years of life

Kull I, Almqvist C, Lilja G, Pershagen G, Wickman M. *J Allergy Clin Immunol* 2004; **114**: 755–60

BACKGROUND. The evidence for a preventive effect of breast-feeding on asthma and other allergic diseases in childhood is inconclusive. The aim of this study was to investigate the effect of breast-feeding on asthma and sensitization to airborne allergens among children up to 4 years of age. A birth cohort of 4089 children was followed. Exposure data were collected at 2 months and 1 year of age. The total dose of breast milk was estimated by combining periods of exclusive and partial breast-feeding. Outcome data were collected at 1, 2 and 4 years of age. The response rate at 4 years was 90%, and 73% participated in a clinical investigation, including blood sampling for analysis of specific immunoglobulin E (IgE) and lung function testing.

INTERPRETATION. Exclusive breast-feeding for 4 months or more reduced the risk of asthma at the age of 4 years (odds ratio 0.72; 95% confidence interval [CI] 0.53–0.97). A duration of 3 months or more of partial breast-feeding seemed to offer additional protection; exclusive breast-feeding for 3–4 months combined with partial breast-feeding for 3 months or more resulted in an odds ratio of 0.44 (95% CI 0.21–0.87). The effects tended to be stronger in children without heredity for allergy (*P* interaction = 0.36). The authors concluded that breast-feeding reduces the risk of asthma during the first 4 years of life.

Comment

The strengths of this study include a large sample, prospective information on breast-feeding and the development of allergy, an excellent questionnaire response rate (90% at 4 years) and an acceptable proportion of children returning for further investigations (73%). The problems are that not all known confounding factors were adjusted for and the asthma diagnosis was based on a questionnaire definition.

The reduction in asthma for exclusive breast-feeding for 4 months or more was significant, with an additional protective effect of continued partial breast-feeding. However, it is difficult to diagnose asthma with certainty before the age of 4 years as diagnosis relies on a history of recurrent wheeze. The authors not only used a diagnostic label of asthma but they also attempted to phenotype this into early, persistent and late-onset asthma, which is not appropriate at the age of 4 years. This is early childhood wheezing, which was reduced, as has been suggested earlier in a meta-analysis [**2**]. Whether breast-feeding protects against asthma remains in doubt, as the outcome of longer-term follow-up studies is less promising. A follow-up of another large birth cohort from the Isle of Wight showed prevention of wheeze in early life by exclusive breast-feeding [**17**], but the effect was lost when these children were seen at 10 years and objective tests, such as lung function and bronchial challenge, were performed [**18**].

The mechanism of the protective effect of exclusive breast-feeding is not clear but it may involve a combination of the avoidance of highly allergenic foods, such as cows' milk and egg, the presence in the breast milk of immune modulators such as immunoglobulins, cytokines or omega-3 fatty acids, or alteration of the infant's intestinal microflora. A combined effect of reducing early exposure of the immune system to food allergens while increasing the exposure to intestinal bacteria and protecting infants from detrimental viral infections may result in the development of the immune system away from allergy-promoting Th2 responses.

House dust mite avoidance in primary prevention

To prevent the development of allergy, allergen avoidance has to be instituted before sensitization has occurred. The specific type of aeroallergens may vary depending on the climatic and economic situation. For example, HDM is the most important allergen in humid climates and pet allergens assume importance in cold countries, while cockroach allergen is the major sensitizing agent in crowded, inner city areas. Several large prospective studies have instituted HDM avoidance measures during pregnancy, at birth and later in childhood, and assessed children for asthma and allergic manifestations.

Effect of mite-impermeable mattress encasings and an educational package on the development of allergies in a multinational randomized, controlled birth-cohort study—24 months results of the Study of Prevention of Allergy in Children in Europe

Horak F Jr, Matthews S, Ihorst G, *et al.*; the SPACE Study Group. *Clin Exp Allergy* 2004; **34**: 1220–5

BACKGROUND. Sensitization to HDM is an important risk factor for the development of asthma and allergic disease in childhood. Higher levels of HDM allergen are linked to increased sensitization to HDM. The aim was to study the effect of mite-impermeable mattress encasings and an educational package on the development of allergies in a newborn cohort. Six hundred and ninety-six newborns at high risk of developing allergies were enrolled in three European countries (Germany, Austria and the UK) in a randomized, controlled birth-cohort study. Children were assigned to an intervention and a control group. Intervention measures included the use of mite-impermeable mattress encasings for the child's bed and a simple educational package on allergen avoidance. The control group received basic information about allergies. Children were followed up at the ages of 6, 12, 18 and 24 months.

INTERPRETATION. A total of 80.9% of the children were followed up to the age of 24 months. No difference between the control and the intervention group was found in the prevalence of sensitization to HDM (control versus intervention group: 8.4 vs 6.1%;

$P = 0.33$) or the development of symptoms or allergic diseases. In this study, HDM avoidance did not show a protective effect against the development of sensitization to HDM or symptomatic allergy in children at the age of 24 months.

Comment

The Study on the Prevention of Allergy in Children in Europe (SPACE) recruited three childhood cohorts (newborn infants, toddlers and schoolchildren) at high risk of developing sensitization to dust mite. This paper describes the effect of simple HDM avoidance measures (dust mite-impermeable covers and an educational package) in the newborn cohort. These measures were intended to be easily implemented, inexpensive, and socially acceptable in different countries and cultures. The primary aim was to reduce sensitization to HDM, which, it was hoped, would have an impact on the development of asthma and allergy. This was a well-designed RCT with an adequate sample size. There was a high level of compliance with the use of mattress covers, which were handed over to the parents. However, compliance with other environment measures, such as the removal of carpets, was variable as these were advised but not implemented by study personnel. The outcome was disappointing as no preventive effect was observed in either sensitization or allergic disease up to the age of 2 years (Table 10.1). A limitation of the study was that HDM allergen levels were not measured. Thus, it is not clear whether HDM levels were not reduced or whether a reduction in HDM level was achieved but had no effect on the development of allergy in the children.

Table 10.1 Sensitization and symptoms in the intervention and control groups in the first 24 months of life (cumulative prevalence)

	Control group		**Intervention group**		***P***
	(%)	**(*n*)**	**(%)**	**(*n*)**	
Sensitization to mites	8.4	311	6.1	330	0.33
Nocturnal cough	12.5	313	12.8	327	0.98
Recurrent wheezing	10.7	337	10.5	342	1.00
Asthma	3.6	334	5.3	340	0.38
Eczema	21.1	342	18.8	346	0.52
Rhinitis	28.3	315	25.6	328	0.51

Source: Horak *et al.* (2004).

Early life environmental control: effect on symptoms, sensitization, and lung function at age 3 years

Woodcock A, Lowe LA, Murray CS, *et al.*; NAC Manchester Asthma and Allergy Study Group. *Am J Respir Crit Care Med* 2004; **170**: 433–9

BACKGROUND. The authors investigated whether environmental control during pregnancy and early life affects sensitization and lung function at the age of 3 years. High-risk children (*n* = 251) were pre-natally randomized to stringent environmental control (active) or no intervention (control). Questionnaires, skin testing and IgE and specific airway resistance (sRaw) measurements were completed at the age of 3 years.

INTERPRETATION. Children in the active group were significantly more frequently sensitized compared with control subjects (at least one allergen by skin tests, risk ratio 1.61; 95% CI 1.02–2.55; $P = 0.04$; mite by IgE, risk ratio 2.85; 95% CI 1.02–7.97; $P = 0.05$). However, sRaw was significantly better in the active group (geometric mean [95% CI] 1.05 [1.01–1.10] vs 1.19 [1.13–1.25] kPa/s; $P < 0.0001$, active versus control). Maximal flow at functional residual capacity was measured using rapid thoracic compression at the age of 4 weeks in a subgroup. Prospective lung function data (at infancy and 3 years) were obtained in 32 children (14 active and 18 control). There was no difference in infant lung function between the groups, but at 3 years sRaw was significantly lower in the active group compared with the control children ($P = 0.003$). Stringent environmental control was associated with an increased risk of mite sensitization but better results for some measurements of lung function in high-risk children at the age of 3 years.

Comment

This study had several strengths. It was a randomized, controlled study with mothers recruited pre-natally, and intervention measures were employed during the last trimester of pregnancy and continued after birth. The environment control measures were comprehensive, including allergen-impermeable covers for the maternal and child's beds, a high-filtration vacuum cleaner, vinyl flooring, weekly hot washing of bed linen and washable soft toys. Mite and animal allergen levels were measured. In addition to questionnaire information, the skin-prick test was done and specific IgE levels and lung function were measured. The intervention failed to influence the development of allergic symptoms. Unfortunately, lung function could only be performed successfully in 50% of the participants, but showed significantly reduced sRaw in the active group.

The outcome of this study is puzzling. The allergen levels were reduced in the active group and yet sensitization was greater, particularly as determined by mite-specific IgE. It is hypothesized that low levels may induce sensitization, whereas higher levels induced tolerance. Alternatively, it is possible that stringent measures, as applied in this study, removed a protective factor such as endotoxins. However, the findings are contradictory to those of other intervention studies in which atopic sensitization was prevented or no difference was observed, with the reduction in allergen exposure [19,20]. The higher atopic sensitization in the active group did not, however, result in more allergic symptoms, as no difference was observed in asthma or atopic dermatitis between the two groups. Contrary to expectation, lung function was better in the active group by the age of 3 years, although, there was no difference in infancy. We can only hypothesize that the environment control may have altered exposures, either *in utero* or post-natally, to influence the development of the lungs in early childhood. It remains to be seen whether the deficit in lung function in the placebo group persists and translates into increased morbidity in later life.

Multifaceted intervention

In the primary prevention of atopy, avoidance of food allergens in early life has met with variable success and avoidance of HDM allergen has generally been disappointing. It has been suggested that a more comprehensive environmental intervention, involving both food and HDM allergen avoidance, would have greater success. Alternatively, combining allergen avoidance with another preventive strategy, such as dietary supplementation, may be useful. The first study, assessing the effect of a multifaceted environmental intervention, was the Isle of Wight primary prevention study. In this study, high-risk children avoided both food and HDM during the first year of life. A recent publication demonstrated reduction in both atopy and asthma up to the age of 8 years in children receiving intervention [19].

The Canadian Childhood Asthma Primary Prevention Study: outcomes at 7 years of age

Chan-Yeung M, Ferguson A, Watson W, *et al. J Allergy Clin Immunol* 2005; **116**: 49–55

BACKGROUND. Avoidance of any one of the individual risk factors associated with childhood asthma has not been successful in preventing its development. The purpose of this study was to determine the effectiveness of a multifaceted intervention programme for the primary prevention of asthma in high-risk infants at 7 years of age. Five hundred and forty-five high-risk infants with an immediate family history of asthma and allergies were prospectively randomized into intervention and control groups pre-natally. Intervention measures introduced before birth and during the first year of life included avoidance of house dust, pets and environmental tobacco smoke, and encouragement of breast-feeding with delayed introduction of solid foods. Assessment of outcomes at 7 years consisted of examination by paediatric allergists, bronchial hyper-responsiveness (BHR) using methacholine inhalation tests, and allergy skin tests.

Interpretation. At 7 years, 469 of the 545 children were contacted and 380 returned for further assessment. The prevalence of paediatric allergist-diagnosed asthma was significantly lower in the intervention group than in the control group (14.9 vs 23.0%; adjusted risk ratio 0.44; 95% CI 0.25–0.79). The prevalence of allergic rhinitis, atopic dermatitis, atopy (defined as a positive skin test reaction to any common allergen) and BHR were not significantly different between the two groups. In summary, the multifaceted intervention programme was effective in reducing the prevalence of asthma in high-risk children at 7 years of age.

Comment

This study used a multifaceted programme of intervention in at-risk infants during the first year of life. This included (i) breast-feeding, (ii) delayed introduction of solids, (iii) reduction of HDM allergen with mite-impermeable mattress covers and application of benzyl benzoate foam to carpets and soft furnishing, and (iv) measures to reduce pet allergen exposure and environmental tobacco smoke. Unfortunately, mite and pet allergens were not measured to assess objectively whether these environmental avoidances had an effect in reducing allergen exposure.

This study showed a reduction in asthma and wheeze, but not atopy, up to the age of 2 years [21]. At 7 years, 380 of the 545 subjects originally recruited (70%) attended for full assessment. This showed that there was a significant reduction in asthma but not in objective tests, i.e. atopy, lung function or BHR. As the intervention was not blinded, a reporting bias in symptoms by parents and children cannot be excluded. However, there was no effect on atopic dermatitis or allergic rhinitis; if there had been a reporting bias it would have been reflected in apparent reductions in other allergy symptoms. Secondly, the reduction in asthma, but not atopy or atopic dermatitis and allergic rhinitis, is consistent in previous follow-up reports of this study. The mechanism of reduction in asthma remains uncertain, as it does not seem to be related to IgE-mediated immune responses. To some extent, it is in line with the findings of Woodcock *et al.* (reviewed earlier in this chapter), who found an improvement in lung function but not atopy in the children receiving the intervention. Thus, it seems possible to reduce clinical manifestations of asthma with environmental control in early life without influencing atopy.

The PREVASC study: the clinical effect of a multifaceted educational intervention to prevent childhood asthma

Schonberger HJ, Dompeling E, Knottnerus JA, *et al.* *Eur Respir J* 2005; **25**: 660–70

Background. As asthma is the most common chronic disease in childhood, much attention is directed towards primary prevention. The clinical effectiveness of a multifaceted educational prevention programme was studied. A total of 476 high-risk children were recruited during the pre-natal period by general practitioners and

randomized to either (i) a control group, receiving usual care, or (ii) an intervention group, in which families received instruction from nurses on how to reduce exposure of newborns to mite, pet and food allergens, and passive smoking. A total of 443 infants were followed up for 2 years.

INTERPRETATION. At 2 years of age, the intervention group ($n = 222$) had less asthma-like symptoms, including wheezing, shortness of breath and night-time cough, than the control group ($n = 221$). No significant differences in total and specific IgE were found between the groups. During the first 2 years of life, the incidence of asthma-like symptoms was similar in the two groups. In conclusion, the intervention used in this study was not effective in reducing asthma-like symptoms in high-risk children during the first 2 years of life, although it was modestly effective at 2 years. Follow-up is necessary to confirm whether the intervention can actually prevent the development of asthma.

Comment

This randomized controlled trial included high-risk children (on the basis of family history of asthma), and a multifaceted environmental control programme was instituted. The environmental intervention consisted of reduction in exposure to mite, pet and food allergens and environment tobacco smoke, both pre- and post-natally. The HDM allergen avoidance measures were comprehensive and included mite-impermeable covers for bedding, hot washing of bed linen, removing textile floor coverings and reducing humidity from 3 months pre-natally up to the age of 2 years. Breast-feeding was recommended, and hydrolysed milk formula was provided as supplementation or after weaning, up to the age of 6 months. The measure taken to avoid pet allergens and smoking was simply the provision of appropriate advice. The environment control was successful in reducing the level of mite, cat and dog allergens in the intervention group (Fig. 10.1). However, this had no effect on sensitization to these allergens.

The main strength of this study is the prospective information available from the general practitioners' records throughout the 2 years of assessment, as the study was based in primary care. This highlights an important aspect of the follow-up of assessment in these studies. Prevalence at 2 years (point prevalence) of asthma-like symptoms was less in the intervention group at 2 years, and this study would have reported a positive outcome if the assessment had been confined to 2 years. However, when the prevalence of reported symptoms throughout the first 2 years of life was evaluated (period prevalence), no significant difference was observed. There could be several explanations for this discrepancy. Bias in reporting to the study physician is likely, especially as there was no difference in an objective measure—IgE levels. Alternatively, it is possible that the intervention had no effect on infantile wheeze during the first year of life, which may be aetiologically different, whereas a significant difference appeared by the age of 2 years. Further follow-up of this cohort would clarify this issue. Despite the negative outcome of intervention measures, exposure to mite and food allergens and tobacco smoke (independently of group allocation) was associated with asthma symptoms. Either the level of

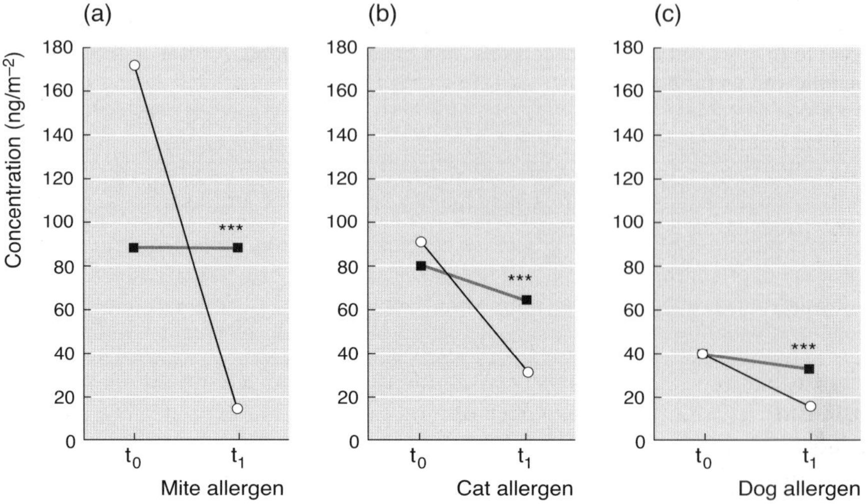

Fig. 10.1 Effectiveness of the Prevention of Asthma in Children (PREVASC) programme on exposure to mite and pet allergens. Median overall concentrations of (a) mite, (b) cat and (c) dog allergens in dust samples of living room, parental and infant mattresses at baseline (t0) and 1 year later (t1) for the intervention group (*circles*) and the control group (*squares*). ***, $P = 0.001$, intervention versus control group after the intervention (t1). Source: Schonberger *et al.* (2005).

reduction achieved in intervention studies is not enough or prenatal exposure, even before the third trimester of pregnancy, is important.

Three-year outcomes of dietary fatty acid modification and house dust mite reduction in the Childhood Asthma Prevention Study

Peat JK, Mihrshahi S, Kemp AS, *et al. J Allergy Clin Immunol* 2004; **114**: 807–13

BACKGROUND. Two factors thought to influence the risk of asthma are the promoting effect of sensitization to HDM and the preventive effect of increased omega-3 fatty acids. Although the avoidance of HDM allergen has been used as a preventive strategy in several trials, the effect of omega-3 fatty acid supplementation in the primary prevention of asthma and allergic disease is not known. This study was designed to assess the effects of dietary supplementation with omega-3 fatty acids and HDM allergen avoidance in children with a family history of asthma. A total of 616 children at high risk of asthma were enrolled antenatally in a randomized controlled trial, and 526 children remained in the trial at age 3 years. The outcomes were symptoms of allergic disease and allergen sensitization.

INTERPRETATION. There was a significant 10.0% (95% CI 3.7–16.4) reduction in the prevalence of cough in atopic children in the active diet group ($P = 0.003$; number needed to treat 10) but a negligible 1.1% (95% CI –7.1 to 9.5) reduction in cough among non-atopic children. There was a 7.2% (95% CI 10.11–14.3) reduction in sensitization to HDM in the active allergen avoidance group ($P = 0.05$; number needed to treat 14). No significant differences in wheeze were found with either intervention. These results suggest that the interventions, which were designed to be used in simple public health campaigns, may have a role in preventing the development of allergic sensitization and airway disease in early childhood.

Comment

Observational studies suggest that a higher intake of oily fish, rich in omega-3 fatty acids, protects against the development of asthma and allergy [22]. A possible mechanism for the protective effect of omega-3 fatty acids is its influence on arachidonic acid metabolism, resulting in reduction in inflammatory mediators such as prostaglandins and thromboxane. These authors evaluated the preventive effect of supplementation with omega-3 fatty acids and the avoidance of HDM allergen, a known risk factor for the development of asthma, in an RCT. This study was designed to assess the separate effects and combined effect of these two interventions. Pregnant women were randomized into four groups: (i) no intervention, i.e. placebo diet and no HDM avoidance; (ii) diet supplementation and no HDM avoidance; (iii) HDM avoidance with placebo diet; and (iv) diet supplementation and HDM avoidance. HDM avoidance measures included mite-impermeable bed covers and the use of acaricidal detergent. Dietary intervention included supplementation of the child's diet with 500 mg tuna fish oil capsules containing 184 mg omega-3 fatty acids and the provision of oils and spreads rich in omega-3 fatty acids. A preliminary report of the 18-month follow-up showed that avoidance of HDM did not have a protective effect, but children randomized to the diet group did benefit in terms of reduced prevalence of wheeze, although not atopy (skin-prick test and serum IgE) or asthma.

Children with diet supplementation had a higher level of omega-3 fatty acids, and those practising HDM avoidance measures showed a reduction in HDM allergen levels. However, there were no between-group differences in IgE levels or the prevalence of wheeze. There was a minor reduction in the occurrence of cough in the diet group and of HDM sensitization in the HDM avoidance group. There was no interaction effect. Although the study was reported as showing benefit, the outcome is disappointing. For example, 14 children were needed to avoid HDM allergen to prevent sensitization in one child and ten children should be given a dietary supplement of omega-3 fatty acid to prevent cough in one child. Moreover, combining the two interventions had no additive effect.

Environment control in secondary prevention

Environmental allergen control is one of the main goals of good asthma management. Patients with allergen sensitivities should receive practical advice on allergen avoidance. Such measures, when strictly applied for a sufficient period of time, can indeed reduce asthma symptoms, the need for medication, and BHR. Ongoing prospective trials in large numbers of patients are being conducted and should enhance our ability to make appropriate recommendations to patients.

Clinical effectiveness of a mite allergen-impermeable bed-covering system in asthmatic mite-sensitive patients

van den Bemt L, van Knapen L, de Vries MP, Jansen M, Cloosterman S, van Schayck CP. *J Allergy Clin Immunol* 2004; **114**: 858–62

BACKGROUND. Exposure to allergens plays a role in the development of BHR and in the chronic inflammatory response seen in asthmatic patients. Reduction of HDM allergens might lead to better lung function and reduction of asthma symptoms. In this RCT, the effect of HDM-impermeable covers on HDM allergen levels, peak flow values and asthma symptoms were measured. Fifty-two allergic asthmatic patients were randomly allocated to use the HDM-impermeable or placebo covers. During the study period, daily peak flow and asthma symptom scores were recorded. Dust samples were taken from the mattresses.

INTERPRETATION. There was a significant reduction in HDM allergen levels on the mattresses after encasing them with HDM-impermeable covers (reduction of 87% in Der p1 in μg/g of dust; $P < 0.001$). Baseline symptoms were so low that no improvement could be established. However, morning peak expiratory flow was significantly higher in the intervention group compared with that seen in the placebo group during the study period ($\beta = 20.2$; $P < 0.01$). The authors concluded that HDM-impermeable covers significantly decreased the level of HDM allergens with a consequent increase in morning peak flow. This study indicates that HDM allergen avoidance measures might have beneficial effects on allergen reduction and asthma outcome.

Comment

Inhalation of HDM allergen causes airway inflammation and BHR. Presuming that most exposure to HDM allergen occurs in bed during sleep, mite-impermeable covers are widely recommended for HDM-allergic asthmatic patients as an established environment control measure. However, RCTs have produced conflicting results. The studies have consistently shown that exposure to HDM allergen is reduced with the application of mite-impermeable mattress, bedding and pillow covers. However, this reduction does not seem to translate easily into clinically meaningful improvements in the symptoms of asthmatic patients, lung function or BHR. This study showed no improvement in the patients' symptoms, which the authors regarded as due to low levels of baseline symptoms, and thus further reduction was not easily achievable. However, other reasons might be the low level of sensitization to HDM of the study subjects and the small sample size, which may have produced false-negative results. The average morning peak flow was improved in the intervention group over the 9 weeks but repeated measures analysis failed to show an overall effect. This study was reported as showing a protective effect. However, as there was no effect on symptoms, evening peak flow or overall peak flow variability, lung function or medication use, it is difficult to accept that HDM avoidance measures led to a clinically meaningful improvement.

Effect of pet removal on pet allergic asthma

Shirai T, Matsui T, Suzuki K, Chida K. *Chest* 2005; **127**: 1565–71

BACKGROUND. Allergen avoidance has been recommended in the management of allergic asthma. Very few studies have assessed the effect of pet removal on pet-allergic asthma. The authors examined the effect of pet removal from homes on pulmonary function testing, BHR and medication use. This was a prospective, controlled but non-randomized and open study. Subjects included 20 symptomatic patients with newly diagnosed pet-allergic asthma who were keeping domestic animals, including hamsters, cats, dogs and ferrets, and were sensitized to these animals. They were treated with inhaled corticosteroids or other medications according to the recommendations, by level of severity, of the Global Initiative for Asthma. Methacholine inhalation tests were performed regularly before and after starting medication. Clinical features were compared between the patients who gave away their pets according to recommendations by the clinician (removal group) and the patients who refused to give away their pets (keeping group).

INTERPRETATION. There were ten patients in both the removal group and the keeping group. After 1 year or more of follow-up with or without pet removal, a 5.9-fold increase in the provocative concentration of methacholine causing a 20% fall in forced expiratory volume in 1 s (FEV_1) was observed in the removal group compared with a 2.3-fold increase in the keeping group ($P = 0.04$). There were no significant differences in the changes in FEV_1 and peak flow variability. No patient received inhaled corticosteroids in the removal group, whereas all but one of the patients needed beclomethasone dipropionate (mean dose 600 μg/day) in the keeping group. This study indicates that the removal of pets from homes reduces BHR in patients with pet-allergic asthma more than optimal pharmacotherapy alone, thereby enabling a decrease in inhaled corticosteroid doses.

Comment

Although the removal of a furry pet is often recommended as a common-sense measure in those with demonstrated allergy to these pets, there are no prospective studies confirming the beneficial effect of this recommendation. This small study is therefore important in providing evidence for a generally recommended environment control measure. Although, the sample size was small, the results are convincing as significant improvements were observed in BHR (Fig. 10.2) and the need for inhaled corticosteroid use. The limitations of this study included its non-randomized (patients chose to remove or keep pets) and non-blinded design, which may have introduced bias, and confounders may have influenced the outcome. However, randomized studies of pet removal are difficult and blindness is impossible in this context. Another limitation was that pet allergen levels were not measured to confirm a reduction in allergens following removal of pets.

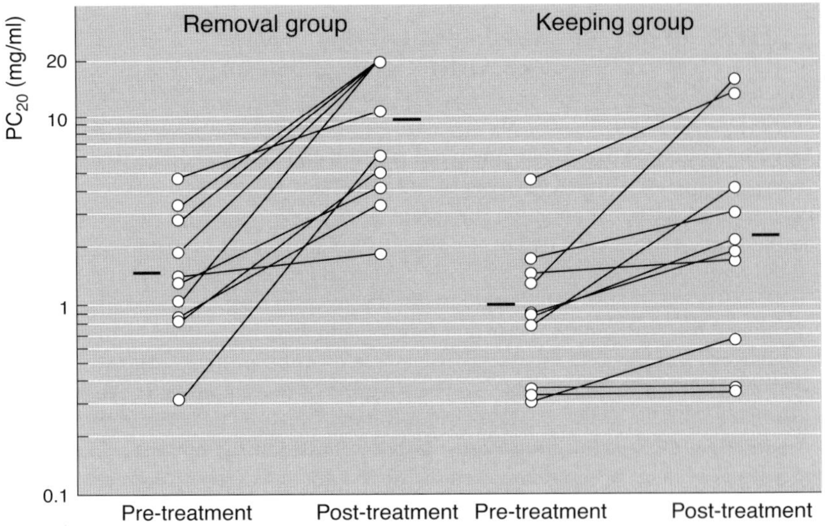

Fig. 10.2 Changes in airway responsiveness to methacholine (PC_{20}: the dose of methacholine that causes a 20% decrease in the patient's baseline FEV_1) in patients with pet allergic asthma in the removal group and the keeping group. Overall, a 5.9-fold increase in the PC_{20} was observed in the removal group in comparison with a 2.3-fold increase in the keeping group, which was statistically significant. Source: Shirai *et al.* (2005).

Results of a home-based environmental intervention among urban children with asthma

Morgan WJ, Crain EF, Gruchalla RS, *et al.*; Inner-City Asthma Study Group. *N Engl J Med* 2004; **351**: 1068–80

BACKGROUND. Children with asthma who live in the inner city are exposed to multiple indoor allergens and environmental tobacco smoke in their homes.

Reductions in these triggers of asthma have been difficult to achieve and have seldom been associated with decreased morbidity from asthma. The objective of this study was to determine whether an environmental intervention tailored to each child's allergic sensitization and environmental risk factors could improve asthma-related outcomes. The authors enrolled 937 children with atopic asthma (age 5–11 years) in seven major US cities in an RCT of an environmental intervention that lasted 1 year (intervention year) and included education and remediation for exposure to both allergens and environmental tobacco smoke. Home environmental exposures were assessed every 6 months and asthma-related complications were assessed every 2 months during the intervention and for 1 year after the intervention.

INTERPRETATION. For every 2-week period, the intervention group had fewer days with symptoms than did the control group, during both the intervention year (3.39 vs 4.20 days; $P<0.001$) and the subsequent year (2.62 vs 3.21 days; $P<0.001$) (Fig. 10.3), as well as greater declines in the levels of allergens at home, such as *Dermatophagoides farinae* (Der f1) allergen in the bed ($P<0.001$) and on the bedroom floor ($P=0.004$), *D. pteronyssinus* in the bed ($P=0.007$) and cockroach allergen on the bedroom floor ($P<0.001$). Reductions in the levels of cockroach allergen and dust-mite allergen (Der f1) on the bedroom floor were significantly correlated with reduced complications of asthma ($P<0.001$). Among inner-city children with atopic asthma, an individualized, home-based, comprehensive environmental intervention decreases

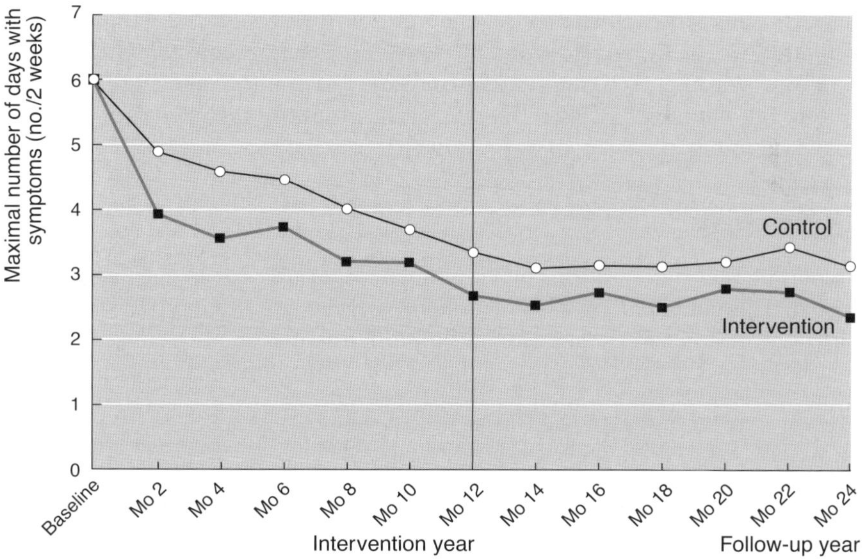

Fig. 10.3 Mean maximal number of days with symptoms for every 2-week period before a follow-up assessment during the 2 years of the study. The difference between the groups was significant in both the intervention year ($P<0.001$) and the follow-up year ($P<0.001$). Source: Morgan *et al.* (2004).

exposure to indoor allergens, including cockroach and dust-mite allergens, resulting in reduced asthma-associated morbidity.

Comment

Children residing in urban environments, often referred to as 'inner cities', suffer from high prevalence of asthma and associated morbidity. It has been suggested that the environment plays an important role in both the prevalence and the severity of asthma in socially deprived inner-city children. It has recently been shown that levels of allergens (mould, pet, cockroach and mouse) and pollutants are high in inner-city homes |**23**|. There have been very few intervention studies in children with asthma in inner cities aimed at improving the control of asthma.

This multicentre RCT, with nearly 1000 children, studied a multifaceted, home-based, environmental intervention to determine whether individualized intervention, tailored to each child's sensitization and risk profile, could improve asthma morbidity. The child's parents/caretakers were provided with the knowledge, motivation, skill, equipment and supplies for a comprehensive programme to reduce exposure to allergens (according to the child's sensitization) and environmental tobacco smoke. The active intervention was for 1 year and monitoring and follow-up continued for another 12 months. The intervention included allergen-impermeable covers, vacuum cleaners with a HEPA (high-efficiency particulate air filter, a HEPA air purifier and pest control for cockroach infestation. A significant reduction in allergen levels and consequent improvement in asthma symptoms and exacerbation was achieved. However, there was no effect on objective measures of peak flow or spirometry. This was an open study, and as improvement occurred in symptoms but not lung function a reporting bias cannot be excluded.

Conclusion

The report by Kull *et al.* confirms previous observations that breast-feeding protects against the development of early childhood wheeze. Another report from this cohort, published in 2005, suggested that atopic dermatitis was also reduced in those who were breast-fed for 4 months or longer |**24**|. Thus, breast-feeding, preferably exclusive, for 4–6 months should be an essential part of any preventative strategy to reduce allergic disease in early childhood. Those infants who are at high risk of atopy may be given hydrolysed formula milk if they are not breast-fed. The newborn cohort of the SPACE study, reported by Horak *et al.*, in which mite-impermeable mattress covers were the main intervention, failed to show any effect on the development of sensitization or allergy. A more comprehensive HDM allergen avoidance intervention by Woodcock *et al.* improved lung function at 3 years but not symptoms or atopic sensitization. The evidence to support a preventive effect of HDM allergen avoidance on the development of sensitization to HDM or respiratory allergy is not compelling. It may be that current methods of allergen reduction are not effective or that reduction in HDM allergen exposure alone is not sufficient. A multifaceted intervention that included breast-feeding, hydrolysed formula and HDM allergen avoidance reduced asthma but not atopic sensitization (Chan-Yeung *et al.*, reviewed above). Two other studies, using a multifaceted environment control intervention and/or dietary supplementation, failed to show a clinically meaningful benefit (Schonberger *et al.* and Peat *et al.*, reviewed above).

Environment control to reduce exposure to HDM allergen in the secondary prevention of asthma and allergy remains a contentious issue. The most commonly used intervention – bed covers – reduces the level of HDM allergen in dust but this may not be effective in reducing symptoms or improving lung function in asthma |**14**|. Studies showing a beneficial effect and those unable to find a benefit continue to appear in the literature. Improvement in morning peak flow, but not symptoms, was reported by van den Bemt *et al.* (reviewed above). If patients can be persuaded to remove their pets, it may result in significant benefits in terms of improvement in BHR and a reduction in the need for inhaled steroids (Shirai *et al.*, reviewed above). In an ideal situation, each subject's home should be assessed for environmental exposure so that an individualized environmental control programme can be instituted, which has been shown to be beneficial (Morgan *et al.*, reviewed above). In summary, allergen avoidance should remain an essential part of the management of allergic diseases.

References

1. Warner JO. The early life origins of asthma and related allergic disorders. *Arch Dis Child* 2004; **89**: 97–102.
2. Schoetzau A, Filipiak-Pittroff B, Franke K, Koletzko S, Von Berg A, Gruebl A, Bauer CP, Berdel D, Reinhardt D, Wichmann HE; German Infant Nutritional Intervention Study Group. Effect of exclusive breast-feeding and early solid food avoidance on the incidence of atopic dermatitis in high-risk infants at 1 year of age. *Pediatr Allergy Immunol* 2002; **13**: 234–42.
3. Gdalevich M, Mimouni D, Mimouni M. Breast-feeding and the risk of bronchial asthma in childhood: a systematic review with meta-analysis of prospective studies. *J Pediatr* 2001; **139**: 261–6.
4. Sears MR, Greene JM, Willan AR, Taylor DR, Flannery EM, Cowan JO, Herbison GP, Poulton R. Long term relation between breast-feeding and development of atopy and asthma in children and young adults: a longitudinal study. *Lancet* 2002; **360**: 901–7.
5. Kramer MS, Kakuma R. Maternal dietary antigen avoidance during pregnancy and/or lactation for preventing or treating atopic disease in the child. *Cochrane Database Syst Rev* 2003; (**4**): CD000133.

6. von Berg A, Koletzko S, Grubl A, Filipiak-Pittroff B, Wichmann HE, Bauer CP, Reinhardt D, Berdel D; German Infant Nutritional Intervention Study Group. The effect of hydrolyzed cow's milk formula for allergy prevention in the first year of life: the German Infant Nutritional Intervention Study, a randomized double-blind trial. *J Allergy Clin Immunol* 2003; **111**: 533–40.

7. Koopman LP, van Strien RT, Kerkhof M, Wijga A, Smit HA, de Jongste JC, Gerritsen J, Aalberse RC, Brunekreef B, Neijens HJ; Prevention and Incidence of Asthma and Mite Allergy (PIAMA) Study. Placebo-controlled trial of house dust mite-impermeable mattress covers: effect on symptoms in early childhood. *Am J Respir Crit Care Med* 2002; **166**: 307–13.

8. Mihrshahi S, Peat JK, Marks GB, Mellis CM, Tovey ER, Webb K, Britton WJ, Leeder SR; Childhood Asthma Prevention Study. Eighteen-month outcomes of house dust mite avoidance and dietary fatty acid modification in the Childhood Asthma Prevention Study (CAPS). *J Allergy Clin Immunol* 2003; **111**: 162–8.

9. Kalliomaki M, Salminen S, Poussa T, Arvilommi H, Isolauri E. Probiotics and prevention of atopic disease: 4-year follow-up of a randomised placebo-controlled trial. *Lancet* 2003; **361**: 1869–71.

10. Jaakkola JJ, Gissler M. Maternal smoking in pregnancy, fetal development, and childhood asthma. *Am J Public Health* 2004; **94**: 136–40.

11. Cook DG, Strachan DP. Health effects of passive smoking. 3. Parental smoking and prevalence of respiratory symptoms and asthma in school age children. *Thorax* 1997; **52**: 1081–94.

12. Arshad SH. Primary prevention of asthma and allergy. *J Allergy Clin Immunol* 2005; **116**: 3–14.

13. Halken S, Host A, Niklassen U, Hansen LG, Nielsen F, Pedersen S, Osterballe O, Veggerby C, Poulsen LK. Effect of mattress and pillow encasings on children with asthma and house dust mite allergy. *J Allergy Clin Immunol* 2003; **111**: 169–76.

14. Woodcock A, Forster L, Matthews E, Martin J, Letley L, Vickers M, Britton J, Strachan D, Howarth P, Altmann D, Frost C, Custovic A; Medical Research Council General Practice Research Framework. Control of exposure to mite allergen and allergen-impermeable bed covers for adults with asthma. *N Engl J Med* 2003; **349**: 225–36.

15. Terreehorst I, Hak E, Oosting AJ, Tempels-Pavlica Z, de Monchy JG, Bruijnzeel Koomen CA, Aalberse RC, Gerth van Wijk R. Evaluation of impermeable covers for bedding in patients with allergic rhinitis. *N Engl J Med* 2003; **349**: 237–46.

16. Mimouni Bloch A, Mimouni D, Mimouni M, Gdalevich M. Does breastfeeding protect against allergic rhinitis during childhood? A meta-analysis of prospective studies. *Acta Paediatr* 2002; **91**: 275–9.

17. Tariq S, Matthews S, Stevens M, Hakim E, Arshad SH. The prevalence of and risk factors for atopy in early childhood: a whole population birth cohort study. *J Allergy Clin Immunol* 1998; **101**: 587–93.

18. Arshad SH, Kurukulaaratchy RK, Fenn M, Matthews S. Early life risk factors for current wheeze, asthma and bronchial hyper-responsiveness at 10 years of age. *Chest* 2005; **127**: 502–8.

19. Arshad SH, Bateman B, Matthews SM. Primary prevention of asthma and atopy during childhood by allergen avoidance in infancy: a randomised controlled study. *Thorax* 2003; **58**: 489–93.

20. Brunekreef B, Smidt J, de Jongste J, Neijens H, Gerritsen J, Postma D, Aalberse R, Koopman L, Kerkhof M, Wilga A, van Strien R. The prevention and incidence of asthma and mite allergy (PIAMA) birth cohort study: design and first results. *Pediatr Allergy Immunol* 2002; **13**: 55–60.

21. Becker A, Watson W, Ferguson A, Dimich-Ward H, Chan-Yeung M. The Canadian asthma primary prevention study: outcomes at 2 years of age. *J Allergy Clin Immunol* 2004; **113**: 650–6.

22. Schwartz J, Weiss ST. Dietary factors and their relation to respiratory symptoms; the second National Health and Nutrition Examination Survey. *Am J Epidemiology* 1990; **132**: 67–76.

23. Brugge D, Vallarino J, Ascolillo L, Osgood ND, Steinbach S, Spengler J. Comparison of multiple environmental factors for asthmatic children in public housing. *Indoor Air* 2003; **13**: 18–27.

24. Kull I, Bohme M, Wahlgren CF, Nordvall L, Pershagen G, Wickman M. Breast-feeding reduces the risk for childhood eczema. *J Allergy Clin Immunol* 2005; **116**: 657–61.

11

Immunotherapy

ANTHONY WILLIAMS, RICHARD BARETTO,
MAMIDIPUDI T KRISHNA

Introduction

Specific immunotherapy (SIT) is an immunomodulatory treatment that is employed in the treatment of patients with allergic diseases, including patients with life-threatening allergic reactions to stinging insects and those with allergic rhinitis and/or allergic asthma. This treatment involves administration of specific allergen, commencing with a minute dose and gradually building up the dosage to a level that is therapeutically efficacious and which the patient is able to tolerate. Allergen is conventionally administered either subcutaneously (SCIT) or sublingually (SLIT). One of the concerns is the potential for inducing life-threatening allergic reactions following administration. The balance between the side effects of a treatment and its therapeutic potential are key to its acceptability and widespread use.

Studies published over the last decade have shown that systemic life-threatening reactions are rare when this treatment is delivered in a specialist centre and when patient selection criteria are carefully followed. Therapeutic advantages, in addition to symptom control, have been specifically ascribed to SIT when undertaken in children with rhinitis. Such studies have suggested that early treatment could block the development of asthma and prevent newer sensitizations [1,2]. Furthermore, in patients with summer hay fever due to grass pollen allergy, administration of SCIT for 3 years has been shown to induce symptomatic benefit for 3–5 years following treatment [3]. In patients undergoing venom immunotherapy (VIT), success rates of 95–100 and 75–80% have been reported for wasp and bee sting allergy respectively [4].

The precise mechanisms underlying the efficacy of SIT/VIT are unclear but studies have highlighted the role of immunoglobulin (Ig) G_4 allergen-specific blocking antibodies, skewing of the immune response to a Th1 phenotype, the development of allergen-specific regulatory T cells and the reduction of effector cells in the target organ [5].

Recent developments include an increasing number of studies investigating the safety and efficacy of SLIT in allergic rhinitis. In addition, new immunomodulatory

© Atlas Medical Publishing Ltd

treatments, including anti-IgE monoclonal antibody, peptide immunotherapy, CpG DNA vaccines and chimeric human allergen fusion proteins, are currently undergoing clinical trials.

In this chapter, we will review some important papers relating to the efficacy and safety of SIT and novel immunomodulatory therapies for allergic diseases published in 2004–2005.

Safety

Twelve-year survey of fatal reactions to allergen injections and skin testing: 1990–2001

Bernstein DI, Wanner M, Borish L, Liss GM; Immunotherapy Committee, American Academy of Allergy, Asthma and Immunology. *J Allergy Clin Immunol* 2004; **113**: 1129–36

BACKGROUND. Allergen immunotherapy has proven to be effective in the management of allergic disease and is the only treatment that is able to modify the natural course of the disease. Its wider applicability for the treatment of allergic disease has, in part, been limited by its perceived safety profile. This study follows up previous fatal reaction surveys undertaken in the USA for the periods 1959–1984 and 1985–1989.

INTERPRETATION. Survey returns concerning the occurrence of fatal (and near-fatal) immunotherapy reactions were received from approximately 25% of clinical entities in North America staffed with American Academy of Asthma, Allergy and Immunology (AAAAI) members. There were 41 fatal immunotherapy reactions over this period, with an estimate of 3.4 deaths per year, equating to one directly reported fatal reaction per 6 850 000 injections. Fatal immunotherapy reactions were estimated to have occurred in 1.7% of clinical practices over this time. Further details were collected on 17 of the 20 directly reported fatal reactions. Two of these occurred during home administration and 60% arose during maintenance treatment. In six of the patients a non-standardized allergen was used in formulating the extract. Fifteen of the 17 patients were receiving injections with a mixture of several allergens. No cases of concomitant β-blocker usage were recorded and only a single case was associated with a dosing error. In three cases the reaction started after 30 min of observation and 15 of the 17 fatal reactors had a diagnosis of asthma. Adrenaline was not administered to three of the 17 patients. The cause of death was recorded as upper airway oedema in five patients, asthma in six patients and shock in six patients. A single case of a skin-test fatality was identified. This occurred in a young woman with asthma and food allergy following the use of a scratch-test allergy panel to 90 allergens.

Comment

This study builds upon previous studies suggesting an incidence rate of fatal reactions of 1 in 2.5 million injections. Recent immunotherapy practice parameters suggest a waiting time of 20–30 min after injection but acknowledge that reactions may occur outside this time-frame, as demonstrated in this study. The timely administration (<5 min) of adrenaline was undertaken in only two-thirds of patients. However, the timely administration of intramuscular/ intravenous adrenaline was recorded in only one of the 17 cases (Table 11.1). Fatal reactions to immunotherapy, as practised in North America, appear to occur at approximately the same incidence as in the 1980s despite the adoption of recommendations to improve safety and some indirect evidence that these recommendations are being adhered to. Continued efforts to improve the safety of immunotherapy should be encouraged and the risk of fatal reactions should be considered to be extremely rare.

Immunotherapy safety: a prospective multicentric monitoring study of biologically standardised therapeutic vaccines for allergic diseases

Moreno C, Cuesta-Herranz J, Fernandez-Tavora L, Alvarez-Cuesta E. *Clin Exp Allergy* 2004; **34**: 527–31

BACKGROUND. The safety of immunotherapy has been a constraint on this form of treatment for allergic disease. Although retrospective survey studies of fatal reactions have been undertaken in North American practices, few European studies have been reported concerning fatal and non-fatal reactions to immunotherapy. Immunotherapy in Europe is normally undertaken with biologically standardized, commercially available single-allergen extracts. The authors of this study undertook a prospective multicentre evaluation of all systemic reactions to SCIT, graded according to the European Academy of Allergy and Clinical Immunology (EAACI) immunotherapy position paper, in adult patients with rhinitis and/or asthma over a 1-year period.

INTERPRETATION. A total of 423 patients completed the trial (488 entered) and 58 (11.9%) developed a local adverse reaction. Only 18 patients (3.7%) developed a systemic reaction. Only three patients (0.6%) developed a grade III reaction. There were no registered fatal reactions, anaphylactic shock or life-threatening occurrences after the administration of 17 526 injections. Of the 53 systemic reactions (0.3% of all doses), 36 were experienced by just five patients. Forty per cent of systemic reactions would have been prevented if all patients experiencing their third systemic reaction had been withdrawn. There was a higher frequency of systemic reactions in asthmatic patients than in non-asthmatic patients (0.46–0.06%; $P < 0.001$).

Comment

This study was limited to dust and pollen allergens in adult patients with rhinitis with or without asthma and thus represents the major group of individuals at

Table 11.1 Treatment of fatal reactions to immunotherapy injections

Patient	Administration site	Time from reaction to initiation of adrenaline	Initial dose of adrenaline	Total dose of adrenaline	Route administration of adrenaline	Cardiopulmonary resuscitation	Intubation attempted	Time of intubation after respiratory failure
1	Allergist	>30 min	2 mg	2 mg	IV	Yes	Yes	40 min
2	Allergist	Immediate terbutaline*	None	None	NA	Yes	Yes	Unknown
3	PCP	10–20 min	Unknown	Unknown	Unknown	Yes	Yes	Unknown
4	PCP	Unknown	Unknown	Unknown	IM, SL	Yes	Yes	Unknown
5	Home†	None	None	None	NA	Unknown	Unknown	Unknown
6	Allergist	Immediate	0.3–0.5 mg	Unknown	IM	Yes	Yes	25 min
7	Allergist	Immediate	0.3–0.5 mg	0.6 mg	Unknown	Yes	Yes	Unsuccessful
8	Allergist	0–3 min	0.3–0.5 mg	Unknown	SQ, IV	Yes	Yes	10 min
9	Work clinic	None	None	None	NA	Unknown	Unknown	Unknown
10	Allergist	Immediate	0.3 mg	0.6 mg	SQ	Yes	Yes	5 min
11	PCP	0–3 min	0.3–0.5 mg	1.2 mg	SQ	Yes	Yes	1 min
12	Allergist	Immediate	0.3–0.5 mg	Unknown	SQ	Yes	Yes	Unsuccessful
13	Allergist	Immediate	0.3–0.5 mg	0.9 mg	SQ	No	Yes	30 min
14	Allergist	Immediate	0.3–0.5 mg	0.6 mg	SQ, IV	Yes	Yes	Unsuccessful
15	Allergist	Immediate	0.3–0.5 mg	Unknown	SQ, IV, IT	Yes	Yes	3–5 min
16	Home†	Immediate	Unknown	Unknown	Unknown	Yes	Yes	Unknown
17	PCP	20–30 min	0.3–0.5 mg	0.6 mg	SQ	No	Yes	Unknown

IV, intravenous; NA, not applicable; PCP, primary care physician; IM, intramuscular; SL, sublingual; SQ, subcutaneous, IT, intratracheal.
*Terbutaline, 0.3–0.5 mg, administered subcutaneously in lieu of adrenaline.
†Injection administered in patient's home.
Source: Bernstein *et al.* (2004).

whom immunotherapy is targeted. Interestingly, most of the systemic reactions occurred during the maintenance phase of immunotherapy (35 vs 18). This feature should highlight the need for continued vigilance in the follow-up of patients after they have reached and been successfully maintained on the maximal dose of immunotherapy. The compliance to immunotherapy of over 80% and the systemic side-effect rate of about 4% are important measures for informing patients of the risks and benefits of this form of treatment in routine practice.

Post-marketing survey on the safety of sublingual immunotherapy in children below the age of 5 years

Rienzo VD, Minelli M, Musarra A, *et al. Clin Exp Allergy* 2005; **35**: 560–4

BACKGROUND. The increasing prevalence of allergic disease in the Western world has led to the concept of the 'allergic march' to describe the evolving spectrum of disease that often begins in childhood. The use of allergen immunotherapy in children has the potential of altering the natural course of allergic disease. However, concerns regarding the safety of using this treatment in children are an obstacle to attenuating the allergic march. The study of Di Rienzo and colleagues reviews the safety of SLIT in children between the ages of 3 and 5 years.

INTERPRETATION. A total of 126 children with a confirmed diagnosis of IgE-mediated allergy (60% rhinitis and asthma, 27% rhinitis only and 13% asthma only) were followed up for at least 2 years across four Italian centres. Immunotherapy was prescribed for allergies to mites (62%), grasses (22.2%), *Parietaria* (11.9%), *Alternaria* (2.4%) and olive (1.5%). SLIT was given in drops under the tongue, held there for 1–2 min and then swallowed. Most children were treated with a single relevant allergen, with maintenance given three times a week. The cumulative dose was 3.25–7 times greater than the equivalent SCIT dose. Thirty-nine thousand doses were given and side effects were reported in seven children (5.6% of patients and 2/10 000 doses). Mild oral itching occurred in two children and no action was needed. Abdominal pain occurred after 45 min in a third child and no action was needed. Two children manifested diarrhoea alone and two children diarrhoea and abdominal pain. These four patients were told to refrain from swallowing and to expel the antigen, and thus the problems disappeared without discontinuing the treatment. No side effects were recorded during the maintenance period.

Comment

Subcutaneous immunotherapy below the age of 5 years is considered a relative contraindication because of the difficulty in treating severe side effects, and the proven safety of alternative forms of immunotherapy in this age group is therefore to be welcomed. Previous studies have demonstrated the efficacy of SLIT in children, in particular its potential to prevent the development of asthma. The rate of side effects in this study, 7% per patient, was similar to those in previous surveys by this group. It is also noteworthy that the dosages used in this study were the same as dosages previously shown to be efficacious in *Parietaria* and grass allergy. The safety profile of SLIT in children of this age should encourage others to explore the therapeutic advantages of modulating allergy in this age group.

Efficacy

Efficacy of sublingual swallow immunotherapy in children with severe grass pollen allergic symptoms: a double-blind placebo-controlled study

Bufe A, Ziegler-Kirbach E, Stoeckmann E, *et al. Allergy* 2004; **59**: 498–504

BACKGROUND. The variables of patient subgroup selection and positive bias study reporting make it difficult to analyse the wider applicability of a new treatment modality. This study is important as it reviews the safety and efficacy of single-allergen SLIT in children with a mean age of 9 years who had severe seasonal rhinoconjunctivitis (with or without asthma) over a 3-year period. It highlights the requirement to view the results of each appropriately conducted study in the context of the study group under consideration.

INTERPRETATION. A total of 161 children were randomized during the first year to placebo or SLIT with a grass pollen extract. A sublingual–swallow delivery was undertaken over a build-up phase of 3 weeks and maintenance treatment was given daily thereafter. The cumulative dosage was approximately 10 times that of an equivalent 3-year SCIT regime. No statistically significant difference in the clinical index between the placebo and SLIT groups was seen after 1 year. Immunological changes – increases in specific IgG_1 and IgG_4 – were seen in the SLIT group after the first year, and subsequently in all children following the open study. A subgroup analysis showed a statistically significant improvement in the clinical index only after 3 years for the group of children with the most severe disease. Interestingly, in those who improved clinically there was no correlate of improvement in their skin-prick test responses. The symptom improvement amounted to a change of approximately 30% in the subgroup of 29 children.

Comment

This study highlights the importance of dissecting clinical variables within a study. The identification of a responder group only among the most severely affected individuals provides a note of caution for the adoption of widespread immunotherapy in individuals with disease of different severity scores, on the basis of positive studies reported in tertiary-centre trials of often severely affected individuals. In addition, the change in immunological parameters with SLIT are encouraging with regard to the potential benefit of such treatments in modulating the allergic march, but, notably, there appeared to be no correlation of this with any direct clinical symptomatic benefit. Finally, the benefits achieved with SLIT may take longer to develop, as seen with the 3-year time-point for efficacy identified in this trial.

Randomized controlled trial of high-dose sublingual immunotherapy to treat seasonal allergic rhinitis

Smith H, White P, Annila I, Polle J, Andre C, Frew A. *J Allergy Clin Immunol* 2004; **114**: 831–7

Background. Many immunotherapy studies are undertaken in tertiary hospital centres, which may select individuals with more severe or complex allergic disease. This study enrolled patients from a community setting and assessed the safety and efficacy of SLIT undertaken in a general practice setting.

Interpretation. Adult patients (aged 18–60 years) with seasonal grass pollen rhinitis poorly controlled with nasal steroids with or without antihistamines were enrolled in a double-blind placebo-controlled trial of 1 or 2 years of SLIT. The dose of allergen used was approximately 300 times the SCIT dose. Safety studies showed that 70% of actively treated and 44% of placebo-treated patients described at least one side effect. Buccal (oral itching) and nasal side effects were more frequent in SLIT-treated subjects. Only 14% of side effects occurred during the maintenance dose phase and all were within the actively treated group. Importantly, seven patients withdrew from the study during year 1 because of side effects and all were in the actively treated group. Four of these had systemic non-life-threatening reactions, including three with transient breathlessness and throat tightness. Efficacy was demonstrable only in subjects who had undertaken 2 years of treatment. This benefit was restricted to a reduction in rhinorrhoea and nasal sneezing.

Comment

In both this study and that of Bufe and colleagues, the placebo group showed a large improvement, illustrating the difficulty in assessing subjective symptoms and the impact of new treatments upon them within the context of allergic disease. The side effects noted were generally mild and well tolerated, supporting the potential of SLIT to be undertaken in a community setting, a feature that is less easily envisaged for SCIT. Future studies demonstrating a modest symptomatic improvement in individuals taking antihistamines and nasal steroids concurrently should perhaps also include an economic evaluation as well as assessments of safety and efficacy when deciding where and how such therapies should be introduced into new treatment programmes.

Effect of tree pollen specific, subcutaneous immunotherapy on the oral allergy syndrome to apple and hazelnut

Bucher X, Pichler WJ, Dahinden CA, Helbing A. *Allergy* 2004; **59**: 1272–6

BACKGROUND. Specific immunotherapy is a recognized specific treatment for pollen allergy, but for food allergy no equivalent treatment exists. Approximately 50% of individuals with tree pollen allergy experience symptoms following the ingestion of fresh fruits and vegetables, such as apple, cherry and hazelnut. This constellation of symptoms has been termed the 'oral allergy syndrome' and is believed to relate to cross-reactivity of IgE against epitopes in pollens and those found in certain fresh fruits and vegetables. Previous studies have shown improvement in these symptoms in monosensitized individuals following birch immunotherapy. This study analysed polysensitized individuals treated with tree pollen extract SCIT for sensitivity to apple and hazelnut after 18 months of treatment.

INTERPRETATION. Fifteen adults treated with birch pollen SCIT were compared with twelve control individuals who had the oral allergy syndrome. Following a mean duration of 18 months of treatment, ten of the 15 actively treated patients reported an improvement compared with two in the control group. All patients in the SCIT group reported an improvement in their respiratory symptoms during the pollen season. Objectively, there was no difference in the skin-prick test results between the two groups, whilst specific IgG_4 was significantly elevated only within the treatment group. In oral provocation studies, 87% of the treated group tolerated a significantly higher quantity of apple ($P < 0.001$) compared with only one in the control group. The average tolerated quantity increase from 12.6 to 32.6 g of apple.

Comment

This study highlights the relative efficacy of SCIT in influencing pollen-related food allergy. It also highlights the fact that in food allergy a successful outcome may relate more to a change in the dose of food that induces symptoms rather than to a cure of the food allergy. The relative effect in this study may relate to the polysensitized nature of the patients or to the underlying specific allergen component that characterized each patient and their cross-reactive potential. This study shows that immunotherapy for tree pollen allergy can have an impact on associated food allergy to apple, but this effect is limited and lacks any predictive pre-treatment phenotype in the patients.

Clinical efficacy of sublingual and subcutaneous birch pollen allergen-specific immunotherapy: a randomized, placebo-controlled, double-blind, double-dummy study

Khinchi MS, Poulsen LK, Carat F, Andre C, Hansen AB, Malling H-J. *Allergy* 2004; **59**: 45–53

BACKGROUND. The role of immunotherapy in the treatment of allergic disease is undisputed whilst the relative efficacy of SLIT compared with SCIT remains unresolved. This study was the first to compare the clinical efficacy and safety of SLIT and SCIT in a placebo-controlled, double-blind, double-dummy study.

INTERPRETATION. This 3-year study randomized 71 adult birch pollen-allergic patients with disease that was uncontrolled by conventional pharmacotherapy for at least 2 years. Clinical efficacy was assessed at the end of the first year in 19 patients treated with SCIT, 14 treated with SLIT and 19 given placebo. The cumulative dose of allergen was 175 times greater in the group given SLIT than in the group given SCIT. A statistically significant change in the rhinosinusitis score and medication usage was seen between each of the actively treated groups and the placebo group, but not between the two actively treated groups (Fig. 11.1). SLIT diminished the median disease severity to 50% and SCIT decreased it to 33%. Grade 2 adverse reactions occurred in all three groups, with no significant differences. Five systemic reactions of grade 3 and one grade 4 reaction were seen in the SCIT group and one grade 3 reaction in the placebo group. All reactions responded to rescue medications and there were no withdrawals secondary to these reactions.

Comment

This study fulfilled the criteria for a conclusive study and demonstrates that a clinically relevant amelioration of symptoms was obtained by both active treatments, with no significant difference between these two groups. However, this does not equate to there being no difference between the two treatments as the risk of a type-2 statistical error is notable because of the limited number of patients. SLIT has fewer significant side effects and this may become important if larger studies support the comparable clinical efficacies of the two treatments.

Sublingual immunotherapy for allergic rhinitis: systematic review and meta-analysis

Wilson DR, Torres Lima M, Durham SR. *Allergy* 2005; **60**: 4–12

BACKGROUND. Sublingual immunotherapy has been proposed as an alternative to SCIT. Whilst most allergists agree that this form of allergen immunotherapy has fewer significant side effects than SCIT and therefore has the potential of treating more patient groups, i.e. children, debate continues over its clinical efficacy compared with

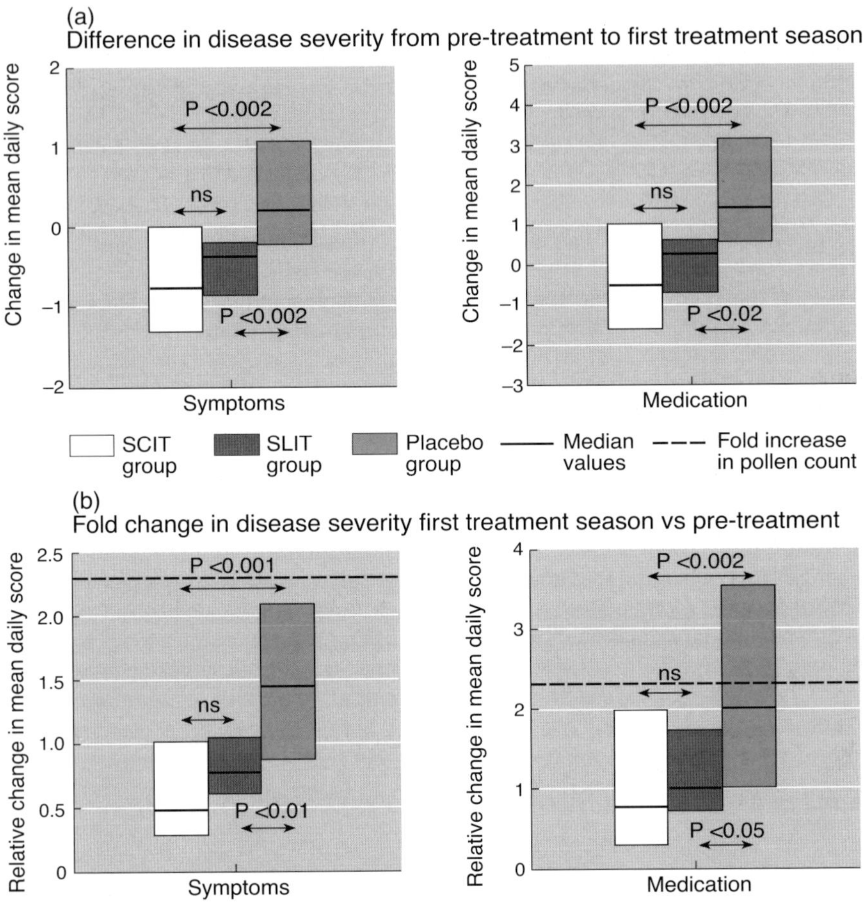

Fig. 11.1 Estimation of clinical efficacy by the subtraction method (a) and the ratio method (b) in the first treatment birch pollen season. The graphs indicate medians and 95% confidence intervals. Source: Khinchi *et al.* (2004).

SCIT. This article reviews the data on the clinical end-points of symptom scores and medication usage within the context of meta-analysis.

Interpretation. The trials included in this meta-analysis were collected from the Cochrane Controlled Clinical Trials Register, Medline and Scisearch. Twenty-two studies were included in the analysis, having met the entry criteria of being randomized, blinded, placebo-controlled trials, with data collected on symptom scores and medication usage in adults or children with confirmed allergic rhinitis. Within these studies, the range of allergens administered included house dust mite (6), grass (5), *Parietaria* (5), *Olea* (2), ragweed, cat, tree and *Cupressus* (each one). Seventeen studies used the sublingual–swallow method, three used the sublingual–spit method and two used sublingual tablets. Unfortunately, it was not possible to determine the dose of allergen administered (in micrograms of major allergen) in most of the trials. Analysis was performed by the method of standardized mean differences (SMD) with 95% confidence intervals. Data on 484 SLIT recipients were pooled and compared with data on 475 controls for their symptom scores. Significant effects of SLIT upon symptoms were found (SMD –0.42; $P = 0.002$). For medication scores, 405 SLIT patients were compared with 398 controls and a significant reduction in medication use was identified (SMD –0.43; $P = 0.00003$). Importantly, none of the studies reported significant side effects during the treatment.

Comment

Although such meta-analyses, especially in immunotherapy trials, are prone to heterogeneity between studies, such a review provides a framework for assessing a new treatment modality when clear end-points are defined. The overall statistically favourable response to SLIT is encouraging for future studies in well-defined, large cohorts prescribed specific doses of allergen immunotherapy to assess whether such treatment has a clinically relevant effect on symptoms and possible long-term modulating effects on asthma or new allergic sensitizations. The limitations of the review are clearly stated throughout the article and caution is needed in interpreting any subgroup analysis within this format of review.

Outcomes of allergy to insect stings in children, with and without venom immunotherapy

Golden DBK, Kagey-Sobotka A, Norman PS, Hamilton RG, Lichtenstein LM. *N Engl J Med* 2004; **351**: 668–74

BACKGROUND. Venom allergy is a recognized cause of anaphylaxis in sensitized individuals, sometimes leading to death. Venom immunotherapy is an established treatment for individuals identified as being at highest risk of venom-induced anaphylaxis in children and adults. This study asked whether there was any evidence that children could outgrow this allergy and whether venom immunotherapy in childhood had long-term benefits.

INTERPRETATION. A total of 1033 patients were initially contacted in a retrospective study and 50% agreed to complete the questionnaire. The mean age of the children at the time of their first reaction was 8 ± 3 years and the mean time to follow-up was 18 ± 5 years. The incidence of stings in this group over this time period was 43%. Within the children who had previously experienced a systemic reaction, a further systemic reaction occurred less frequently in the immunotherapy-treated group (2 of 64; 3%) compared with untreated children (19 of 111; 17%; $P = 0.007$). The incidence of systemic reactions in those children with only a previous local reaction was 7% (3 of 40) over this time period. Interestingly, the number of individuals with previous mild cutaneous reactions treated with VIT who subsequently experienced new systemic reactions did not differ significantly from the corresponding number among similar patients who did not receive VIT. However, a statistically significant increase in the percentage of individuals experiencing a further systemic reaction was identified between those who had previously had a moderate to severe reaction compared with those with a mild reaction, within the group not given immunotherapy. No deaths could be identified in the records of the 520 patients who responded to the questionnaire or in the National Death Index for those who did not respond.

Comment

This study shows that most children do outgrow their venom allergy but approximately 20% have a systemic reaction up to 32 years later. Additionally, the benefit of immunotherapy is long-lived, suggesting long-term modulatory effects of immunotherapy in children. The relapse rate of 5% amongst children (average duration of treatment, 3.5 years) is lower than the reported 15% in adults, suggesting that treatment may not need to be continued beyond 3–5 years. Importantly, this study confirms that the 60% of affected children with only mild reactions have a very low risk of subsequent reactions. The rate of systemic reactions in those with only local reactions was similar to previously reported values of 4–10%. The recommendation for venom immunotherapy to prevent future severe reactions only in children with moderate to severe reactions now appears to be based on evidence.

Vaccination with genetically engineered allergens prevents progression of allergic disease

Niederberger N, Horak F, Vrtala S, *et al. Proc Natl Acad Sci USA* 2004; **101** (Suppl 2): 14677–82

Background. Immunotherapy is an effective treatment for allergic disease. It is the only treatment modality that is able to modify the natural course of the disease. Current difficulties in immunotherapy relate to its safety profile and specificity for the dominant allergen in different individuals. The authors of this paper attempted to overcome the safety and specificity limitations of SCIT by using a recombinant, genetically modified birch pollen allergen (Bet v1) vaccine on individuals previously shown to have IgE reactivity to recombinant Bet v1 allergen by component-resolved diagnostics.

Interpretation. This study of 124 patients in a double-blind, placebo-controlled trial set out to establish the mechanisms underlying vaccination with genetically modified allergens. Within the actively treated group, significant elevations of IgG_1, IgG_2 and IgG_4 were seen in those treated with either the recombinant trimer or Betv1 fragments. This response was qualitatively different from responses to previous SCIT practices in which IgG_4 has been induced, suggesting that genetically modified allergen immunotherapy establishes a greater Th1 effect than those achieved by natural allergen extract vaccines. Common epitopes were shown in food allergens associated with the oral allergy syndrome. Importantly, the therapy-induced antibodies were shown to inhibit basophil histamine release approximately 10-fold following pre-seasonal treatment. This treatment was able to reduce the IgE boosting of memory responses to pollen that normally occurs during the seasonal exposure.

Comment

This was the first clinical trial of a genetically engineered recombinant allergen vaccine for the treatment of allergic disease. The study convincingly showed the nature of the immunological responses induced by this form of vaccination. However, information on the extent of any clinical response was, surprisingly, absent from the report and the assertion that allergic disease progression is prevented is not substantiated by this mechanistic study. This first study will now allow the clinically relevant end-points of safety and efficacy to be analysed within subsequent larger studies.

Newer approaches

Construction of hevein (Hev b 6.02) with reduced allergenicity for immunotherapy of latex allergy by comutation of six amino acid residues on the conformational IgE epitopes

Karisola P, Mikkola J, Kalkkinen N, *et al. J Immunol* 2004; **172**: 2621–8

BACKGROUND. Certain allergen-driven diseases are not suitable for immunotherapy because of safety concerns regarding their administration to sensitized patients. Latex allergy is one such condition which is becoming more prevalent and for which no specific treatment exists. This study attempts to define regions on the major latex allergen hevein (Hev b 6.02) that contribute to IgE reactivity and to modify these without disrupting the conformation of the protein, so that such a hypo-allergenic variant may be used in subsequent immunotherapy trials of latex-allergic patients.

INTERPRETATION. Single-nucleotide substitutions were established in the hevein gene by site-directed mutagenesis following a bioinformatic approach with sequence alignment of hevein-like proteins, NMR (nuclear magnetic resonance) structure and position-specific rotamer analysis. Inhibition ELISA (enzyme-linked immunosorbent assay) using sera from 26 latex-allergic patients identified six single-residue mutants able to reduce IgE binding by 80% in over 25% of the patients. Combinatorial mutants with different combinations of these six single-residue changes were then constructed and analysed. The most consistent and strongest inhibition of IgE binding was obtained with a mutant containing all six mutations. Follow-up skin testing in four patients showed that this combinatorial mutant abrogated skin-prick test reactivity in all patients.

Comment

This is an important study for demonstrating one of the current approaches to engineering hypo-allergenic vaccines in clinical settings where immunotherapy may lead to anaphylactic side effects. Previous studies have looked at the use of deletion mutants, protein fragments and linear epitopes for aeroallergens. This study has furthered previous work on the natural rubber latex allergen hevein. Through an informed and directed mutagenesis approach they identify single-residue hevein mutants that have reduced IgE reactivity. A combinatorial approach leads to a hevein protein that is hypo-allergenic by skin-prick testing in latex-allergic patients. Such recombinant, engineered, hypo-allergenic proteins may then become candidates for immunotherapy trials in allergic patients.

The co-seasonal application of anti-IgE after pre-seasonal specific immunotherapy decreases ocular and nasal symptom scores and rescue medication use in grass pollen allergic children

Rolinck-Werninghaus C, Hamelmann E, Keil T, *et al.*; Omalizumab Rhinitis Study Group. *Allergy* 2004; **59**: 973–9

BACKGROUND. The recent introduction of novel drugs for the management of allergic disease necessitates the integration of such approaches with conventional treatments to assess whether there are any efficacy or safety benefits to be gained with these agents. Anti-IgE monoclonal antibody treatment is one such example. This study analyses the effect of this new therapy alone or with SCIT in the treatment of grass pollen rhinosinusitis.

INTERPRETATION. This prospective, randomized, double-blind, placebo-controlled, multicentre study compared the efficacy of pre-seasonal grass pollen immunotherapy alone or in combination with anti-IgE therapy against monotherapy with anti-IgE or allergen-irrelevant SCIT, in mild to moderately symptomatic subjects between the ages of 6 and 17. The only statistically effective therapies in this study were anti-IgE monotherapy and combined SCIT and anti-IgE treatment. Surprisingly, pre-seasonal SCIT monotherapy was not effective within the first season after treatment. Combination treatment reduced the proportion of days with rescue medication by 90% and led to the absence of ocular symptoms in 27% of patients.

Comment

This study was the first comparative clinical study of SCIT and anti-IgE therapy in mild to moderate grass pollen allergy of children/young adults. It is important because it highlights the different effects of such treatments in the first season of treatment. The failure of SCIT to produce a clinically relevant response in the first year has been noted previously, especially in patients of a milder phenotype and when pollen levels are generally lower. However, the additive effect of SCIT with respect to the anti-IgE therapy suggests that beneficial effects of SCIT can even be achieved in these circumstances when IgE-mediated processes are suppressed. This study also includes some information on the economics of treatment, recognizing that this combination treatment is an expensive approach to a common condition that may have important consequences for health economies. The average cost of combination treatment over a 24-week period was €9196 compared with €425 for SCIT alone or €8771 for anti-IgE monotherapy. For polysensitized individuals or those with food or latex allergy, where SCIT is either unsafe or ineffective, such costs may have to be accepted if this form of combination treatment is shown to overcome these current barriers of efficacy and safety.

A chimeric human–cat fusion protein blocks cat-induced allergy

Zhu D, Kepley CL, Zhang K, Terada T, Yamada T, Saxon A. *Nat Med* 2005; **11**: 446–9

BACKGROUND. The specific treatment of allergy has previously relied upon allergen avoidance and immunotherapy. These approaches have been used predominantly in venom and aero-allergen-driven disease when previous food allergy immunotherapy has been unsuccessful. Emerging complementary treatments for allergic disease have recently included anti-IgE therapy and engineered allergen immunotherapy to reduce side effects or improve specificity. This study describes a novel approach to specific immunotherapy using a chimeric IgG–allergen protein to engage the inhibitory FcγRIIb receptor on basophils and mast cells in addition to specific IgE, to block allergen-induced signalling.

INTERPRETATION. The cDNA for a Fel d1 construct containing both chain 1 and chain 2 was cloned next to the CH3γ domain of a human IgGγ1 constant region through a glycine/serine linker. This chimeric fusion protein was expressed and shown to bind to both FcγRIIb on basophils and IgE from cat-allergic patient sera. The fusion protein was shown to inhibit Fel d1-mediated histamine release from sensitized human basophils in a dose-dependent manner. This inhibition was concurrent with the inhibition of tyrosine phosphorylation of Syk (splenic tyrosine kinase) and ERK (extracellular signal regulated kinase) that normally follows binding of Fel-d1 to IgE. The fusion protein blocked *in vivo* reactivity in FcεRIα-transgenic mice passively sensitized with IgE and in mice actively sensitized against Fel d1 (Fig. 11.2). Importantly, no histamine release was induced by the fusion protein.

Comment

This study describes a new approach to the modulation of allergen-specific disease. The use of a chimeric molecule that engages both 'stimulatory'-specific IgE and an inhibitory IgG receptor to inhibit the signalling pathway of mast cells and basophils provides a rationale for targeting other allergens in this manner. The inclusion of both the allergen that may lead to a protective immune response, as seen with

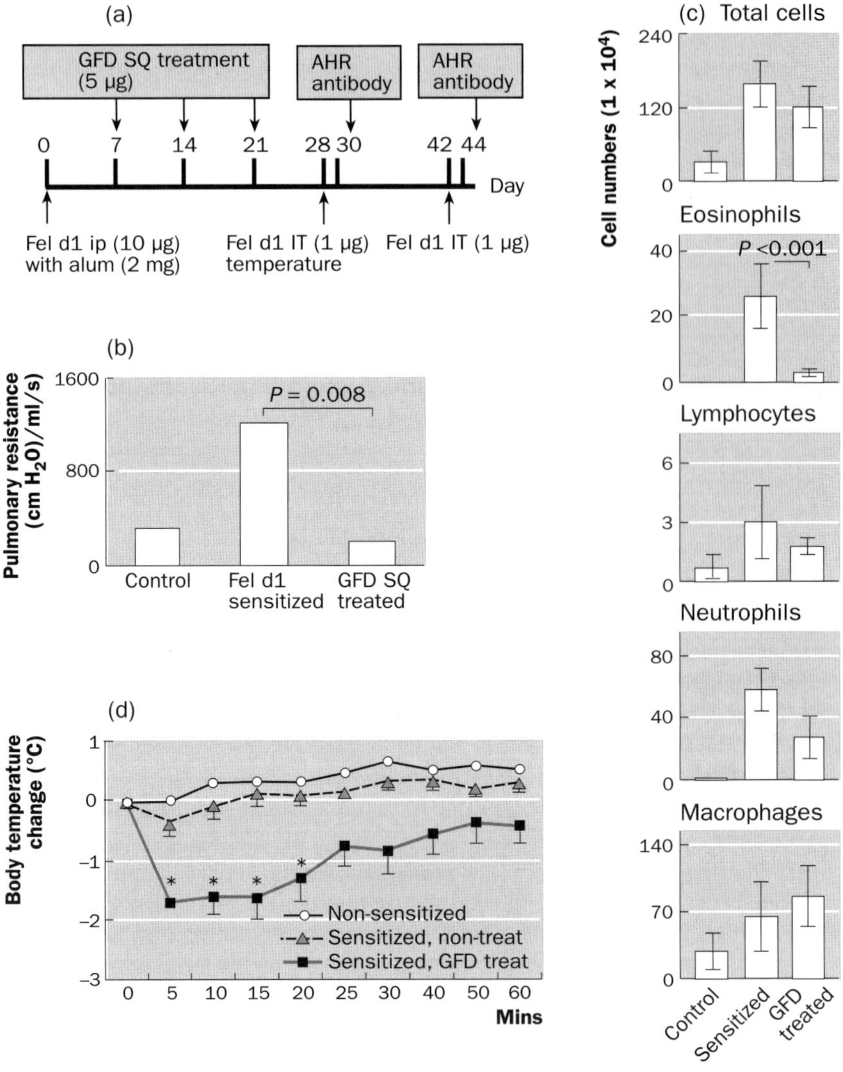

Fig. 11.2 GFD (Human IgG Fel d1 fusion protein) blocks the Fel d1-induced allergic response in mice. (a) Schematic diagram of the experimental protocol. (b) Inhibitory effect of GFD on Fel d1-induced airway hyper-responsivesness (AHR). The numbers represent the average values from three measurements of airway resistance.
(c) Inhibitory effect of GFD Fel d1-induced pulmonary eosinophilic inflammation. Total and differential numbers of bronchoalveolar lavage fluid cells were counted. (d) Inhibitory effect of GFD on Fel d1-induced systemic allergic reactivity, evidenced as core body temperature. Changes in core body temperature were measured at 5-min intervals immediately after Fel d1 challenge. *Statistically significant difference between the two conditions, $P < 0.05$. Source: Zhu *et al.* (2005).

standard immunotherapy regimes, and an inhibitory component to counter allergen-induced side effects may provide a safer treatment for allergies such as those to food and latex, which have so far precluded successful immunotherapy approaches.

Conclusion

There is little doubt that specific allergen immunotherapy is effective in the treatment of allergic rhinitis due to seasonal allergens such as grass and tree pollens and house dust mite and allergy to cat dander. VIT is the only treatment currently available for the prevention of life-threatening bee and wasp sting allergy. Although there is some evidence from recent studies that early institution of immunotherapy may halt the progression to asthma and the development of newer sensitizations, further studies are required to confirm this.

Studies addressing the safety of immunotherapy suggest that life-threatening reactions occur rarely and that the benefits clearly outweigh such small risks. It is prudent to assess each patient carefully and to ensure that patients with uncontrolled asthma are not enrolled into such programmes unless they have suffered from severe allergic reactions to insect stings, when a different approach must be used for patient selection. It is important that SCIT is carried out by well-trained and experienced staff and that appropriate recommendations are adopted to minimize the likelihood of a severe adverse reaction.

SCIT and SLIT are currently licensed treatments for allergic rhinitis due to pollen and dust mite sensitivity. Recent studies have clearly demonstrated that SLIT is effective and safe and that it can be self-administered by patients at home (i.e. without medical supervision). Anti-IgE monoclonal antibody has been shown to be effective in seasonal allergic rhinitis and the combination of this with SCIT seems to exert a synergistic influence, albeit at a cost. Novel approaches, including the modification of allergens to make them less allergenic whilst preserving immunogenicity, CpG DNA vaccines, peptide immunotherapy and chimeric fusion proteins, are potentially safer approaches that may now be tested in clinical trials for efficacy and long-term benefits.

References

1. Di Rienzo V, Marcucci F, Puccinelli P, Parmiani S, Frati F, Sensi L, Canonica GW, Passalacqua G. Long-lasting effect of sublingual immunotherapy in children with asthma due to house dust mites: a ten-year prospective study. *Clin Exp Allergy* 2003; **33**:

206–10.

2. Purello-D'Ambrosio F, Gangemi S, Merendino RA, Isola S, Puccinelli P, Parmiani S, Ricciardi L. Prevention of new sensitizations in monosensitized subjects submitted to specific immunotherapy or not: a retrospective study. *Clin Exp Allergy* 2001; **31**: 1295–302.
3. Durham SR, Walker SM, Varga EM, Jacobson MR, O'Brien F, Noble W, Till SJ, Hamid QA, Nouri-Aria KT. Long-term clinical efficacy of grass-pollen immunotherapy. *N Engl J Med* 1999; **341**: 468–75.
4. Sturm G, Krank B, Rudolf C, Aberer W. Rush Hymenoptera venom immunotherapy: a safe and practical protocol for high-risk patients. *J Allergy Clin Immunol* 2002; **110**: 928–33.
5. Till FJ, Francis JN, Nouri-Aria K, Durham SR. Mechanisms of immunotherapy. *J Allergy Clin Immunol* 2004; **113**: 1025–34.

12

Bronchodilators including phosphodiesterase-4 inhibitors

BRETT PEREIRA

Introduction

Asthma is a chronic inflammation of the airways caused by environmental factors in genetically predisposed individuals. Episodic airway obstruction and reversible bronchial hyper-responsiveness to non-specific irritants are the hallmarks of this disease, the prevalence of which has increased worldwide despite advances in therapy.

Most asthmatic patients are atopic, i.e. they have a genetic predisposition to produce high levels of immunoglobulin E (IgE) against environmental antigens and to mount an allergic inflammatory response. Inflammation is indeed central in the pathogenesis of asthma and there is a consensus that every patient with persistent asthma, regardless of disease severity, should use a daily controller medication. The main classes of drugs for asthma consist of: (i) bronchodilators—long-acting β_2-agonists (LABAs), anticholinergic agents and theophylline and its derivatives; and (ii) anti-inflammatory agents—corticosteroids, antileukotrienes, cromones and anti-IgE. Inhaled corticosteroids are by far the most effective treatment available for the control of asthma. However, concerns regarding long-term administration and steroid resistance have encouraged the search for new asthma therapies.

Bronchodilators that relax airway smooth muscle are often needed for the relief of acute symptoms in asthma. β_2-agonists, one of the oldest classes of drugs used in medicine, act by mimicking the effects of adrenaline. They bind to specific receptors expressed along the surface of the bronchial smooth muscle cells. This binding activates a cascade of events that elevates cyclic adenosine monophosphate (AMP) levels, leading to a decrease in intracellular calcium, smooth muscle relaxation and bronchodilation.

The β_2-agonists, including salbutamol, terbutaline, fenoterol, reproterol, are effective in producing rapid reversal of bronchoconstriction. Although terbutaline and salbutamol are widely used, they have a relatively short duration of action. Whether taken by inhalation or by mouth, the duration of bronchodilation achieved with a single dose of either drug does not exceed 4–6 h. This imposes limitations for patients who require continuing bronchodilator therapy to reverse airway narrowing

© Atlas Medical Publishing Ltd

and long-term protection from bronchospasm, such as patients with nocturnal asthma. Long-acting versions, including salmeterol and formoterol, have been found to be of benefit in producing bronchodilation that lasts more than 12 h. Compared with salmeterol and salbutamol, formoterol is a full agonist at the β_2 receptor; it produces more than 80% of maximal β_2-receptor activation and also has a rapid onset of action [1]. Compared with formoterol, salmeterol is a partial agonist at the β_2 receptor and does not result in maximal bronchodilation [2]; hence it is appropriate for use as a regular LABA but not for rapid reversion of airflow obstruction or for treatment of acute symptoms of asthma. Studies with the longer-acting β_2-agonists (formoterol 12 μg twice daily and salmeterol 50 μg twice daily) have shown that both improve lung function and increase overall asthma control when used regularly in combination with an inhaled corticosteroid (ICS). Regular use of these agents has also been shown to reduce the ICS dose requirement and hence the potential for side effects associated with prolonged high-dose ICS therapy [3].

Treatment with combination inhalers containing a corticosteroid and an LABA is becoming the gold standard therapy for asthma. There have been concerns regarding the safety of β_2-agonists, especially when used alone (i.e. without concomitant ICS) and also regarding tachyphylaxis to the bronchoprotective and the bronchodilator activity [4]. The latter occurs with all β_2-agonists, although this can be attenuated with corticosteroid therapy. The significance of such tachyphylaxis has been much debated and concerns have arisen recently over tolerance to regular long-acting β_2-agonist therapy. Two Cochrane systematic reviews have found that LABAs are more effective than regular short-acting β_2-agonists, and are as effective as theophylline with fewer side effects [5]. β_2-agonists have played a significant role in the treatment of asthma since they were first introduced nearly half a century ago. They have shown a continuous evolution, with compounds offering progressively increasing selectivity, combined with faster onset and longer duration of action.

β_2-agonists, including long-acting β agonists

Tachyphylaxis to LABA

Rapid onset of tolerance to beta-agonist bronchodilation

Haney S, Hancox RJ. *Respir Med* 2005; **99**: 566–71

BACKGROUND. Regular use of β-agonists has been known to lead to tolerance to their bronchodilator effects. It is not known how quickly tolerance develops or how long it lasts after stopping β-agonist therapy.

INTERPRETATION. Bronchodilator tolerance occurs after even a single dose and reaches a maximum after 1 week of regular formoterol. Sensitivity recovers 3 days after stopping treatment.

Comment

Regular use of β-adrenergic drugs may result in a reduction in the protective effect afforded by these bronchodilators against bronchoconstrictor stimuli. Tachyphylaxis to the effect of LABA has been shown to occur after regular use of formoterol in exercise-induced bronchospasm [6].

In this study ten subjects with stable asthma were followed for 2 weeks without β-agonists and after baseline methacholine challenge. The response to inhaled salbutamol (100, 100, 200 μg at 5-min intervals) was then measured. This procedure was repeated 24 h after one dose and 24 h after 3, 7 and 14 days of inhaled formoterol 12 μg twice daily, and 3 and 5 days after formoterol was discontinued. The use of β-agonists was not permitted in the intervals between testing. Bronchodilator tolerance, assessed by a reduction in the area under the salbutamol dose–response curve, occurred after one dose of formoterol (28% reduction; 95% confidence interval [CI] 12–45%), increased up to 1 week and plateaued between 1 and 2 weeks (58% reduction; 95% CI 38–78%). Three days after stopping formoterol, the response to salbutamol was similar to baseline. The first dose of formoterol provided significant bronchoprotection to methacholine (1.6 doubling doses; $P = 0.007$). This diminished with regular treatment and by 2 weeks the PD_{20} (the dose of methacholine producing a 20% fall in forced expiratory volume in 1 s [FEV_1]) was not significantly different from baseline. Further studies are necessary to see whether longer-term use of formoterol is also associated with tachyphylaxis to the effect of bronchodilator, whether this affects the other parameters of asthma control, and whether as-required use would restore this protection against bronchoconstriction.

Asthma control on LABA/ICS combination therapy

Can guideline-defined asthma control be achieved? The Gaining Optimal Asthma ControL study

Bateman ED, Boushey HA, Bousquet J, *et al.*; the GOAL Investigators Group. *Am J Resp Crit Care Med* 2004; **170**: 836–44

BACKGROUND. For most patients, asthma is not controlled as defined by guidelines; whether this is achievable has not been prospectively studied. It is also not known whether combination therapy is more likely to achieve this than an increased dose of ICS.

INTERPRETATION. Control was achieved more rapidly and at a lower corticosteroid dose with salmeterol/fluticasone than with fluticasone. This study confirms that the goal of guideline-derived asthma control was achieved in most of the patients.

Comment

A 1-year, randomized, stratified, double-blind, parallel-group study of 3421 patients with uncontrolled asthma compared fluticasone propionate and salmeterol/fluticasone in achieving two rigorous, composite, guideline-based measures of control – totally and well-controlled asthma – using measures that included the following asthma outcomes: peak expiratory flow rate (PEF), rescue medication use, symptoms, night-time awakenings, exacerbations, emergency visits, and adverse events. The definitions of control were derived from the treatment goals of the Global Initiative for Asthma/National Institutes of Health guidelines, with equal weighting given to each of the criteria. During the run-in period, patients continued on their usual dose (if any) of ICS treatment and were then randomized to one of three strata based on their ICS dose during the 6 months before screening: stratum 1, no ICS; stratum 2, 500 μg or less of beclomethasone dipropionate daily or equivalent; stratum 3, >500 to 1000 μg of beclomethasone dipropionate daily or equivalent. Treatment was stepped up until total control was achieved (or a maximum of 500 μg corticosteroid twice a day was reached) for a period of 12 weeks, and patients remained on the dose at which they achieved totally controlled asthma or the maximum dose of study medication until the end of the 1-year double-blind treatment period. Control was assessed over an 8-week period before each clinic visit at weeks 12, 24, 36 and 52. Significantly more patients in each stratum (previously corticosteroid-free, low- and moderate-dose corticosteroid users) achieved control with salmeterol/fluticasone than with fluticasone. In phase I, totally controlled asthma was achieved in 42 and 31% of patients for salmeterol/fluticasone and fluticasone respectively in stratum 1 (odds ratio [OR] 1.71; 95% CI 1.30–2.24; $P<0.001$), 32 and 20% in stratum 2 (OR 2.07; 95% CI 1.56–2.76; $P<0.001$), and 19 and 8% in stratum 3 (OR 2.90; 95% CI 1.98–4.26; $P<0.001$) and 690 (41%) vs 468 (28%) at 1 year for salmeterol/fluticasone and fluticasone respectively. In each stratum, the proportion of patients achieving control at the same or a lower dose of inhaled corticosteroid was greater for those treated with salmeterol/fluticasone and control was achieved earlier. Across all strata, 68 and 76% of the patients receiving salmeterol/fluticasone and fluticasone respectively were on the highest dose at the end of treatment. Interestingly, mean annual rates of exacerbations requiring oral corticosteroids and/or hospitalization or emergency visits were low in both treatment groups and lower in the combination therapy group. This study suggests that salmeterol/fluticasone achieves sustained control of asthma, as defined by a composite of relevant clinical goals of treatment, in more patients, more rapidly and at a lower dose of inhaled corticosteroids than fluticasone alone.

This study was mainly symptom-driven and had a high degree of compliance, which may or may not reflect actual clinical practice as some patients may be reluctant to increase medication for occasional symptoms to achieve complete absence of symptoms.

Fixed versus adjustable LABA/ICS combination therapy

The CONCEPT trial: a 1-year, multicentre, randomized, double-blind, double-dummy comparison of a stable dosing regimen of salmeterol/fluticasone propionate with an adjustable maintenance dosing regimen of formoterol/budesonide in adults with persistent asthma

Fitzgerald J, Boulet L, Follows R. *Clin Ther* 2005; **27**: 393–406

BACKGROUND. A patient-driven, adjustable maintenance dosing approach to asthma therapy, in which the dose is adjusted by patients according to the severity of their symptoms, was compared with a fixed-dose regimen.

INTERPRETATION. In this adult population with persistent asthma, stable dosing of salmeterol/fluticasone 50/250 μg twice daily resulted in significantly greater increases in symptom-free days and days free of rescue medication, as well as reducing the exacerbation rate, compared with adjustable maintenance dosing of formoterol/budesonide 6/200 μg. The results suggest that there is a minimum daily amount of maintenance therapy necessary to prevent exacerbations in adults with persistent asthma.

Comment

A previous study had suggested that adjustable maintenance therapy with budesonide/formoterol reduced exacerbations and reliever medication usage compared with fixed-dose salmeterol/fluticasone [7].

It is important to see whether the findings of that study can be reproduced. Participants were allocated to receive either a stable dose of salmeterol/fluticasone or an adjustable maintenance dose of formoterol/budesonide. The intent-to-treat population comprised 688 patients (344 per treatment arm) with a mean age of 45 years and a mean baseline FEV_1 of 81% of the predicted normal value. After 4 weeks of stable dosing, 581 patients (295 salmeterol/fluticasone, 286 formoterol/budesonide) continued beyond visit 3 into the remaining 48-week treatment period. As this was a double-blind, double-dummy trial in adult patients with symptomatic asthma that was not controlled by therapy with 200–500 μg/day of ICS plus a long-acting β_2-agonist, or with >500 to 1000 μg/day ICS alone, all participants were given two inhalers (Turbuhaler and Diskus). During the first 4 weeks, all participants received one inhalation of salmeterol/fluticasone 50/250 μg (via Diskus) and two inhalations of placebo (via Turbuhaler) or two inhalations of formoterol/budesonide 6/200 micrograms (via Turbuhaler) and one inhalation of placebo (via Diskus), twice daily. Rescue medication, in the form of the oral corticosteroid and salbutamol, was permitted as needed by all participants. During weeks 5–52, those eligible to continue the trial (no night-time awakenings, rescue medication with salbutamol for <2 days) were instructed to reduce the dose from the formoterol/budesonide or placebo Turbuhaler to one inhalation twice daily, and then to one inhalation per day (week 16 onwards). The dosage was increased as indicated by the presence or absence of nocturnal awakenings due to asthma, frequency of rescue medication use, and changes in morning PEF. The primary end-point was the percentage of symptom-free days. Other parameters included daily asthma symptom scores, morning PEF, percentage of days free of rescue medication use, daily rescue medication use, percentage of night awakenings due to asthma, percentage of weeks with well-controlled asthma, and number of exacerbations requiring oral corticosteroids or emergency department visits/hospitalizations.

During weeks 1–52, participants receiving salmeterol/fluticasone experienced a higher proportion of symptom-free days compared with those taking formoterol/budesonide (median 58.8 and 52.1%, respectively; $P = 0.034$). This equated to an average of 24 additional symptom-free days for the salmeterol/fluticasone group. The incidence of asthma exacerbations requiring oral steroids or an emergency department visit/hospitalization was 47% lower with salmeterol/fluticasone compared with formoterol/budesonide (adjusted annual mean rate 0.18 vs 0.33; $P = 0.008$) (39 vs 61 patients). Interestingly, the percentages of symptom-free and rescue medication-free days were high in both groups. In real life, however, patients may still take treatment depending on symptoms alone, i.e. they may increase medication with increased symptoms and reduce treatment when asymptomatic. The incidence of adverse events was similar in the two groups. This was a well-conducted study over a period of 1 year and after ensuring stability in the run-in period. This study is applicable to adults with persistent asthma and is at variance with the previous study of adjustable maintenance dosing in asthma, suggesting that patients may not be as aware of the need to increase their medication appropriately as previously thought, because of persistent low levels of airway inflammation.

LABA therapy as required

Formoterol used as needed in patients with intermittent or mild persistent asthma

Chuchalin A, Kasl M, Bengtsson T, Nihlen U, Rosenborg J. *Respir Med* 2005; **99**: 461–70

BACKGROUND. Formoterol is a full β_2-agonist with rapid onset of action and when used as required it may fulfil the need for rapid bronchodilation.

INTERPRETATION. Formoterol 4.5 μg used as needed was at least as effective and safe as terbutaline 0.5 mg used as needed in intermittent and mild persistent asthma.

Budesonide/formoterol combination therapy as both maintenance and reliever medication in asthma

O'Byrne PM, Bisgaard H, Godard PP, *et al. Am J Resp Crit Care Med* 2005; **171**: 129–36

BACKGROUND. Asthma control is improved by combining inhaled corticosteroids with long-acting β_2-agonists but patients still require reliever medication for breakthrough symptoms. Periodic fluctuations in symptoms and airway inflammation are characteristics of asthma, which means that treatment requirements, especially reliever use, can vary over time.

INTERPRETATION. Using budesonide/formoterol for both maintenance and relief reduces the risk and rate of severe asthma exacerbations and the need for systemic steroids and improves asthma symptoms, nocturnal awakenings and lung function compared with traditional fixed dosing regimens, therefore reducing the morbidity and potentially the mortality of asthma.

Comment

Chuchalin *et al.* conducted two double-blind, 12-month, parallel-group, non-inferiority trials comparing as-needed use of formoterol 4.5 μg and terbutaline 0.5 mg via a dry-powder inhaler. One trial was in 675 patients with intermittent asthma and one was in 455 patients with mild persistent asthma; the patients were 6–87 years of age. The authors assessed PEF, symptoms, rescue medication use, exacerbations and airway responsiveness, and safety. Formoterol 4.5 μg was found to be as effective as terbutaline 0.5 mg with regard to morning PEF, methacholine sensitivity, exacerbation rates and the use of rescue medication. Both treatments were safe and well tolerated.

O'Byrne *et al.* studied 2760 patients with asthma (FEV_1 60–100% of predicted with ≥12% reversibility), aged 4–80 years. They were randomized to the following study treatments: 925 patients to budesonide/formoterol maintenance + relief; 909 to budesonide/formoterol + short-acting β-agonist (SABA); and 926 to budesonide + SABA. The patients received terbutaline 0.4 mg as SABA with budesonide/formoterol 80/4.5 μg twice a day (budesonide/formoterol + SABA), budesonide 320 μg twice a day (budesonide + SABA), or budesonide/formoterol 80/4.5 μg twice a day with 80/4.5 μg as needed (budesonide/formoterol maintenance + relief). Children used a once-at-night maintenance dose. The risk of a severe exacerbation requiring medical intervention was reduced by 45% with budesonide/formoterol for maintenance and relief compared with patients using a 4-fold higher maintenance dose of budesonide with SABA for relief. Moreover, the times to second and third exacerbations were significantly prolonged with budesonide/formoterol for maintenance and relief compared with the 4-fold higher maintenance dose of budesonide with SABA. This suggests that budesonide/formoterol for maintenance and relief is also effective in patients with more severe asthma who experience repeat exacerbations. The combination as maintenance and reliever also reduced the rate of severe exacerbations and improved symptoms, awakenings and lung function compared with both fixed-dosing regimens. The authors suggest that it is the timing of the increase in ICS dose – resulting from as-needed use of budesonide/formoterol in response to symptoms – rather than the total inhaled dose of ICS that improves efficacy. This would require a well-informed, motivated patient with the perception to adjust medication from the first onset of symptoms, rather than after a medication review by his own doctor, and puts the patient in greater control of his asthma. Importantly, no additional drug-related adverse events were identified with the use of extra budesonide/formoterol for relief in addition to maintenance in this study. Both studies reinforce the view that formoterol's rapid onset of action makes it a suitable reliever medication and, in combination with ICS, may allow improved control of asthma at the time of need in both children and adults.

Both these studies show that the as-required use of formoterol, either alone or in combination with ICS, is a viable option for patients with mild asthma on reliever alone or regular ICS respectively, and further studies of the most effective regimen in the latter group would be beneficial.

Once-daily LABA/ICS combination

The 24 h duration of bronchodilator action of the budesonide/formoterol combination inhaler

Masoli M, Williams M, Weatherall M, Beasley R. *Respir Med* 2006; **100**: 20–5

BACKGROUND. The duration of the bronchodilator action of the long-acting β-agonist formoterol when administered in the evening had not been investigated.

INTERPRETATION. The single evening administration of formoterol from the combination budesonide/formoterol inhaler resulted in a duration of bronchodilation of at least 24 h.

The 24 h duration of bronchodilator action of the salmeterol/fluticasone combination inhaler

Masoli M, Weatherall M, Ayling J, Williams M, Beasley R. *Respir Med* 2005; **99**: 545–52

BACKGROUND. The duration of bronchodilator action of the long-acting β-agonist salmeterol when administered in the evening and its effect of attenuating the circadian rhythm in airway tone over 24 h had not been investigated.

Interpretation. The single evening administration of salmeterol/fluticasone via the Accuhaler™ resulted in a duration of bronchodilation of at least 24 h, with the abolition of the accentuated biphasic circadian variation in airway tone observed in asthma.

Comment

Previous studies have shown that once-daily administration of ICS is as effective as a twice-daily regimen in patients with mild to moderate asthma.

In these two studies the same group of authors investigated whether a single evening dose of formoterol, administered from the combination budesonide/formoterol Turbuhaler, or a single evening dose of salmeterol, administered from the combination salmeterol/fluticasone Accuhaler, significantly attenuated the circadian rhythm in airway tone over 24 h.

Twenty and 18 subjects with mild to moderate asthma (mean FEV_1 84% of predicted) participated in double-blind, placebo-controlled, crossover studies of the respective drug combinations. Subjects inhaled, in random order, placebo or budesonide/formoterol (2 × 100/6 μg) and placebo, salbutamol (200 μg) or salmeterol/fluticasone (50/100 μg) administered in the evening (2000 h) on separate occasions. Lung function measurements, including FEV_1, specific airway conductance (sGaw) and maximum expiratory flow at 25–75% of vital capacity ($MEF_{25-75\%}$), were assessed at baseline, at 1 h and subsequently every 4 h after dosing for 24 h.

Compared with placebo, budesonide/formoterol and salmeterol/fluticasone significantly improved the three measures of airway function throughout the 24-h period, with a difference in FEV_1 at 24 h of approximately 200 ml and with attenuation of the biphasic pattern of the circadian rhythm in airway tone. Placebo was used to confirm the marked circadian variation in airway calibre that occurs in asthma and to confirm attenuation in the treatment arms.

The lung function measures suggest bronchodilation at airways of varying calibre. These studies suggest that both combination LABA/ICS products were effective in providing bronchodilation for 24 h when administered in the evening and would need studies to compare the effect against twice daily standard dosing regimens, especially in the longer term. If confirmed in larger studies, this once daily/evening dosing regimen would have significant benefit not just in terms of cost–benefit but also in patient compliance.

Phosphodiesterase-4 inhibitors

Theophylline has been shown to have an anti-inflammatory and immunomodulatory effect when used in low doses. Inflammatory cells, such as eosinophils and T-lymphocytes, contain several phosphodiesterase enzymes. These are a family of enzymes involved in the degradation of cyclic adenosine monophosphate (cAMP), which is a natural modulator of inflammation and a potential target for new anti-inflammatory therapeutic agents. The anti-inflammatory effect of theophylline is believed to be due to its effect on the phosphodiesterase (PDE)-4 isoenzyme. Phosphodiesterases hydrolyse the second messenger cAMP to 5′-adenosine monophosphate, rendering it inactive. Inhibition of PDE4 activity results in maintenance of appropriate cAMP levels, resulting in downregulation of the inflammatory processes in cells involved in the pathophysiology of asthma. The PDE4 isoenzyme has localized activity in the lung, and PDE4 inhibitors, such as roflumilast and cilomilast, block cAMP hydrolysis in the airways. This has led to the development of new phosphodiesterase inhibitors with greater selectivity in enhancing the beneficial effects whilst minimizing the side effects associated with theophyllines. The inflammatory response is highly sensitive to levels of cAMP, and, by preventing the breakdown of cAMP, PDE4 inhibitors are associated with a natural anti-inflammatory activity. PDE4 inhibitors are being shown to be effective in some phase III clinical trials of asthma and chronic obstructive pulmonary disease, but the presence of dose-limiting side effects such as arteritis in animals continues to hamper their development. The therapeutic ratio for PDE4 inhibitors is thought to be related to the selectivity of receptor subtypes for relative effects on PDE4B (anti-inflammatory) and PDE4D (emesis). Roflumilast has a better safety and tolerability profile than cilomilast, an agent which was discontinued in trials for asthma in 2003 but has recently been licensed for chronic obstructive pulmonary disease. New approaches to improve the therapeutic ratio and the safety of these compounds are being looked at, including the synthesis of small molecules with a broader PDE specificity. The development of dual-specificity compounds that inhibit PDE4 and PDE1, PDE3, PDE5 or PDE7 could be beneficial in the treatment of chronic inflammatory lung diseases, and are also being investigated [8].

Oral phosphodiesterase-4 inhibitor versus inhaled corticosteroid

Comparison of roflumilast, an oral anti-inflammatory, with beclomethasone dipropionate in the treatment of persistent asthma

Bousquet J, Aubier M, Sastre J, Izquierdo JL, *et al. Allergy* 2006; **61**: 72–8

BACKGROUND. Roflumilast is an oral, once-daily PDE4 inhibitor with anti-inflammatory activity in development for the treatment of asthma. Roflumilast was compared with inhaled beclomethasone dipropionate in patients with asthma.

INTERPRETATION. Once-daily, oral roflumilast 500 μg was comparable with inhaled twice-daily beclomethasone dipropionate (400 μg/day) in improving pulmonary function and asthma symptoms, and reducing the use of rescue medication in patients with asthma.

Comment

The authors compared the efficacy and safety of once-daily oral roflumilast 500 μg with those of beclomethasone dipropionate 200 μg twice daily (400 μg/day) in patients aged 12–70 years with stable persistent asthma and FEV_1 55–80% of predicted. This was a randomized, double-blind, double-dummy, parallel-group, multicentre, non-inferiority study. After a single-blind placebo baseline period of 1–3 weeks, eligible patients were randomized to receive either (i) an oral roflumilast 500 μg tablet once daily in the morning and two puffs of placebo administered via a metered dose inhaler in the morning and in the evening for 12 weeks; or (ii) an oral placebo tablet once daily in the morning and beclomethasone dipropionate 400 μg daily administered with a metered dose inhaler as two 100-μg puffs delivered in the morning and in the evening for 12 weeks. Lung function was tested at baseline and weeks 3, 6, 9 and 12. Salbutamol was permitted as rescue medication, but all other respiratory medications, including ICS, anticholinergic agents, theophylline and inhaled long-acting β-agonists were withdrawn at the start of the study. Four hundred and ninety-nine patients with FEV_1 50–85% were followed for 12 weeks. Lung function and adverse events were monitored. Roflumilast and beclomethasone dipropionate both significantly improved FEV_1, by 12% (270 ± 30 ml) and 14% (320 ± 30 ml) respectively (P<0.0001 versus baseline), and forced vital capacity (P<0.0001 versus baseline), with no significant difference between the two drugs. Roflumilast and beclomethasone dipropionate consistently improved morning and evening PEF. This study suggests that roflumilast could potentially be an oral alternative in patients with stable asthma who do not tolerate ICS or have poor compliance. Poor compliance with ICS therapy, lack of response to ICS and inadequate patient techniques for administering inhaled medications are associated with poor asthma control. An oral PDE4 inhibitor would address these issues and aid compliance. Longer-term studies are needed to see if this effect is sustained without deterioration in asthma control. Long-term placebo-controlled studies of roflumilast in asthma together with post-marketing surveillance will be necessary to further characterize its place in management and its tolerability.

Anticholinergic treatment

Anticholinergic agents have a demonstrated role in combination with β_2-agonists in the treatment of acute severe asthma and there is a suggestion that they may benefit stable asthmatics, particularly those who have the Arg/Arg genotype [9].

A Cochrane review concluded that there was no justification for routinely introducing anticholinergic agents as part of add-on treatment for patients whose asthma is not well controlled on standard therapies but did not exclude the possibility that there could be a subgroup of patients who derived some benefit and that a trial of treatment in individual patients was justified [10]. The use of anticholinergic therapy for wheeze in children under the age of 2 years was also not advocated, although the authors recognized that parents using these agents at home were able to identify benefits [11].

Glycopyrrolate causes prolonged bronchoprotection and bronchodilatation in patients with asthma

Hansel TT, Neighbour H, Erin EM, Tan AJ, *et al. Chest* 2005; **128**: 1974–9

BACKGROUND. Anticholinergic agents, including nebulized glycopyrrolate, a potent but non-selective muscarinic receptor blocker, have been found to be effective bronchodilators in patients with chronic obstructive pulmonary disease, who have limited reversibility. The effect in asthmatic patients has not been studied.

INTERPRETATION. Each glycopyrrolate dose provided significantly more protection against methacholine challenge than placebo at all time-points, and against ipratropium bromide at 12, 24 and 30 h.

Comment

The authors investigated the duration of protection against the constrictor effects of inhaled methacholine of a single dose of inhaled nebulized racemic glycopyrrolate (0.5, 1.0 and 2.0 mg) compared with ipratropium bromide (0.5 mg) and placebo in twelve patients with mild to moderate asthma with FEV_1 ≥70% of predicted in a double-blind, five-way, crossover study. All subjects received three single doses of glycopyrrolate (0.5 mg, 1 mg and 2 mg), one dose of ipratropium bromide (0.5 mg) and one dose of placebo. Because of the potentially long duration of action of glycopyrrolate, each treatment day was separated by a washout period of at least 7 days. Pairwise analyses of the primary efficacy variable (log PC_{20} [concentration of methachline required to produce a 20% drop in FEV1]/log 2) showed that there were no statistically significant differences among the active-treatment study arms and placebo prior to dosing. After treatment, each glycopyrrolate dose provided significantly more protection against methacholine challenge than placebo at all time-points, and against ipratropium bromide at all time-points from 2 to 30 h.

There was not a clear dose response since glycopyrrolate at doses of 0.5, 1.0 or 2.0 mg caused bronchoprotection for up to 30 h, suggesting that even the lowest dose of glycopyrrolate in this study exerted maximal cholinergic blockade, and in fact 2.0 mg of glycopyrrolate had only half the effect of 0.5 and 1 mg. It remains to be seen whether significant bronchodilatation would be achieved in subjects with more severe reversible airway obstruction or with lower doses and regular use of glycopyrrolate. Further studies are indicated to see if this is potentially a useful drug in the treatment of asthma.

References

1. Tattersfield AE, Löfdahl CG, Postma DS, Eivindson A, Schreurs AG, Rasidakis A, Ekstrom T. Comparison of formoterol and terbutaline for as-needed treatment of asthma: a randomised trial. *Lancet* 2001; **357**: 257–61.
2. Tattersfield AE. Clinical pharmacology of long-acting beta2-receptor agonists. *Life Sci* 1993; **52**: 2161–9.
3. Masoli M, Weatherall M, Holt S, Beasley R. Moderate dose inhaled corticosteroids plus salmeterol versus higher doses of inhaled corticosteroids in symptomatic asthma. *Thorax* 2005; **60**: 730–4.
4. Nelson HS. Is there a problem with inhaled long-acting beta-adrenergic agonists? *J Allergy Clin Immunol* 2006; **117**: 3–14.
5. Walters JAE, Wood-Baker R, Walters EH. Long-acting beta2-agonists in asthma: an overview of Cochrane systematic reviews. *Resp Medicine* 2005; **99**: 384–95.
6. Garcia R, Guerra P, Feo F, Galindo PA, Gomez E, Borja J, Fernandez-Pacheco R. Tachyphylaxis following regular use of formoterol in exercise-induced bronchospasm. *J Investig Allergol Clin Immunol* 2001; **11**: 176–82.
7. Aalbers R, Backer V, Kava TT, Omenaas ER, Sandstrom T, Jorup C, Welte T. Adjustable maintenance dosing with budesonide/formoterol compared with fixed-dose salmeterol/fluticasone in moderate to severe asthma. *Curr Med Res Opin* 2004; **20**: 225–40.
8. Giembycz MA. Life after PDE4: overcoming adverse events with dual-specificity phosphodiesterase inhibitors. *Curr Opin Pharmacol* 2005; **5**: 238–44.

9. Kanazawa H. Anticholinergic agents in asthma: chronic bronchodilator therapy, relief of acute severe asthma, reduction of chronic viral inflammation and prevention of airway remodeling. *Curr Opin Pulm Med* 2006; **12**: 60–7.

10. Westby M, Benson M, Gibson P. Anticholinergic agents for chronic asthma in adults. *Cochrane Database Syst Rev* 2004 (**3**): CD003269.

11. Everard ML, Bara A, Kurian M, Elliott TM, Ducharme F, Mayowe V. Anticholinergic drugs for wheeze in children under the age of two years. The *Cochrane Database Syst Rev* 2005 (**3**): CD001279.

13

Corticosteroids and asthma

SURESH BABU, JAYMIN MORJARIA

Introduction

The introduction of adrenocorticotrophic hormone back in 1949 paved the way for corticosteroids as the mainstay of therapy for asthma [1]. It is now more than 50 years since the introduction of corticosteroids, but with the recognition of asthma as an inflammatory disorder of the airways, these drugs continue to enjoy their place as the cornerstone of asthma treatment. However, the discovery of various adverse effects of corticosteroids has led to the investigation of newer molecules that have a lower side-effect profile but maintain therapeutic efficiency.

Research into newer corticosteroids is looking at steroids that are metabolized locally, so that there is less risk of systemic absorption from the respiratory tract. These are known as soft steroids. Earlier steroids in this category, butixocort 21-propionate and tipredane, proved to have poor efficacy in clinical studies because they are metabolized before they exert any anti-inflammatory action. However, new soft steroids, such as ciclesonide, appear to be more promising and corticosteroids that are inactivated in plasma are now in development [2]. Systemic adverse effects of corticosteroids are largely mediated through DNA binding; however, it may be possible to dissociate the anti-inflammatory effects from the adverse effects. Several dissociated corticosteroids have now been synthesized, and a separation between transactivation (DNA binding) and transrepression (transcription factor inhibition) has been demonstrated in gene reporter systems and in intact cells *in vitro* [3,4]. It is likely that in future, the use of these novel dissociated corticosteroids would be able to exert their pharmacological effects without the adverse effects previously associated with these medications.

Efficacy of inhaled corticosteroids

Although the efficacy of inhaled corticosteroids (ICS) in asthma has long been established, some issues need clarification, such as the optimal dose, the dose–response relationship and the efficacy versus safety issue (risk/benefit). It is also important to study whether ICS are effective in specific risk groups, such as smokers, and in specific phenotypes, such as infantile wheezers and subjects with

© Atlas Medical Publishing Ltd

cough variant asthma. A systemic review and two original articles address the issues of the dose of fluticasone and its effectiveness in asthmatics who smoke.

Inhaled fluticasone at different doses for chronic asthma in adults and children

Adams NP, Bestall JC, Jones PW, Lasserson TJ, Griffiths B, Cates C. *Cochrane Database Syst Rev* 2005; (**3**): CD003534

BACKGROUND. Inhaled fluticasone propionate is a high-potency ICS used for the management of asthma. The authors assessed the efficacy and safety outcomes of the use of inhaled fluticasone propionate at different nominal daily doses in the treatment of chronic asthma, and they tested for the presence of a dose–response effect.

INTERPRETATION. Forty-three randomized double-blind studies were included in this analysis. The effects of fluticasone were dose-dependent but relatively small. At dose ratios of 1:2, there were significant differences in favour of the higher dose in morning peak flow across the low dose range. Patients with moderate disease achieved levels of asthma control on medium doses of fluticasone (400–500 µg/day) similar to those achieved at high doses (800–1000 µg/day). High-dose fluticasone propionate did not lead to clear improvements in symptoms compared with the lower dose and increased the risk of a hoarse voice and fungal mouth infections. In people with severe asthma, very high doses of fluticasone propionate (2000 µg/day) appeared to allow more people on oral steroids to stop or reduce their dose of oral steroid tablets compared with lower doses of fluticasone propionate (1000–1500 µg/day).

Comment

This analysis was a quantitative synthesis of all the available randomized clinical trial evidence with fluticasone propionate in asthma. Fluticasone propionate is an effective treatment for chronic asthma when administered over a wide range of daily doses. Although a shallow dose–response effect is evident for a number of measures of asthma control where oral steroids are not given, the findings of this analysis suggest that most children and adults with mild to moderate asthma do not achieve clinically worthwhile additional improvements at higher doses (more than 500 µg/day) compared with lower doses (up to 200 µg/day). The dose–response effect in people with more severe asthma may be greater, higher doses of fluticasone propionate (over 500 µg/day) conferring greater benefit than 200 µg/day or a lower dose. Patients with severe asthma who are dependent on oral steroids gain clinically worthwhile benefit in terms of cessation of oral steroids and reduction in the daily dose of prednisolone on very high doses of fluticasone propionate (2000 µg/day). People who cannot be weaned off oral steroids using lower doses should have a trial of fluticasone propionate at 2000 µg/day.

Can guideline-defined asthma control be achieved? The Gaining Optimal Asthma Control study

Bateman ED, Boushey HA, Bousquet J, *et al.*; GOAL Investigators Group. *Am J Respir Crit Care Med* 2004; **170**: 836–44.

Background. The goal of asthma control is total and effective control of asthma symptoms with no side effects of medications. The important question is whether this is achievable. This study was designed as a 1-year, stratified, randomized, double-blind, parallel-group study comparing the efficacy and safety of individual, predefined, stepwise increases in salmeterol/fluticasone propionate with fluticasone propionate alone in achieving two predefined composite measures of asthma control.

Interpretation. The study population comprised 3421 patients with uncontrolled asthma. The results demonstrate that, in most patients with uncontrolled asthma across a wide range of severities, comprehensive guideline-defined control can be achieved and maintained. More patients achieved both totally controlled and well-controlled asthma with combination inhaled salmeterol/fluticasone more rapidly and at a lower dose of corticosteroid than with inhaled fluticasone alone. Patients who achieved control recorded very low rates of exacerbations and near-maximal health status scores. Furthermore, in stepping up treatment in an attempt to achieve guideline-defined total control, even those patients who did not attain stringent definitions of control showed considerable improvements in health status and a reduction in exacerbation rates.

Comment

This study shows that guideline-defined asthma control is achievable in patients with poorly controlled asthma and that the combination of salmeterol/fluticasone achieves this control more rapidly with a lower dose of ICS.

Efficacy of low and high dose inhaled corticosteroid in smokers versus non-smokers with mild asthma

Tomlinson JE, McMahon AD, Chaudhuri R, Thompson JM, Wood SF, Thomson NC. *Thorax* 2005; **60**: 282–7

Background. Unfortunately, smoking is as common in asthmatics, as it is in the general population. It is believed that asthmatic patients who smoke are less sensitive to ICS than those who do not smoke. This study looked at the efficacy of inhaled corticosteroid treatment when given for a longer duration and at different doses in smokers and non-smokers.

Interpretation. Ninety-five individuals with mild asthma were recruited to a multicentre, randomized, double-blind, parallel group study comparing inhaled beclomethasone at doses of 400 or 2000 μg daily for 12 weeks in smokers and non-smokers. The primary end-point was the change in morning peak expiratory flow (PEF).

There was a considerable difference between the morning PEF measurements of smokers and non-smokers with asthma. Among those receiving 400 µg daily, there was a significant difference between the mean morning PEF in smokers and non-smokers and in the number of asthma exacerbations. However, smaller differences were found between smokers and non-smokers receiving 2000 µg inhaled beclomethasone daily.

Comment

This study showed that smokers with asthma had a reduced therapeutic response to ICS over a 3-month period compared with non-smokers. Furthermore, this reduced response was particularly marked in those receiving a low dose of inhaled corticosteroid. Participants receiving 2000 µg daily of inhaled beclomethasone had improved morning PEF measurements, although the change was greater for non-smokers (Fig. 13.1). The results of this study are similar to those of earlier studies which found that the efficacy of ICS was dampened in asthmatic smokers [5,6]. Therefore, asthmatics who smoke would need a higher dose of ICS to control their asthma because they are relatively insensitive to ICS.

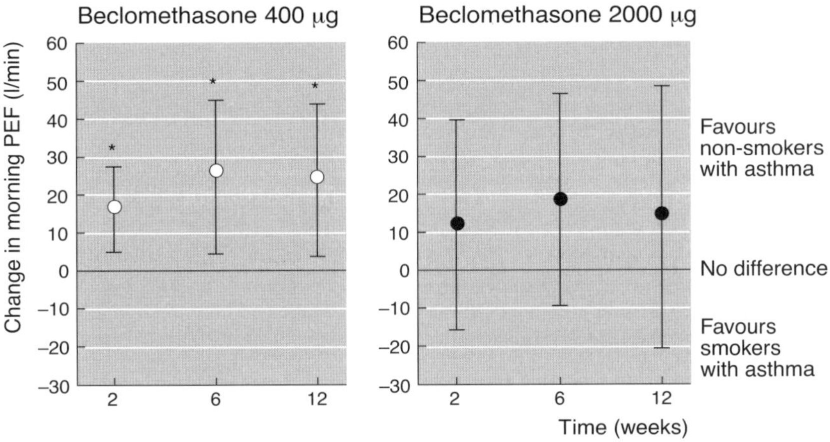

Fig. 13.1 Mean (95% confidence interval) difference between non-smokers and smokers with asthma in change in morning PEF (l/min) on different doses of inhaled beclomethasone. **P*<0.01 for smokers with asthma versus non-smokers with asthma. Source: Tomlinson *et al.* (2005).

Randomized trial of inhaled beclomethasone dipropionate versus theophylline for moderate asthma during pregnancy

Dombrowski MP, Schatz M, Wise R, *et al.*; National Institute of Child Health and Human Development Maternal–Fetal Medicine Units Network; National Heart, Lung, and Blood Institute. *Am J Obstet Gynecol* 2004; **190**: 737–44

Background. This study was undertaken to compare the efficacy of inhaled beclomethasone dipropionate with that of oral theophylline for the prevention of asthma exacerbation(s) requiring medical intervention in pregnant women with moderate asthma.

Interpretation. In this trial 199 patients were enrolled to receive oral theophylline and 199 to receive inhaled beclomethasone. There was no significant difference in the proportion of asthma exacerbations among the cohort receiving beclomethasone and that receiving theophylline. The beclomethasone cohort had significantly lower incidences of discontinuing study medications caused by adverse effects. There were no significant differences in treatment failure, compliance, or the proportion with PEF less than 80% of predicted. There were no significant differences in maternal or perinatal outcomes.

Comment

This study concluded that the treatment of moderate asthma with inhaled beclomethasone versus oral theophylline resulted in similar rates of asthma exacerbations and similar obstetric and perinatal outcomes. Studies have shown that the use of ICS is safer in pregnancy when compared with oral steroids, which were associated with prematurity and the likelihood of pre-eclampsia (see Schatz *et al.*, reviewed below) [7]. It is therefore important to have good control of asthma during pregnancy. The need to monitor serum levels of theophylline and its adverse effect profile make ICS a safer and easier alternative for the management of asthma during pregnancy.

Safety of inhaled corticosteroids

While the efficacy of ICS is not in doubt, safety concerns following long-term use continue to influence decision-making when prescribing ICS to vulnerable groups such as children and pregnant mothers. However, these concerns are being addressed by ongoing and new studies of ICS in mild to moderate persistent asthma.

Long-term safety of once-daily budesonide in patients with early-onset mild persistent asthma: results of the Inhaled Steroid Treatment as Regular Therapy in Early Asthma (START) study

Sheffer AL, Silverman M, Woolcock AJ, Diaz PV, Lindberg B, Lindmark B. *Ann Allergy Asthma Immunol* 2005; **94**: 48–54

BACKGROUND. The START study is a worldwide, randomized, prospective study to investigate early intervention with ICS in order to evaluate the safety and tolerability of long-term treatment with once-daily budesonide therapy in patients with recent-onset mild persistent asthma.

INTERPRETATION. Patients aged 5–66 years with mild persistent asthma for less than 2 years and no previous regular corticosteroid treatment received budesonide or placebo once daily for 3 years, in addition to their usual asthma therapy. It was found that 3 years of treatment with budesonide once daily (200 or 400 μg) is safe and well tolerated in children and adults with newly detected mild persistent asthma.

Comment

ICS are the mainstay of asthma treatment and the recommended dosage schedule for ICS is twice a day. From this study it is difficult to evaluate the efficacy of once-daily treatment with budesonide in patients with mild persistent asthma. However, the authors of this study found that an ICS was well tolerated in both adults and children with mild persistent asthma and that there were minimal adverse effects.

Use of inhaled corticosteroids during pregnancy and risk of pregnancy induced hypertension: nested case–control study

Martel MJ, Rey E, Beauchesne MF, *et al. BMJ* 2005; **330**: 230

BACKGROUND. Asthma is a common condition among pregnant women and the use of oral corticosteroids has been associated with an increased risk of pre-eclampsia [8]. This study was designed to evaluate whether the use of ICS during pregnancy increases the risk of pregnancy-induced hypertension and pre-eclampsia among asthmatic women.

INTERPRETATION. This nested case–control study included a total of 4593 pregnancies in 3505 women with asthma between 1990 and 2000. The primary objective was to study whether the use of ICS during pregnancy increases the risk of pregnancy-induced hypertension. The use of ICS from conception until the date of outcome was not associated with an increased risk of pregnancy-induced hypertension (adjusted odds ratio 1.02; 95% confidence interval 0.77–1.34) or pre-eclampsia (1.06; 0.74–1.53). No significant dose–response relation was observed between ICS and pregnancy-induced hypertension or pre-eclampsia. Oral corticosteroids were significantly associated with the risk of pregnancy-induced hypertension (adjusted odds ratio 1.57; 1.02–2.41), and a trend was seen for pre-eclampsia.

Comment

This study provides evidence that the use of ICS during pregnancy is safe and is not associated with an increased risk of pre-eclampsia, whereas oral corticosteroids were associated with an increased risk. Furthermore, there was no significant association with increasing doses of ICS and the development of pre-eclampsia.

The relationship of asthma medication use to perinatal outcomes

Schatz M, Dombrowski MP, Wise R, *et al.*; Maternal–Fetal Medicine Units Network, The National Institute of Child Health and Development; The National Heart, Lung and Blood Institute. *J Allergy Clin Immunol* 2004; **113**: 1040–5

BACKGROUND. The use of any medication in pregnancy is fraught with side effects both for the mother and for the baby. Because asthma is a common condition and there is a need for good asthma control during pregnancy, it is necessary to collect data regarding the safety of contemporary asthma medications during pregnancy. In this observational cohort study, asthmatic patients with all levels of severity were enrolled and monitored. Perinatal outcome variables included gestational hypertension, preterm births, low birth weight, small-for-gestational-age infants, and major malformations.

INTERPRETATION. The study concluded that the use of inhaled β-agonists, inhaled steroids and theophylline does not appear to increase perinatal risks in pregnant asthmatic women but that the mechanism of the association between maternal oral corticosteroid use and prematurity remains to be determined.

Comment

This study provides evidence to support the management of asthma with ICS during pregnancy as this treatment is not associated with significant perinatal risks. Furthermore, this study stresses the need for good asthma control as the use of oral steroids during an exacerbation can be associated with prematurity. It is not clear, however, whether oral corticosteroids cause the prematurity directly or whether they serve as a marker for asthma severity or poor asthma control, which may be the real cause of prematurity. In combination with the Martel *et al.* study (above), the results of this study provide evidence that the use of oral corticosteroids is associated with an increased maternal and fetal risk |9| and that ICS are a safer option.

Inhaled corticosteroids for asthma exacerbation

Acute exacerbation of asthma represents a major event in the lives of asthmatic patients. It has an adverse effect on quality of life, there is the risk of adverse effects from the oral corticosteroids that are often used to treat these exacerbations, and it has a major impact on health economics. Thus, effective prevention of asthma exacerbation remains a primary target for various new and old therapeutic strategies. The successful use of ICS to prevent and treat asthma exacerbation would be a significant advance, with improvement in quality of life and a reduction in adverse effects from systemic steroids.

Doubling the dose of inhaled corticosteroid to prevent asthma exacerbations: randomised controlled trial

Harrison TW, Oborne J, Newton S, Tattersfield AE. *Lancet* 2004; **363**: 271–5

BACKGROUND. The management of asthma in the community involves patient education to avoid the triggers, doubling the dose of inhaled steroids and increasing the use of rescue medications during an exacerbation in order to prevent unnecessary hospital visits. This randomized, controlled study looks at whether doubling the dose of corticosteroid in isolation is effective when asthma deteriorates.

INTERPRETATION. Three hundred and ninety patients with asthma who were at risk of an exacerbation monitored their morning peak flow and asthma symptoms for up to 12 months. When peak flow or symptoms started to deteriorate, subjects added an active or placebo corticosteroid inhaler to their usual corticosteroid for 14 days to produce a doubling of the dose or no change in dose. The primary outcome was the number of individuals starting oral prednisolone in each group. It was concluded that doubling the dose of inhaled steroids when asthma starts to deteriorate does not prevent asthma exacerbation requiring a course of oral steroid.

Comment

It is a general belief among physicians that doubling the dose of ICS during an exacerbation reduces the necessity for oral steroids in asthma. In this study, doubling the dose of ICS led to a small reduction in the mean maximum fall in peak flow but there was no difference in the lowest peak flow recorded, the increase in symptom scores or the highest symptom score recorded in comparison with patients who remained on the same dose. Doubling the dose of ICS had no effect on the time taken for peak flow or symptom scores to return to the baseline values. Furthermore, controls who had a fall in peak flow of 15% or more before starting the study inhaler were more likely to need oral prednisolone than were those with a smaller reduction. These results could have an important impact on asthma self-management, and this is in agreement with the recent British Thoracic Society guidelines on asthma management |**10**|. Although this study provides evidence that doubling the dose of ICS does not alter the need for oral steroids, the authors did not investigate the specific dose of ICS that may or may not be effective in preventing the need for oral steroids, or whether increasing the dose of ICS reduces the dose of oral steroids in patients having an asthma exacerbation.

Doubling the dose of budesonide versus maintenance treatment in asthma exacerbations

FitzGerald JM, Becker A, Sears MR, Mink S, Chung K, Lee J; Canadian Asthma Exacerbation Study Group. *Thorax* 2004; **59**: 550–6

BACKGROUND. This study was similar to the study of Harrison and colleagues (reviewed above), which looked at doubling the dose of ICS during an asthma exacerbation. This study investigated whether doubling the dose of budesonide in patients on regular inhaled budesonide would be beneficial during an asthma exacerbation.

INTERPRETATION. In a 6-month double-blind, randomized, placebo-controlled, parallel-group, multicentre trial, 290 patients were randomized to treatment with either a continued maintenance dose of ICS or doubling the dose at the time of an exacerbation. The study concluded that, in patients who regularly take an inhaled corticosteroid, doubling the maintenance dose may not affect the pattern of the exacerbation.

Comment

The results of this study are similar to those of the earlier study (Harrison *et al.*, reviewed above) which did not show any effect on asthma exacerbation of doubling the dose of ICS during an exacerbation. The pattern of β_2-agonist use, mean symptom scores and nocturnal awakenings was similar in the two arms of the study at the time when the patients had an exacerbation (Fig. 13.2). There were no significant differences in the three major criteria for triggering an asthma exacerbation (changes in PEF, increased bronchodilator use, nocturnal awakenings). Furthermore, There was no difference in outcome between patients who were switched from other ICS to budesonide ($n = 40$) compared with patients who were already taking budesonide. The study concludes that, if patients routinely comply with maintenance ICS, doubling the dose of ICS may not alter the course of an asthma exacerbation. Studies with repeated low-dose allergen exposure in patients with mild allergic asthma have shown that worsening of the airway inflammation precedes deterioration of asthma symptoms and asthma control [11]. Hence, the ideal time for doubling the dose of ICS may be earlier than the predicted fall in PEF or forced expiratory volume in 1 second (FEV_1). Future studies should investigate ways to recognize worsening airway inflammation before a reduction in PEF or an increase in symptoms has occurred, in an attempt to pre-empt exacerbation. Further studies are also needed to assess the optimal dose of ICS before it can be concluded that an increase in the dose of ICS is unlikely to be of benefit during an asthma exacerbation.

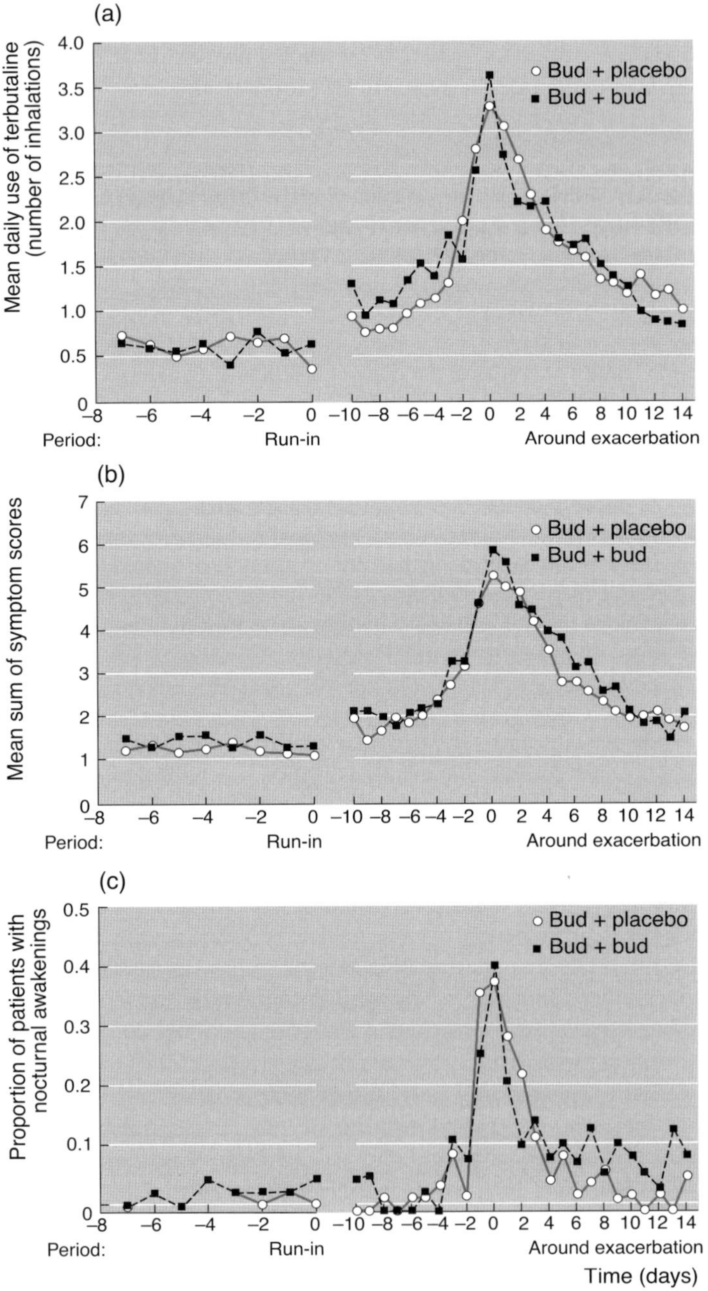

Fig. 13.2 Pattern of (a) short-acting β_2-agonist use, (b) symptom scores and (c) nocturnal awakenings around the time of the exacerbation. Bud, budesonide. Source: FitzGerald *et al.* (2004).

Comparison of inhaled fluticasone with intravenous hydrocortisone in the treatment of adult acute asthma

Rodrigo GJ. *Am J Respir Crit Care Med* 2005; **171**: 1231–6

BACKGROUND. The role of oral and inhaled corticosteroids in the management of acute asthma is well known. This study compared the effects of inhaled fluticasone propionate with those of intravenous hydrocortisone in patients with acute severe asthma.

INTERPRETATION. One hundred and six patients with acute severe asthma were assigned in a double-blind, randomized manner to receive fluticasone propionate by means of a metered-dose inhaler into a spacer device in a dose of two puffs at 10-min intervals (3000 μg fluticasone propionate/h), or intravenous hydrocortisone. In addition, all patients received four puffs of albuterol and ipratropium bromide each hour. Primary outcome measures were improvement in pulmonary function (FEV_1 or PEF) and admission rate. The use of repeated doses of inhaled fluticasone was more effective than the use of intravenous hydrocortisone and was associated with an early improvement. This therapeutic benefit was particularly evident in patients with the most severe obstruction.

Comment

Studies that had compared oral versus inhaled corticosteroids in the management of acute asthma have found no significant differences between the two forms of administration [12]. ICS have been compared with oral corticosteroids in children [13,14]. This study compared the use of intravenous corticosteroids with ICS in adult patients with acute severe asthma. The authors found that inhaled fluticasone improved both FEV_1 and PEF (Fig. 13.3) in patients with acute asthma. The differences were also significant in the subgroup of patients who had an FEV_1 of <1 l at presentation. This is interesting as it is believed that in patients with low FEV_1 the inspiratory pressures may not be adequate to produce an effective inhalation to carry the medications into the airways, but the treatment with β_2-agonist could have produced enough bronchodilation to show the improvement. It may be too early to use this as a routine therapeutic option in emergencies, and further randomized trials with a larger population are required to confirm these results.

Intermittent use of inhaled corticosteroids

It is well known that compliance with ICS treatment is poor in patients with mild to moderate asthma. This may be a result of the lack of persistent symptoms and (in the patient's mind) the need for regular therapy or the fear of adverse effects of steroids, or both. If asthma can be effectively treated with ICS given as required, this would empower the patient with control of their asthma (therapy directed by

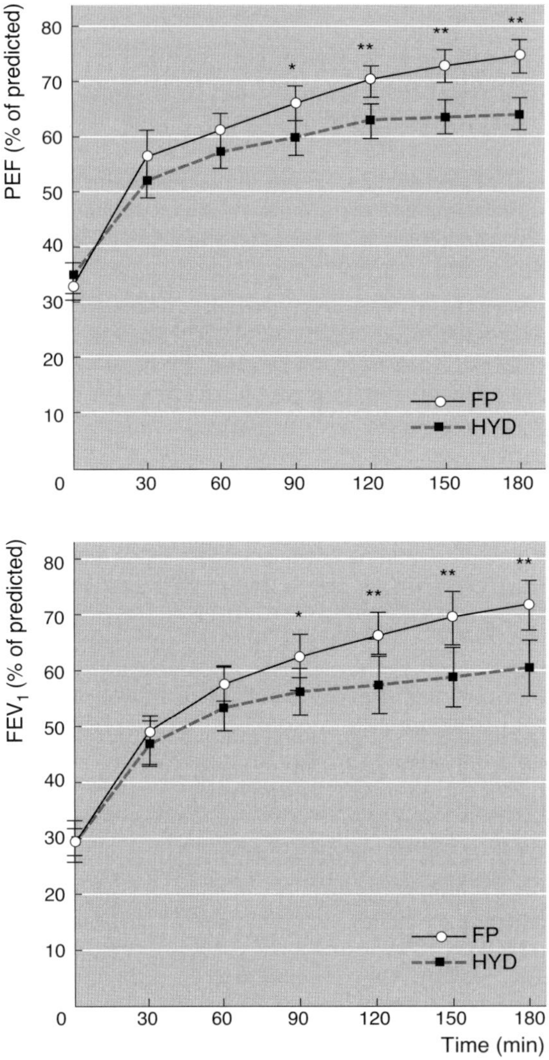

Fig. 13.3 PEF and FEV_1 values (% predicted) after the administration of fluticasone propionate (FP) or hydrocortisone (HYD). Data points are mean values, and the brackets represent the 95% confidence interval. *P<0.05; **P<0.01. Source: Rodrigo (2005).

symptoms) and has the potential for reducing adverse effects with a smaller overall dose of corticosteroid.

Daily versus as-needed corticosteroids for mild persistent asthma

Boushey HA, Sorkness CA, King TS, *et al.*; National Heart, Lung, and Blood Institute's Asthma Clinical Research Network. *N Engl J Med* 2005; **352**: 1519–28

BACKGROUND. The guidelines for asthma management recommend the use of regular ICS in patients with mild persistent asthma, but in clinical practice it has been observed that patients often do not feel the need to use their ICS regularly, which may lead to poor compliance. One possible reason is that because there are no symptoms the patients are not reminded to use their medications. Hence, the use of intermittent ICS during worsening of asthma may be an option that could be considered in these subgroups of asthmatics.

INTERPRETATION. In a double-blind, randomized trial, 225 patients with mild persistent asthma were evaluated during a 1-year period to assess the efficacy of an intermittent short course of inhaled corticosteroid treatment guided by a symptom-based action plan alone, or added to daily treatment with either inhaled budesonide or oral zafirlukast. The primary outcome was morning PEF. The three treatments produced similar increases in morning PEF (7.1–8.3%; approximately 32 l/min; $P = 0.90$) and similar rates of asthma exacerbations. Thirty exacerbations of symptoms warranting treatment with prednisone occurred in 25 (11.1%) patients, an overall rate of 0.13 per patient-year. The proportion of patients who had one or more exacerbations did not differ significantly among the groups. The authors concluded that it may be possible to treat mild persistent asthma with short, intermittent courses of inhaled or oral corticosteroids taken when symptoms worsen.

Comment

The use of ICS during asthma worsening rather than on a regular basis in patients with mild persistent asthma could serve as a useful therapeutic option in patients who are not troubled regularly by their asthma. In this trial patients received instruction in a symptom-based asthma treatment plan for taking open-label budesonide (800 µg twice daily) for 10 days or prednisone (0.5 mg/kg of body weight per day) for 5 days if their asthma symptoms worsened. After completing the run-in period, the patients were assigned to one of three parallel treatment groups: (i) twice-daily oral placebo and inhalation of 200 µg of budesonide; (ii) twice-daily oral zafirlukast (20 mg) and inhalation of placebo; or (iii) twice-daily oral and inhaled placebo. The primary outcome variable was the change from baseline in the 2-week average morning PEF. Other objective outcome variables were the change from baseline in FEV_1 before bronchodilator use, FEV_1 after treatment with 540–720 µg of albuterol, morning PEF during the period of intense combined therapy, and FEV_1 after the period of intense combined therapy. The primary outcome, the change in morning PEF from the final 2 weeks of the run-in period to the final 2 weeks of the year of treatment, did not differ significantly among the groups. Compared with intermittent therapy or daily zafirlukast therapy, daily budesonide therapy produced greater improvements in pre-bronchodilator FEV_1 and bronchial reactivity. Kaplan–Meier curves showed no significant differences among the groups, whether they were plotted as the time to a first event ($P = 0.39$ by the log-rank test) or allowed multiple events per patient ($P = 0.24$) (Fig. 13.4). The 12-month Kaplan–Meier exacerbation rates for the budesonide and intermittent treatment groups were 16.1 and 11.3% respectively, resulting in an average difference of +4.8 percentage points (the positive sign indicates more exacerbations in the budesonide group). The clinical implications of this trial may be enormous: intermittent use of ICS may have a huge impact on the health economics of asthma management but its long-term effects on airway physiology and the need for effective control of airway inflammation will need to be further investigated. Whether this approach to treatment would be possible in a community situation, as opposed to a well-controlled clinical trial, needs to be investigated in order to evaluate adherence to this form of asthma management.

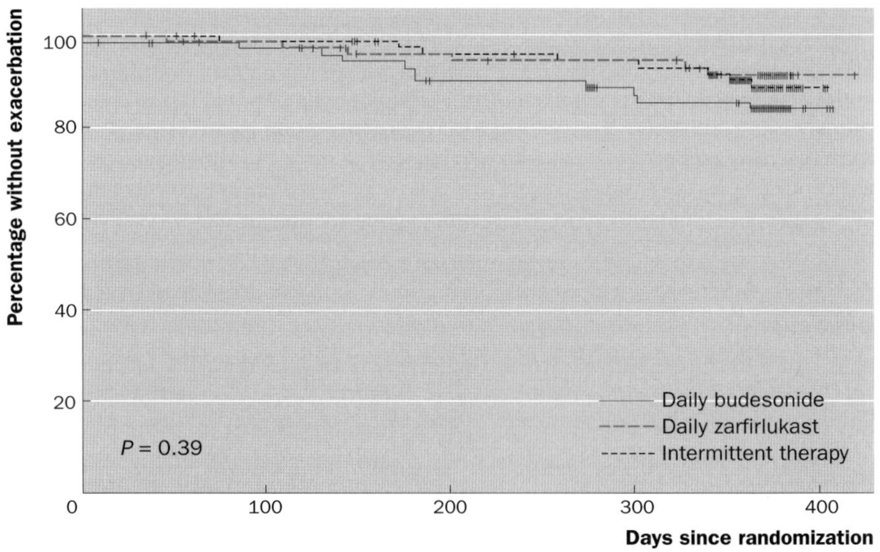

Fig. 13.4 Kaplan–Meier estimates of the time to a first exacerbation of asthma. There was no significant difference among the groups ($P = 0.39$). Source: Boushey *et al.* (2005).

Efficacy and safety of budesonide/formoterol single inhaler therapy versus a higher dose of budesonide in moderate to severe asthma

Scicchitano R, Aalbers R, Ukena D, *et al. Curr Med Res Opin* 2004; **20**: 1403–18

BACKGROUND. This study evaluated the efficacy and safety of a novel asthma management strategy – budesonide/formoterol for both maintenance and symptom relief (Symbicort Single Inhaler Therapy) – compared with a higher maintenance dose of budesonide in patients with moderate to severe asthma.

INTERPRETATION. In this randomized, double-blind, parallel-group study, symptomatic patients with asthma received either budesonide (160 μg, two inhalations twice daily) plus terbutaline 0.4 mg as needed or a daily maintenance dose of budesonide/formoterol (160/4.5 μg, two inhalations once daily) with additional inhalations of budesonide/formoterol 160/4.5 μg as needed. It was found that single-inhaler therapy with budesonide/formoterol had the potential to provide a complete asthma management approach with one inhaler, demonstrating a high level of efficacy in patients with moderate to severe asthma.

Comment

Among the long-acting β_2-agonists, formoterol, as opposed to salmeterol, has a rapid onset of action and a linear dose–response curve. The investigator took advantage of these properties of formoterol to assess whether the combination inhaler containing budesonide and formoterol can be used as regular maintenance therapy as well as to alleviate symptoms. The budesonide/formoterol group had 45% fewer severe exacerbations requiring medical intervention per patient compared with the budesonide group ($P<0.001$). Patients treated with budesonide/formoterol had fewer hospitalizations/emergency room treatments (15 and 25 events, respectively, and fewer treatment days with systemic steroids: 1776 days and 3177 days, respectively) compared with patients in the budesonide group. Patients receiving single-inhaler therapy with budesonide/formoterol used less as-needed medication compared with patients in the budesonide group (0.90 vs 1.42 inhalations/day; $P<0.001$). The mean daily ICS dose was lower in the budesonide/formoterol group than in the budesonide group (466 vs 640 μg/day).

This study shows that the addition of a long-acting β_2-agonist to an ICS is more beneficial than increasing the dose of the ICS (Fig. 13.5). This can also reduce the adverse effects of ICS in the treatment of asthma, because the total dose of inhaled steroid used by the group receiving budesonide plus formoterol (using this as a single dose plus prn [as and when required]) was less than the group receiving only budesonide (who used this as a regular twice-a-day maintenance therapy. One of the significant aspects of this study was the reduction in the number of severe

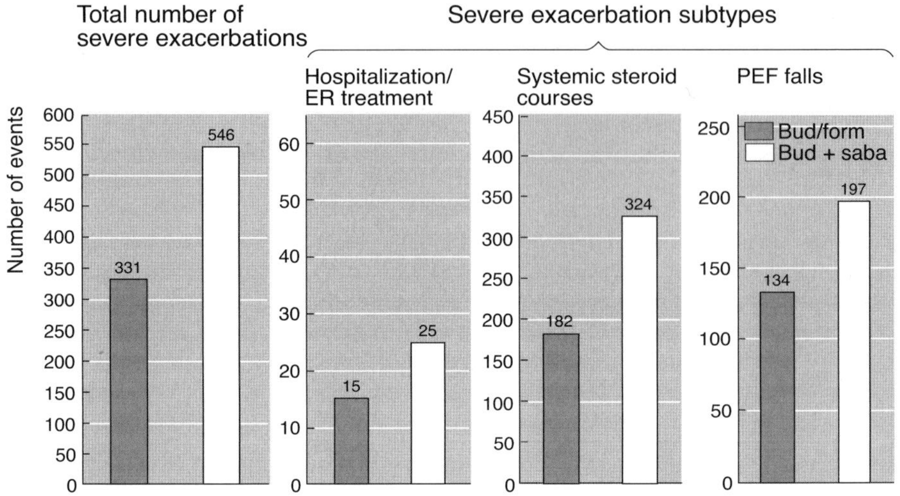

Fig. 13.5 Single-inhaler therapy with budesonide plus formoterol resulted in fewer hospitalizations/emergency room treatments during the study compared with the group receiving only budesonide (15 and 25 events respectively [descriptive statistics]). Patients receiving single-inhaler therapy with budesonide plus formoterol required 142 fewer courses of systemic steroids than patients receiving only budesonide (182 vs 324 courses, respectively). Source: Scicchitano *et al.* (2004).

exacerbations by a ratio of 10:1 in favour of the group receiving budesonide plus formoterol.

Budesonide/formoterol combination therapy as both maintenance and reliever medication in asthma

O'Byrne PM, Bisgaard H, Godard PP, *et al. Am J Respir Crit Care Med* 2005; **171**: 129–36

BACKGROUND. The combination of a long-acting β_2-agonist (LABA) with ICS improves asthma control. This has been shown in various clinical trials |15| and is now part of the asthma management guidelines |10,16|. As asthma is characterized by variable airflow limitation, periodic fluctuations in symptoms are usually treated with reliever medications. This study looked at a combination inhaler containing both an ICS and an LABA for both regular maintenance therapy and as needed. The authors believed that this strategy provides additional anti-inflammatory therapy and rapid symptom relief if symptoms appear.

INTERPRETATION. In this double-blind, randomized, parallel-group study, 2760 patients with asthma, aged 4–80 years and with FEV_1 60–100% of predicted, received either budesonide/formoterol 80/4.5 μg twice a day or budesonide 320 μg twice a day with terbutaline 0.4 mg as reliever medication or budesonide/formoterol 80/4.5 μg twice a day with budesonide/formoterol 80/4.5 μg as needed (maintenance + relief). Children used a once-nightly maintenance dose. The authors concluded that using budesonide/formoterol for both maintenance and relief reduces the risk and rate of severe asthma exacerbations and the need for systemic steroids and improves asthma symptoms, nocturnal awakenings and lung function compared with traditional fixed dosing regimens, therefore reducing the morbidity and potentially the mortality of asthma.

Comment

This study demonstrated that a budesonide/formoterol combination for maintenance and relief was beneficial and reduced asthma exacerbations in adults and children compared with doubling the dose of budesonide or the addition of a long-acting β_2-agonist to budesonide in a fixed dose while using a short-acting β_2-agonist for rescue.

One of the concerns of the last two studies was the overuse of a long-acting β_2-agonist as a reliever. There are not very many data on the overuse of long-acting β_2-agonists and one has to be cautious because patients with severe asthma tend to overuse reliever medications during worsening control of asthma. Furthermore, with this combination there is the possibility of overuse of the ICS, which can also be deleterious in the long run. Although these studies showed that it was safe to use the combination of LABA with ICS as a reliever medication, the consequences of over-medicating oneself with LABA have not been looked at adequately.

Newer inhaled corticosteroids

A number of new steroids are being investigated with the aim of maintaining the excellent efficacy of ICS while improving the short- and long-term safety profile. One of these, ciclesonide, has recently been approved for use in asthma patients. HFA (hydro fluro alkane) ciclesonide has a lung deposition rate of 50–60%. High lipophilicity and the formation of a local depot prolong the pulmonary duration of action, justifying the once-daily administration of ciclesonide. High protein binding and rapid clearance reduces systemic interactions. In long-term studies, ciclesonide at doses as high as 1280–1600 μg/day did not suppress biochemical markers of adrenal function. Since ciclesonide is not being activated in the oropharynx, the incidence of local adverse effects is comparable to that of placebo |**17–19**|.

Maintenance of asthma control by once-daily inhaled ciclesonide in adults with persistent asthma

Chapman KR, Patel P, D'Urzo AD, *et al.* *Allergy* 2005; **60**: 330–7

BACKGROUND. Ciclesonide is an inhaled corticosteroid that is converted to an active metabolite, desisobutyryl ciclesonide, in the lungs, thereby minimizing effects on endogenous cortisol |20|. The goal of finding newer, safer corticosteroids for the management of asthma has led to the development of this novel corticosteroid.

INTERPRETATION. This 12-week, double-blind, randomized, parallel-group, placebo-controlled study evaluated the efficacy and safety of ciclesonide in adults with persistent asthma. Efficacy was monitored with asthma symptom scores, rescue medication use, morning and evening PEF measurements, spirometry, and the probability of study completion without experiencing lack of efficacy. It was concluded that ciclesonide (160 or 640 μg) once daily in the morning maintains asthma control effectively, does not affect cortisol levels, and has an adverse event profile comparable with that of placebo in adults with primarily mild to moderate asthma.

Comment

It has been reported previously that, compared with fluticasone, ciclesonide possesses equivalent anti-inflammatory efficacy, through pulmonary activation,

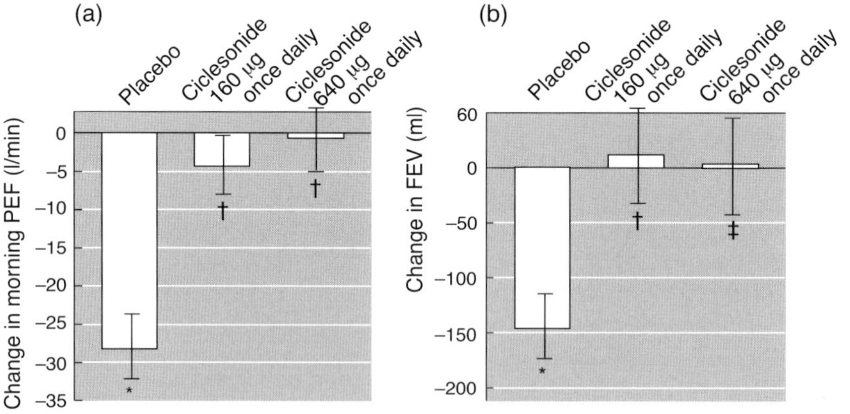

Fig. 13.6 (a) Change in morning PEF from patient diaries following a switch to ciclesonide or placebo therapy. Morning PEF significantly decreased with placebo treatment but remained stable with treatment with either dose of ciclesonide (160 or 640 μg). (b) Change in FEV_1 in patients with stable asthma after switching to ciclesonide or placebo treatment. FEV_1 declined significantly with placebo and was maintained for both doses of ciclesonide. Source: Chapman *et al.* (2005).

with a significantly improved safety profile [21]. Since it has low bioavailability because it is metabolized by the lung, it is believed to cause minimal systemic adverse effects. It was found that the morning PEF and FEV_1 values from patient diaries decreased significantly in patients switched from their usual ICS therapy to placebo but remained stable in patients switched to either dose of ciclesonide (160 or 640 μg; Fig. 13.6). Furthermore, in patients switched to placebo there were significant increases in daily asthma symptoms and the use of rescue medication, with no significant changes from baseline in patients switched to either dose of ciclesonide. Mean changes from baseline in serum and urinary cortisol levels were not statistically significant in any of the treatment groups. Adverse effects were mild, with no reported cases of oral candidiasis. In conclusion, once-daily ciclesonide (160 or 640 μg) was superior to placebo in the maintenance of asthma control in adult patients previously treated with moderate doses of ICS, without any significant adverse effects.

Airway and systemic effects of hydrofluoroalkane formulations of high-dose ciclesonide and fluticasone in moderate persistent asthma

Lee DK, Fardon TC, Bates CE, Haggart K, McFarlane LC, Lipworth BJ. *Chest* 2005; **127**: 851–60

BACKGROUND. The new corticosteroid ciclesonide has been evaluated in various studies to assess its efficacy and adverse effect profile in asthma. However, there are no data comparing the effects of high-dose ciclesonide with those of fluticasone propionate on airway and systemic outcomes in patients with moderate persistent asthma.

INTERPRETATION. The relative effects of 4 weeks of treatment with ciclesonide and fluticasone propionate on airway hyper-reactivity, exhaled nitric oxide levels, lung function, symptoms, and quality of life were compared in 14 patients with moderately persistent asthma. Both drugs significantly improved airway outcomes in terms of methacholine bronchial hyper-responsiveness and exhaled nitric oxide levels. Fluticasone propionate 2000 μg daily but not ciclesonide 1600 μg daily significantly suppressed hypothalamic–pituitary–adrenal (HPA) axis outcomes, overnight 10 h urinary cortisol levels being lower after fluticasone propionate administration than after ciclesonide administration.

Comment

The efficacy of a new medication depends upon comparison with an existing medication that is used in the community for the treatment of a particular condition. ICS, namely beclomethasone, budesonide and fluticasone, have been used in the treatment of asthma. The introduction of newer ICS would depend on the efficacy of the medication in comparison with existing medication. Ciclesonide has been evaluated in various studies [22–24] essentially looking at the adverse effect profile and its effectiveness in asthma. There are no reports of head-to-head comparisons with the standard ICS. This study compared the effects of ciclesonide with those of fluticasone propionate, albeit in a small population of moderately persistent asthmatics. The absence of significant differences between the group receiving fluticasone propionate and the group receiving ciclesonide in airway parameters, including spirometry, PEF, symptoms and Mini-AQLQ (Asthma Quality of Life Questionnaire) score, suggest that ciclesonide could prove to be a useful option in the management of asthma. With regard to safety, the treatment period of 4 weeks may not be adequate to cause significant suppression of the HPA axis and long-term trials are required to evaluate the effects of ciclesonide on the HPA axis.

The findings of these studies, coupled with the results of earlier studies on the pharmacology, pharmacokinetics and efficacy of ciclesonide, indicate great promise for this new inhaled steroid in the treatment of asthma. The higher bioavailability and improved plasma binding of this steroid provide it with greater efficacy and minimal side effects. Furthermore, ciclesonide, with its minimal effect on the HPA axis |**25**|, could be useful in the treatment of children with asthma. However, data on the long-term effects on the HPA axis with ciclesonide are necessary if they are to be considered to be safe medications with no effect on the HPA axis.

Conclusion

Guidelines for the management of asthma suggest the regular use of ICS for asthma control. One recent study looked at daily versus as-needed corticosteroids in patients with mild persistent asthma. This study provided evidence that the use of ICS during worsening of asthma could be useful in patients with mild persistent asthma. This therapy could be potentially beneficial in patients who are not troubled regularly by their asthma. The implications of these results may be significant as they suggest new recommendations for asthma management and also affect the economics of the treatment of patients with mild persistent asthma.

Corticosteroids are the mainstay of the management of asthma. ICS are used regularly for good asthma control. Patients with asthma are usually advised by their physicians to double the dose of their ICS if they have an upper respiratory tract infection of if they feel that their asthma is worsening. Two studies discussed in this chapter looked at doubling the dose of ICS in asthma exacerbations. Interestingly, these studies concluded that doubling the dose of ICS during an exacerbation would not provide any added advantage, such as requiring a lower dose of oral corticosteroids, and would not alter the course of an asthma exacerbation.

The use of corticosteroids in pregnancy has been evaluated in the past, and studies have suggested that ICS are safe in pregnancy whereas oral steroids can be associated with maternal and fetal complications. Two studies looked at this aspect and found that ICS are safer in pregnancy but that poor asthma control can be associated with perinatal complications and maternal complications. These studies suggest the importance of asthma control during pregnancy.

ICS are associated with steroid-related side effects, which include impaired glucose tolerance, osteoporosis, hypertension and thinning of the skin, leading to bruising [26]. Although these are associated with higher doses of ICS, this is a real issue. Hence, researchers are evaluating newer corticosteroids [27–29]. One of these drugs is ciclesonide, which is metabolized locally so that a minimal amount of drug reaches the systemic circulation. Studies have looked at the efficacy of ciclesonide in allergen-induced airway responsiveness and its safety profile. Ciclesonide is effective in reducing airway hyper-responsiveness and has a lesser effect on the hypothalamo-pituitary axis, and is thus a safer ICS. Most studies have confirmed that ciclesonide is an effective ICS in the treatment of asthma. However, there are not enough studies comparing this newer corticosteroid with other standard ICS used in the management of asthma. Comparison of ciclesonide with beclomethasone, budesonide and fluticasone may provide important information on the efficacy of this new steroid in asthma.

Our understanding of asthma has changed significantly in the past few years but this has not translated into many new effective therapies for asthma. Although a lot of research is being carried out into the development of newer therapies of asthma, including biological therapies, ICS remain the backbone of asthma management.

References

1. Brattsand R. Development of glucocorticosteroids with lung selectivity. In: Hargreave FE, Hogg JC, Malo JL, Toogood JH (eds). *Glucocorticoids and mechanisms of asthma.* Amsterdam: Excerpta Medica, 1988; pp 17–38.
2. Taylor DA, Jensen MW, Kanabar V, Engelstatter R, Steinijans VW, Barnes PJ, O'Connor BJ. A dose-dependent effect of the novel inhaled corticosteroid ciclesonide on airway responsiveness to adenosine-5′-monophosphate in asthmatic patients. *Am J Respir Crit Care Med* 1999; **160**: 237–43.
3. Vayssiere BM, Dupont S, Choquart A, Petit F, Garcia T, Marchandeau C, Gronemeyer H, Resche-Rigon M. Synthetic glucocorticoids that dissociate transactivation and AP-1 transrepression exhibit antiinflammatory activity *in vivo. Mol Endocrinol* 1997; **11**: 1245–55.
4. Barnes PJ. Anti-inflammatory actions of glucocorticoids: molecular mechanisms. *Clin Sci (Lond)* 1998; **94**: 557–72.
5. Chaudhuri R, Livingston E, McMahon AD, Thomson L, Borland W, Thomson NC. Cigarette smoking impairs the therapeutic response to oral corticosteroids in chronic asthma. *Am J Respir Crit Care Med* 2003; **168**: 1308–11.

6. Chalmers GW, Macleod KJ, Little SA, Thomson LJ, McSharry CP, Thomson NC. Influence of cigarette smoking on inhaled corticosteroid treatment in mild asthma. *Thorax* 2002; **57**: 226–30.

7. Evans DJ, Taylor DA, Zetterstrom O, Chung KF, O'Connor BJ, Barnes PJ. A comparison of low-dose inhaled budesonide plus theophylline and high-dose inhaled budesonide for moderate asthma. *N Engl J Med* 1997; **337**: 1412–18.

8. Schatz M, Zeiger RS, Harden K, Hoffman CC, Chilingar L, Petitti D. The safety of asthma and allergy medications during pregnancy. *J Allergy Clin Immunol* 1997; **100**: 301–6.

9. Martel MJ, Rey E, Beauchesne MF, Perreault S, Lefebvre G, Forget A, Blais L. Use of inhaled corticosteroids during pregnancy and risk of pregnancy induced hypertension: nested case–control study. *BMJ* 2005; **330**: 230.

10. British Thoracic Society, Scottish Intercollegiate Guidelines Network. British guideline on the management of asthma. *Thorax* 2003; **58**(Suppl 1): i1–94.

11. Babu KS, Arshad SH, Puddicombe SM, Wilson SJ, Holgate S, Davies DE. Repeated low dose allergen exposure up regulates tumour necrosis factor alpha TNF-alpha and adhesion molecules in asthma. *Am J Respir Crit Care Med* 2004; **169**: A551.

12. Cunnington D, Smith N, Steed K, Rosengarten P, Kelly AM, Teichtahl H. Oral versus intravenous corticosteroids in adults hospitalised with acute asthma. *Pulm Pharmacol Ther* 2005; **18**: 207–12.

13. Volovitz B, Bentur L, Finkelstein Y, Mansour Y, Shalitin S, Nussinovitch M, Varsano I. Effectiveness and safety of inhaled corticosteroids in controlling acute asthma attacks in children who were treated in the emergency department: a controlled comparative study with oral prednisolone. *J Allergy Clin Immunol* 1998; **102**(4 Pt 1): 605–9.

14. Devidayal S, Singhi S, Kumar L, Jayshree M. Efficacy of nebulized budesonide compared to oral prednisolone in acute bronchial asthma. *Acta Paediatr* 1999; **88**: 835–40.

15. Pauwels RA, Lofdahl CG, Postma DS, Tattersfield AE, O'Byrne P, Barnes PJ, Ullman A. Effect of inhaled formoterol and budesonide on exacerbations of asthma. Formoterol and Corticosteroids Establishing Therapy (FACET) International Study Group. *N Engl J Med* 1997; **337**: 1405–11.

16. National Asthma Education and Prevention Program. *Guidelines for the diagnosis and management of asthma: Expert Panel Report 2.* Bethesda, MD: US Department of Health and Human Services, Public Health Service, National Institutes of Health, National Heart, Lung, and Blood Institute. NIH publication no. 97–4051, 1997.

17. Ukena D. [Ciclesonide—a new inhaled corticosteroid]. *Pneumologie* 2005; **59**: 689–95 (in German).

18. Hubner M, Hochhaus G, Derendorf H. Comparative pharmacology, bioavailability, pharmacokinetics, and pharmacodynamics of inhaled glucocorticosteroids. *Immunol Allergy Clin North Am* 2005; **25**: 469–88.

19. Rohatagi S, Luo Y, Shen L, Guo Z, Schemm C, Huang Y, Chen K, David M, Nave R, King SP. Protein binding and its potential for eliciting minimal systemic side effects with a novel inhaled corticosteroid, ciclesonide. *Am J Ther* 2005; **12**: 201–9.

20. Reynolds NA, Scott LJ. Ciclesonide. *Drugs* 2004; **64**: 511–19; discussion 520–1.

21. Belvisi MG, Bundschuh DS, Stoeck M, Wicks S, Underwood S, Battram CH, Haddad el-B, Webber SE, Foster ML. Preclinical profile of ciclesonide, a novel corticosteroid for the treatment of asthma. *J Pharmacol Exp Ther* 2005; **314**: 568–74.

22. Langdon CG, Adler M, Mehra S, Alexander M, Drollmann A. Once-daily ciclesonide 80 or 320 μg for 12 weeks is safe and effective in patients with persistent asthma. *Respir Med* 2005; **99**: 1275–85.

23. Agertoft L, Pedersen S. Short-term lower-leg growth rate and urine cortisol excretion in children treated with ciclesonide. *J Allergy Clin Immunol* 2005; **115**: 940–5.

24. Dent G. Ciclesonide (Byk Gulden). *Curr Opin Investig Drugs* 2002; **3**: 78–83.

25. Weinbrenner A, Huneke D, Zschiesche M, Engel G, Timmer W, Steinijans VW, Bethke T, Wurst W, Drollmann A, Kaatz HJ, Siegmund W. Circadian rhythm of serum cortisol after repeated inhalation of the new topical steroid ciclesonide. *J Clin Endocrinol Metab* 2002; **87**: 2160–3.

26. Allen DB, Bielory L, Derendorf H, Dluhy R, Colice GL, Szefler SJ. Inhaled corticosteroids: past lessons and future issues. *J Allergy Clin Immunol* 2003; **112**(3 Suppl): S1–40.

27. Schacke H, Schottelius A, Docke WD, Strehlke P, Jaroch S, Schmees N, Rehwinkel H, Hennekes H, Asadullah K. Dissociation of transactivation from transrepression by a selective glucocorticoid receptor agonist leads to separation of therapeutic effects from side effects. *Proc Natl Acad Sci USA* 2004; **101**: 227–32.

28. Stoeck M, Riedel R, Hochhaus G, Hafner D, Masso JM, Schmidt B, Hatzelmann A, Marx D, Bundschuh DS. *In vitro* and *in vivo* anti-inflammatory activity of the new glucocorticoid ciclesonide. *J Pharmacol Exp Ther* 2004; **309**: 249–58.

29. Belvisi MG, Wicks SL, Battram CH, Bottoms SE, Redford JE, Woodman P, Brown TJ, Webber SE, Foster ML. Therapeutic benefit of a dissociated glucocorticoid and the relevance of *in vitro* separation of transrepression from transactivation activity. *J Immunol* 2001; **166**: 1975–82.

14

Experimental therapies for allergic disorders

JAYMIN MORJARIA, SURESH BABU

Introduction

Bronchial asthma is a disorder of the conducting airways, which exhibit hyper-responsiveness to a wide range of stimuli, ultimately leading to airflow obstruction. Chronic airway inflammation, demonstrable in even mild, asymptomatic asthmatics, is thought to underlie at least a component of the hyper-responsiveness. The current management of asthma therefore focuses on the optimal control of symptoms and the reduction of airway inflammation [1]. Thus, at present the principal treatment for controlling asthma remains corticosteroids.

However, given the significant systemic adverse effects of corticosteroids, newer, more specific and safer therapies are being investigated to target specific mechanisms underlying the airway inflammation. Hence, novel therapies in various severities of asthma are discussed here. Additionally, other novel treatments in allergic diseases are included.

Tumour necrosis factor (TNF α) as a novel therapeutic target in symptomatic corticosteroid-dependent asthma

Howarth PH, Babu KS, Arshad HS, *et al. Thorax* 2005; **60**: 1012–18

Background. Tumour necrosis factor-α (TNF-α) is a major therapeutic target in a range of chronic inflammatory disorders [2] involving neutrophils and its excess production is characterized by a Th1-type immune response. Asthma is regarded as a Th2-type disorder when associated with atopy, but when it becomes more severe and chronic it adopts additional characteristics, including refractoriness to corticosteroids and neutrophil involvement, suggesting an altered inflammatory profile towards a Th1-type response. Etanercept (Enbrel®) is a soluble TNF-α receptor immunoglobulin (Ig) G1–Fc fusion protein. The aim of this open-label, uncontrolled study was to assess the clinical improvement in asthma control and changes in airway hyper-responsiveness to inhaled methacholine and lung function in patients treated with etanercept.

© Atlas Medical Publishing Ltd

Interpretation. Seventeen subjects (five male, twelve female) requiring regular oral and inhaled corticosteroids and nebulized β_2-agonist therapy were enrolled to receive etanercept injections administered subcutaneously twice weekly for 12 weeks. Lung function, asthma symptoms, rescue medication use, induced sputum and airway hyper-responsiveness were assessed before and after treatment. Treatment with etanercept in the 15 subjects who completed the study produced marked and significant improvements in asthma symptoms as measured by Asthma Control Questionnaire (ACQ) scores ($P<0.001$) (Fig. 14.1), lung function (forced expiratory volume in 1 s [FEV_1], forced vital capacity [FVC], and morning and evening peak expiratory flows) and β_2-agonist use. All but one patient completely withdrew from nebulized salbutamol. Of particular significance was the methacholine PC_{20} (the dose of methacholine that causes a 20% decrease in the patient's baseline FEV_1, measured after inhaling normal saline), which revealed an improvement of 2.5 doubling dilutions ($P = 0.033$) (Fig. 14.2). Although reductions in eosinophil and neutrophil numbers were observed in the sputum counts in eight of the eleven subjects, this failed to achieve statistical significance. In summary, blocking the effects of TNF-α was associated with dramatic improvement in the condition of patients with corticosteroid-resistant asthma and only mild adverse effects. Additional experimental studies revealed vital information regarding the link between TNF-α and severe corticosteroid-refractory asthma. Bronchial alveolar lavage fluid from severe asthmatics had a significantly higher median concentration of TNF-α than fluid from either healthy controls or subjects with mild asthma ($P \leq 0.001$). Relative TNF-α mRNA levels were also significantly higher in bronchial biopsies from severe asthmatics than in biopsies from patients with mild asthma ($P = 0.002$). Furthermore, there were significantly greater numbers of TNF-α-immunoreactive cells/mm^2 in bronchial biopsies from subjects with severe asthma than in biopsies from subjects with mild asthma ($P<0.03$).

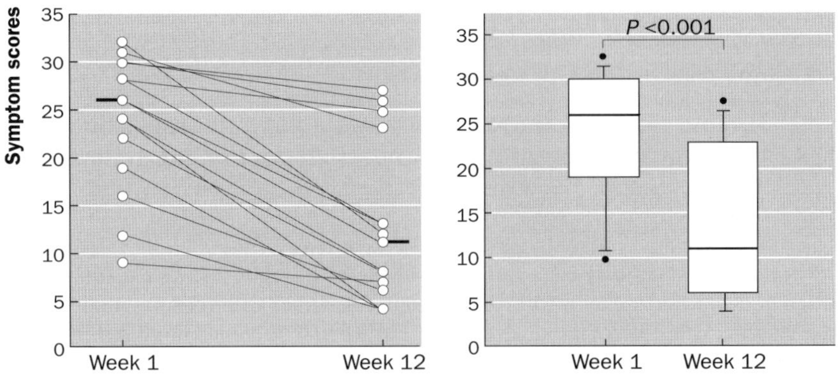

Fig. 14.1 Improvement in asthma control as assessed by Juniper's Asthma Control Questionnaire after 12 weeks of treatment with etanercept. Source: Howarth *et al.* (2005).

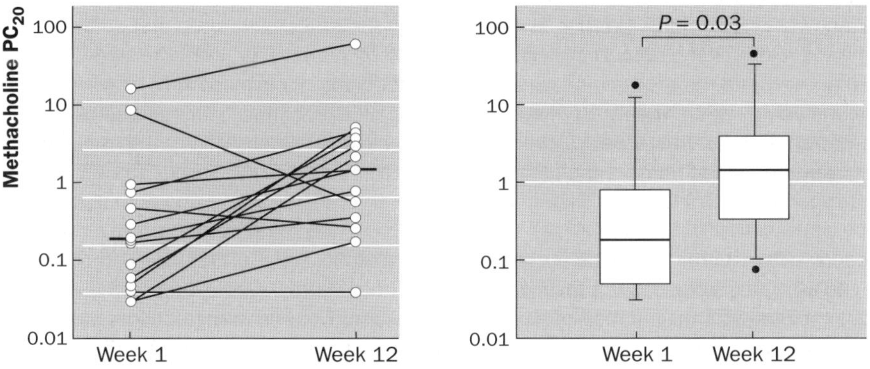

Fig. 14.2 Improvement in airway hyper-responsiveness assessed following methacholine challenge in patients with severe asthma after 12 weeks of treatment with etanercept. Source: Howarth *et al.* (2005).

Comment

The therapeutic options for patients with corticosteroid-refractory asthma are limited, and it is this subgroup of patients that represent a clinical burden that accounts for approximately 30% of the healthcare costs of asthma [3]. Anti-TNF-α therapy is not efficacious in milder forms of asthma (see Rouhani *et al.*, reviewed below). However, this proof-of-concept study highlights that TNF-α-blocking therapies may be a therapeutic option in severe disease. These findings warrant validation in large, randomized, placebo-controlled trials using both the soluble receptor as well as antibody approaches to identify the role of TNF-α blockade and the safety profile of these in severe corticosteroid-dependent asthma, where there remains a large unmet clinical need.

Effect of tumor necrosis factor antagonism on allergen-mediated asthmatic airway inflammation

Rouhani FN, Meitin CA, Kaler M, Miskinis-Hilligoss D, Stylianou M, Levine SJ. *Respir Med* 2005; **99**: 1175–82

BACKGROUND. TNF is a pro-inflammatory cytokine implicated in the pathogenesis of asthmatic airway inflammation [4–9], hyper-reactivity [10] and remodelling [11–13]. The primary aim of the trial was to assess whether TNF antagonism, using a soluble TNF receptor (TNFR:Fc etanercept, Enbrel®), can attenuate eosinophilic airway inflammation in patients with mild to moderate allergic asthma. The secondary outcome measures included the attenuation of pulmonary eosinophilia, Th2-type cytokines, and airway hyper-responsiveness to methacholine. This study was designed as a double-blind, placebo-controlled, randomized trial.

Interpretation. Twenty-six subjects receiving only inhaled β_2 bronchodilator therapy and who demonstrated an FEV_1 of ≥70% of their predicted value and both an early- and a late-phase response to inhalational allergen challenge were recruited prospectively into the study. Injections (etanercept 25 mg or placebo) were administered subcutaneously twice weekly for 2 weeks, followed by a bronchoscopic segmental allergen challenge. Unfortunately, one of the subjects in the etanercept group developed a transient left-sided hemiplegia lasting 36 h, which resulted in the suspension of the trial. Thus, the data from the 21 subjects (placebo 9, etanercept 12) who completed the study were analysed. Subjects in the etanercept group had significantly increased levels of TNF receptor 2 (TNFR2) in the epithelial lining fluid ($P < 0.001$), consistent with delivery of etanercept to the lungs. However, administration of etanercept was not associated with attenuation of airway hyper-responsiveness to methacholine or reduction in pulmonary eosinophilia, but was associated with an elevated level of interleukin (IL)-4 in the epithelial lining fluid ($P = 0.033$) 24 h after segmental allergen challenge.

Comment

This study highlights two important issues. Firstly, that TNF antagonism may not be an effective treatment option for preventing allergen-mediated eosinophilic airway inflammation in mild to moderate asthma. Furthermore, TNF antagonism increased pulmonary IL-4 levels, suggesting that TNF signalling pathways may play a counter-regulatory role in downregulating the functioning of Th2-type T cells. Secondly, although no serious adverse events were described in the etanercept open-label study in patients with severe asthma (see Howarth *et al.*, reviewed above), caution is necessary before administering anti-TNF treatments because of the development of transient hemiplegia in this trial and case reports of new-onset central nervous system demyelinating lesions in patients with inflammatory arthritides and an increase in multiple sclerosis |**14–17**|. Further in-depth and larger studies are necessary to ascertain the safety of such treatments, and increased vigilance of patients already on treatment should be maintained in order to detect any new-onset neurological or other serious adverse events.

The effect of marimastat, a metalloprotease inhibitor, on allergen–induced asthmatic hyper-reactivity

Bruce C, Thomas PS. *Toxicol Appl Pharmacol* 2005; **205**: 126–32

Background. Marimastat is a synthetic broad-spectrum matrix metalloproteinase (MMP) inhibitor. This study assessed the anti-inflammatory effects of marimastat in patients with asthma by reducing TNF-α production *in vivo* by inhibiting MMP activity and hence TNF-α release. The primary aim of the study was to investigate the effects of this MMP inhibitor on allergen-induced hyper-reactivity. The study was designed as a double-blind, placebo-controlled, randomized crossover trial.

INTERPRETATION. Twelve non-smoking steroid-naive subjects with mild asthma (four males and eight females) were recruited to either of two treatment sequences (marimastat 5 mg then placebo, or placebo then marimastat 5 mg), twice daily orally for 8 weeks separated by a 6-week washout period. All subjects underwent an allergen inhalation provocation test to Dermatophagoides pteronyssinus before and after each study phase. Only nine subjects completed the trial; marimastat reduced bronchial hyper-responsiveness to inhaled allergen in these subjects from an allergen PC_{20} of 22.2 to 17.0 allergen units (AU)/ml ($P = 0.02$). Furthermore, the marimastat arm of the study showed a non-significant fall in sputum inflammatory cells, and at this low dose marimastat was well tolerated and no drug-related adverse events were reported.

Comment

TNF-α has been shown to be an important cytokine in the pathogenesis of allergic airway inflammatory responses **[18,19]** and has been shown to be activated by a number of MMPs **[20]**. MMP-9 levels are increased after an allergen challenge and this has been implicated in inflammatory cellular migration and airway remodelling **[21,22]**. However, a naturally occurring inhibitor, tissue inhibitor of metalloproteinase-3 (TIMP-3), can reduce TNF-α production by inhibiting TNF-α-converting enzyme (TACE), which is the enzyme that synthesizes TNF-α. This study suggests that marimastat provides significant protection against allergen hyper-reactivity either by inhibition of TNF-α production or by reducing an alternative effect of MMPs in the airway, or by a combination of both mechanisms. There is a necessity for larger, power-calculated, double-blind, randomized, controlled studies to assess whether marimastat can achieve significant results in other asthma parameters, but the actual mechanisms of action, optimal dosage and efficacy of MMP inhibitors also merit further research. There is also a need for more specific targeting of MMP inhibitors.

Roflumilast, an oral, once-daily phosphodiesterase 4 inhibitor, attenuates allergen-induced asthmatic reactions

van Schalkwyk E, Strydom K, Williams Z, *et al. J Allergy Clin Immunol* 2005; **116**: 292–8

BACKGROUND. Roflumilast is an oral, once-daily inhibitor of phosphodiesterase type 4 (PDE4) that prevents the breakdown of cyclic adenosine monophosphate (cAMP) levels, leading to inhibition of pro-inflammatory signalling. This study investigated the effects of repeated doses of 250 or 500 µg of roflumilast on asthmatic airway responses to allergen.

INTERPRETATION. Twenty-three patients with mild allergic asthma who had an FEV_1 of 70% of predicted value or greater were enrolled in a randomized, double-blind, placebo-controlled, three-period crossover study. Patients received roflumilast (250 or 500 µg) or placebo once daily over three treatment periods of 7–10 days separated by a washout period of 2–5 weeks. An allergen challenge was performed at the end of each

Table 14.1 Treatment differences in the late and early allergen reactions with area under the curve (AUC) analysis

		Late allergen reaction, $AUC_{2–12h}$			**Early allergen reaction, $AUC_{0–2h}$**		
Roflumilast dose	Patients* (*n*)	Point estimate (95% CI)	*P*-value	Reduction (%)	Point estimate (95% CI)	*P*-value	Reduction (%)
Roflumilast 250 μg† vs placebo‡	21	–0.148 (–0.272 to –0.024)	0.0110	27	–0.146 (–0.248 to –0.044)	0.0038	25
Roflumilast 500 μg† vs placebo‡	19	–0.243 (–0.382 to –0.104)	0.0009	43	–0.179 (–0.307 to –0.050)	0.0046	28
Roflumilast 500 μg† vs roflumilast 250 μg‡	19	–0.084 (–0.223 to 0.056)	0.1113	21	–0.015 (–0.118 to 0.089)	0.3851	3

$AUC_{2\text{-}12h}$, area under the curve for FEV_1 between 2 and 12 h; $AUC_{0\text{-}2h}$, area under the curve for FEV_1 between 0 and 2 h; CI, confidence interval.
*This summarizes the per-protocol population. Data for the comparisons between 500 μg of roflumilast versus placebo or 500 μg of roflumilast versus 250 μg of roflumilast were available for only 19 patients.
† Test.
‡ Reference.
Source: van Schalkwyk *et al.* (2005).

treatment, followed by FEV_1 measurements over the ensuing 24 h. Roflumilast had only a modest effect on the early allergen reaction, but demonstrated a more pronounced effect on the late allergen reaction (Fig. 14.3). Attenuation of the late reaction showed a dose-related trend; compared with placebo, 500 and 250 μg of roflumilast resulted in a mean attenuation of 43 and 27%, respectively. Treatment with 250 and 500 μg of roflumilast resulted in a modest yet statistically significant inhibition of the maximum decrease in FEV_1 during the late allergic reaction of 17 and 33%, respectively, compared with placebo (Table 14.1). Moreover, unlike broad-spectrum PDE inhibitors in asthma |**23**|, roflumilast was well tolerated and no serious adverse events were reported.

Comment

This proof-of-concept study on allergen-induced asthmatic responses, along with other human studies in exercise-induced asthma |**24**| and studies in animal models |**25**|, demonstrates that roflumilast has multiple anti-inflammatory effects, including the inhibition of inflammatory cell infiltration and reduction of TNF-α release in the lungs. However, further clinical studies with surrogate markers of inflammation are needed to confirm the anti-inflammatory effects, safety and optimal dosing of roflumilast. As a targeted PDE4 inhibitor, roflumilast may offer earlier benefits compared with corticosteroids and leukotriene receptor antagonists.

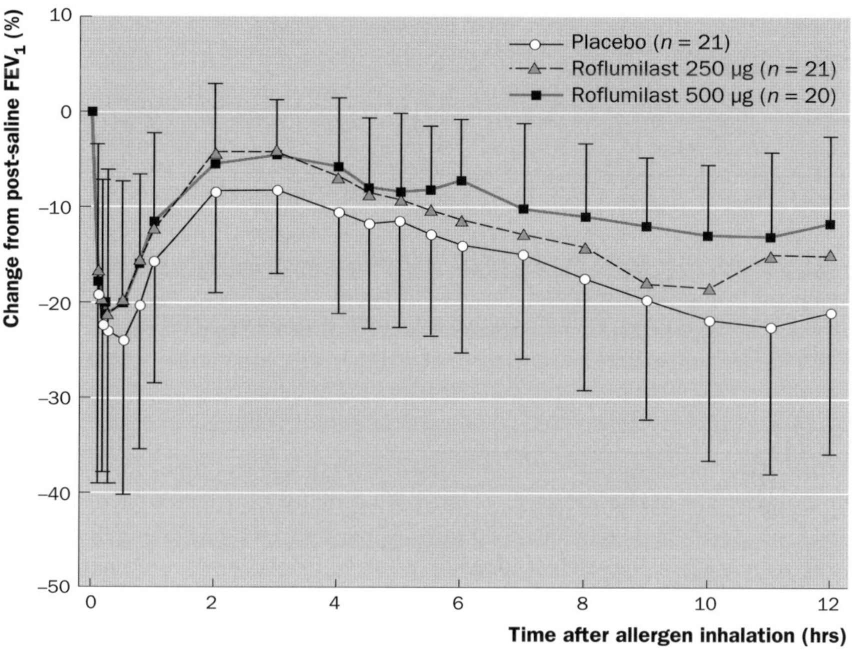

Fig. 14.3 Mean percentage decrease in FEV_1 from post-saline value after allergen challenge. Roflumilast 250 and 500 μg significantly attenuated the early allergen reaction (EAR) (0–2 h) and late allergen reaction (LAR) (2–12 h) compared with placebo. Data are presented for the intent-to-treat population. Source: van Schalkwyk *et al.* (2005).

Treatment of asthma with nebulized lidocaine: a randomized, placebo-controlled study

Hunt LW, Frigas E, Butterfield JH, *et al. J Allergy Clin Immunol* 2004; **113**: 853–9

BACKGROUND. Lidocaine is a local anaesthetic that possesses the ability to potently shorten eosinophil survival [26]. This study assessed the safety and efficacy of nebulized lidocaine in a randomized, placebo-controlled study in patients with mild to moderate asthma.

INTERPRETATION. Fifty subjects were recruited (18 male and 32 female) to receive lidocaine (25) or placebo (25). All the subjects had a pre-bronchodilator FEV_1 of 60–125% of the predicted normal value and were treated daily with inhaled glucocorticoids (but not systemic glucocorticoids) and bronchodilators for at least

2 months. Prior to enrolling in the study, the subjects were monitored for asthma symptoms and peak expiratory flow values, and were maintained on their medications for 2 weeks. At initiation, spirometry, methacholine PD_{20} and complete blood count (including eosinophil count) were performed, and subjects inhaled either nebulized placebo (saline) or lidocaine (4%, 100 mg) four times daily. For the first 3 treatment weeks, all subjects were asked to reduce their inhaled glucocorticoid medications by one-half of the total number of daily sprays each week and at week 4 to discontinue them. The nebulized treatment was continued for a total of 8 weeks with symptom monitoring and the use of bronchodilators. The nebulized lidocaine treatment group showed significant differences in FEV_1, night-time awakenings, asthma symptom scores and blood eosinophils compared with the placebo group. Furthermore, nebulized lidocaine provided effective and safe (no toxicity) therapy in subjects with mild to moderate asthma.

Comment

Glucocorticoids potently alter inflammation [**27,28**]; for example, they shorten eosinophil survival in the presence of pro-inflammatory cytokines such as IL-5, IL-3 and granulocyte–macrophage colony-stimulating factor (GM-CSF) [**26,29**]. The initial interest in the use of lidocaine as an anti-inflammatory treatment in asthma arose from *in vitro* data showing that, like glucocorticoids, lidocaine inhibited cytokine-induced eosinophil activation [**30,31**]. Previous uncontrolled studies in adults [**32**] and children [**33,34**] with asthma, like the present double-blind, randomized, controlled trial, have shown that nebulized lidocaine is a safe and effective steroid-sparing treatment in asthma, although further insight into the mechanism(s) responsible for its efficacy is necessary.

Dual tachykinin NK1/NK2 antagonist DNK333 inhibits neurokinin A-induced bronchoconstriction in asthma patients

Joos GF, Vincken W, Louis R, *et al. Eur Respir J* 2004; **23**: 76–81

BACKGROUND. The sensory neuropeptides substance P and neurokinin A (NKA) are members of the tachykinin family, present within pulmonary sensory nerves and immune cells [35]. In the airways they mainly interact with tachykinin (NK1, NK2) receptors to induce bronchoconstriction, bronchial hyper-responsiveness, mucus secretion, vasodilatation, increased vascular permeability, and attraction and activation of inflammatory cells [36–38]. In this randomized, double-blind, placebo-controlled crossover multicentre trial the effects of a single dose of a dual tachykinin NK1/NK2 receptor, DNK333, were assessed on NKA-induced bronchoconstriction in asthma.

INTERPRETATION. Ten male adult subjects with mild to moderate asthma who were on inhaled bronchodilators with a PC_{20} of less than 8 mg/ml of methacholine underwent an NKA inhalation challenge. Increasing concentrations of NKA (3.3×10^{-9} to 1.0×10^{-6}

mol/ml) were inhaled at 1- and 10-h intervals after a single oral dose of either DNK333 (100 mg) or placebo. DNK333 did not affect baseline lung function but did protect against NKA-induced bronchoconstriction in 15 of the subjects at 1 h but not at 10 h after the dose. The mean $\log_{10}$ provocative concentration causing a 20% fall in FEV_1 for NKA was –5.6 and 6.8 $\log_{10}$ mol/ml at 1 h after DNK333 and placebo respectively. This was equivalent to a difference of 4.08 doubling doses at 1 h, which decreased to a difference of 0.90 doubling doses 10 h after treatment.

Comment

DNK333, compared with other previously studied tachykinin receptor antagonists **[39–41]**, has offered greater bronchoprotection both in animals **[42–44]** and in this double-blind placebo-controlled trial. This study suggests that DNK333 may be an effective agent as an adjunct to bronchodilators prior to the initiation of corticosteroids in patients with asthma. However, there is a need not only for more experimental and clinical studies to be conducted to examine the contributions of each of the NK1 and NK2 receptors, as well as effects in females, but also for the clinical efficacy and safety profiles of DNK333 and future agents from this group of tachykinin receptor inhibitors to be established.

Impact of a soluble phospholipase A2 inhibitor on inhaled allergen challenge in subjects with asthma

Bowton DL, Dmitrienko AA, Israel E, Zeiher BG, Sides GD. *J Asthma* 2005; **42**: 65–71

BACKGROUND. In asthma, the secretory phospholipases A2 (sPLA2) have been implicated in the release of arachidonic acid from cellular membranes, the generation of lysophospholipids, the sPLA2-mediated activation of cellular PLA2 (cPLA2) with increased leukotriene synthesis, and the breakdown of surfactant. In this double-blind, placebo-controlled, random-order crossover study, a potent inhibitor of sPLA2, LY333013, was assessed.

INTERPRETATION. Fifty subjects with atopic asthma were randomly assigned to the study to examine the impact of two doses of LY333013 versus placebo on allergen-induced bronchoconstriction following an inhaled allergen challenge. Forty subjects completed the study with no significant drug-related adverse events of note. However, LY333013 failed to demonstrate any improvement in the area under the FEV_1 response curve (AUC) in both the early phase (0–3 h) and late phase (3–8 h) response following inhaled allergen challenge.

Comment

This study demonstrates that sPLA2 antagonists have no impact on pulmonary function in patients with atopic bronchial asthma.

Anti-interleukin-5 (mepolizumab) therapy for hypereosinophilic syndromes

Garret JK, Jameson SC, Thomson B, *et al.* *J Allergy Clin Immunol* 2004; **113**: 115–19

BACKGROUND. Interleukin-5 is the key cytokine in eosinophil differentiation and growth in the bone marrow [45] and stimulates the release of eosinophils into the peripheral circulation [46]. Thus, it is thought that IL-5 may be involved in the pathogenesis of hypereosinophilic syndromes (HES), a diverse group of poorly treated disorders characterized by sustained peripheral blood and/or tissue eosinophilia. Mepolizumab is a humanized monoclonal antibody to IL-5, and its safety and efficacy were assessed in this open-labelled trial.

INTERPRETATION. Four subjects (two male, two female) with HES defined by peripheral blood and/or tissue eosinophilia were enrolled in the study. Each of the subjects, after the run-in period of 8 weeks, received three intravenous doses (10 mg/kg, maximum 750 mg) of mepolizumab at 4-weekly intervals. The effects of treatment on safety, eosinophil levels (in peripheral blood and/or diseased tissue), pulmonary function and quality of life were measured over a 28-week period. This study demonstrated that the anti-IL-5 therapy was well tolerated and improved peripheral blood eosinophil counts, FEV_1 measurements, a variety of clinical symptoms and quality of life measures. The improvement with mepolizumab was so striking that in one of the subjects with tissue eosinophilia (eosinophilic oesophagitis), treatment with mepolizumab resulted in a 10-fold reduction in tissue eosinophil levels.

Comment

In atopic dermatitis [47] and allergic asthma [48,49] no clinical benefit was achieved with mepolizumab. In asthma, treatment with mepolizumab resulted in reductions in blood and airway eosinophils but did not produce improvements in airway hyper-responsiveness and asthma control [50]. This may have been because the contribution of eosinophils to the pathogenesis of the first two of these conditions may have been different from their contribution to HES. Furthermore, the profound decline in one of the subjects in this study following mepolizumab treatment suggests that this agent may provide relatively more tissue effectiveness in patients with HES. This proof-of-concept study demonstrates that mepolizumab may have clinical utility in HES as well as a potential steroid-sparing benefit, but further evaluation in larger randomized, clinical trials is needed.

Immunotherapy with depigmented glutaraldehyde-polymerized extracts: changes in quality of life

Alvarez-Cuesta E, Aragoneses-Gilsanz E, Martin-Garcia C, Berges-Gimeno P, Gonzalez-Mancebo E, Cuesta-Herranz J. *Clin Exp Allergy* 2005; **35**: 572–8

BACKGROUND. Allergic rhinitis is a very common problem associated with poor quality of life, reductions in social and work activities and poor interpersonal relationships. The main goal of the management of allergic rhinitis is to improve the quality of life. Immunotherapy is a specific therapy for allergic rhinitis and several reports have documented the safety and efficacy of this treatment [51]. Safety has been a key issue in immunotherapy and various modalities are being investigated to make immunotherapy more tolerable and safe to administer. Polymerization of the allergen extracts by gluteraldehyde has been shown to be effective and safe for therapeutic vaccines and modified allergen extracts [52,53]. This double-blind, placebo-controlled prospective study investigated changes related to the patients' quality of life induced by a modified (depigmented glutaraldehyde-polymerized) therapeutic vaccine and the safety of the vaccine.

INTERPRETATION. Fifty-three subjects with a well-documented clinical history of seasonal allergic rhinitis sensitized to *Dactylis glomerata* and *Olea europaea* pollens were included such that 25 subjects received a mixture of *D. glomerata* and *O. europaea* pollen extract and 28 subjects received placebo. A Rhinoconjunctivitis Quality of Life Questionnaire (RQLQ) and dose–response skin-prick test with each allergen extract were conducted before treatment (pollen season of the year 2000) and after 1 year of treatment (pollen season of 2001). All the subjects completed the study, receiving a total of 17 injections during the study period, and no systemic adverse reactions were recorded. Symptom scores ($P<0.001$) and medication requirements ($P<0.001$) were significantly reduced in the group receiving immunotherapy during the pollen season (Fig. 14.4). During the pollen season, patients receiving immunotherapy had significantly greater improvements both in overall RQLQ scores and in five of the seven domains of the Health-Related Quality of Life (HRQOL) questionnaire (sleep, non-hay-fever symptoms, practical problems, nasal symptoms and eye symptoms). Immunotherapy was well tolerated, with no reported systemic reactions.

Comment

Improvement of quality of life with improvements in symptoms and the use of medication is a key point in the treatment of allergic rhinitis. The results of this study are in agreement with previous reports of beneficial effects of immunotherapy with modified vaccines as well as other depigmented modified extracts [52–55]. Future studies are needed to establish (i) the benefits of these therapeutic vaccines, which are tailor-made to the patients' requirement for a combination of allergens (two or more), and (ii) the groups of patients – in terms of disease severity – in which such vaccines may be sufficiently efficacious.

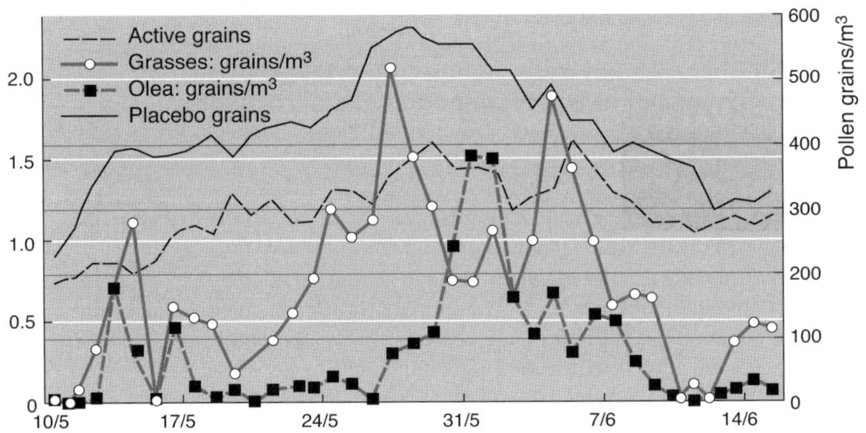

Fig. 14.4 Symptom scores and pollen counts. Source: Alvarez-Cuesta *et al.* (2005).

Conclusion

A number of drugs targeting and neutralizing specific molecules, such as anti-IL-5 and IL-12 agents, have been developed with little if any discernible effect on asthma outcome measures. However, to date the only novel therapeutic biological agent that has been introduced for the treatment of asthma and allergy is a humanized, monoclonal antibody targeted to the C3 domain on the heavy chains of human IgE, omalizumab |**56**|. It is slowly becoming clear that single molecular targets in asthma may not be fruitful and that the disease is heterogeneous, consisting of a series of separate subphenotypes in which individual effector molecules play a dominant role. Illustrations of this already exist in the greater efficacy of anti-leukotriene agents in aspirin-intolerant asthma and the use of omalizumab in the treatment of severe allergic asthma. The future of asthma lies in the identification of heterogeneous biomarkers that could identify disease subtypes, such that asthma treatment can be tailor-made to the patient's requirements.

References

1. New NHLBI guidelines for the diagnosis and management of asthma. National Heart, Lung and Blood Institute. *Lippincott Health Promot Lett* 1997; **2**: 1, 8–9.

2. Feldmann M, Maini MR. Lasker Clinical Medical Research Award. TNF defined as a therapeutic target for rheumatoid arthritis and other autoimmune diseases. *Nat Med* 2003; **9**: 1245–50.
3. Antonicelli L, Bucca C, Neri M, De Benedetto F, Sabbatani P, Bonifazi F, Eichler HG, Zhang Q, Yin DD. Asthma severity and medical resource utilisation. *Eur Respir J* 2004; **23**: 723–9.
4. Gosset P, Tsicopoulos A, Wallaert B, Vannimenus C, Joseph M, Tonnel AB, Capron A. Increased secretion of tumor necrosis factor alpha and interleukin-6 by alveolar macrophages consecutive to the development of the late asthmatic reaction. *J Allergy Clin Immunol* 1991; **88**: 561–71.
5. Gosset P, Tsicopoulos A, Wallaert B, Joseph M, Capron A, Tonnel AB. Tumor necrosis factor alpha and interleukin-6 production by human mononuclear phagocytes from allergic asthmatics after IgE-dependent stimulation. *Am Rev Respir Dis* 1992; **146**: 768–74.
6. Cembrzynska-Nowak M, Szklarz E, Inglot AD, Teodorczyk-Injeyan JA. Elevated release of tumor necrosis factor-alpha and interferon-gamma by bronchoalveolar leukocytes from patients with bronchial asthma. *Am Rev Respir Dis* 1993; **147**: 291–5.
7. Ying S, Robinson DS, Varney V, Meng Q, Tsicopoulos A, Moqbel R, Durham SR, Kay AB, Hamid Q. TNF alpha mRNA expression in allergic inflammation. *Clin Exp Allergy* 1991; **21**: 745–50.
8. Bradding P, Roberts JA, Britten KM, Montefort S, Djukanovic R, Mueller R, Heusser CH, Howarth PH, Holgate ST. Interleukin-4, -5, and -6 and tumor necrosis factor-alpha in normal and asthmatic airways: evidence for the human mast cell as a source of these cytokines. *Am J Respir Cell Mol Biol* 1994; **10**: 471–80.
9. Ackerman V, Marini M, Vittori E, Bellini A, Vassali G, Mattoli S. Detection of cytokines and their cell sources in bronchial biopsy specimens from asthmatic patients. Relationship to atopic status, symptoms, and level of airway hyper-responsiveness. *Chest* 1994; **105**: 687–96.
10. Thomas PS, Yates DH, Barnes PJ. Tumor necrosis factor-alpha increases airway responsiveness and sputum neutrophilia in normal human subjects. *Am J Respir Crit Care Med* 1995; **152**: 76–80.
11. Paulsson Y, Austgulen R, Hofsli E, Heldin CH, Westermark B, Nissen-Meyer J. Tumor necrosis factor-induced expression of platelet-derived growth factor A-chain messenger RNA in fibroblasts. *Exp Cell Res* 1989; **180**: 490–6.
12. Palombella VJ, Mendelsohn J, Vilcek J. Mitogenic action of tumor necrosis factor in human fibroblasts: interaction with epidermal growth factor and platelet-derived growth factor. *J Cell Physiol* 1988; **135**: 23–31.
13. Polosa R, Sapsford RJ, Dokic D, Cacciola RR, Prosperini G, Devalia JL, Holgate ST, Howarth PH, Davies DE. Induction of the epidermal growth factor receptor and its ligands in nasal epithelium by ozone. *J Allergy Clin Immunol* 2004; **113**: 120–6.
14. Day R. Adverse reactions to TNF-alpha inhibitors in rheumatoid arthritis. *Lancet* 2002; **359**: 540–1.
15. Mohan N, Edwards ET, Cupps TR, Oliverio PJ, Sandberg G, Crayton H, Richert JR, Siegel JN. Demyelination occurring during anti-tumor necrosis factor alpha therapy for inflammatory arthritides. *Arthritis Rheum* 2001; **44**: 2862–9.

16. Sicotte NL, Voskuhl RR. Onset of multiple sclerosis associated with anti-TNF therapy. *Neurology* 2001; **57**: 1885–8.

17. TNF neutralization in MS: results of a randomized, placebo-controlled multicenter study. The Lenercept Multiple Sclerosis Study Group and The University of British Columbia MS/MRI Analysis Group. *Neurology* 1999; **53**: 457–65.

18. Casale TB, Costa JJ, Galli SJ. TNF alpha is important in human lung allergic reactions. *Am J Respir Cell Mol Biol* 1996; **15**: 35–44.

19. Thomas PS. Tumour necrosis factor-alpha: the role of this multifunctional cytokine in asthma. *Immunol Cell Biol* 2001; **79**: 132–40.

20. Gearing AJ, Beckett P, Christodoulou M, Churchill M, Clements J, Davidson AH, Drummond AH, Galloway WA, Gilbert R, Gordon JL. Processing of tumour necrosis factor-alpha precursor by metalloproteinases. *Nature* 1994; **370**: 555–7.

21. Kelly EA, Busse WW, Jarjour NN. Increased matrix metalloproteinase-9 in the airway after allergen challenge. *Am J Respir Crit Care Med* 2000; **162**: 1157–61.

22. Lee YC, Lee HB, Rhee YK, Song CH. The involvement of matrix metalloproteinase-9 in airway inflammation of patients with acute asthma. *Clin Exp Allergy* 2001; **31**: 1623–30.

23. Torphy TJ. Phosphodiesterase isozymes: molecular targets for novel antiasthma agents. *Am J Respir Crit Care Med* 1998; **157**: 351–70.

24. Timmer W, Leclerc V, Birraux G, Neuhauser M, Hatzelmann A, Bethke T, Wurst W. The new phosphodiesterase 4 inhibitor roflumilast is efficacious in exercise-induced asthma and leads to suppression of LPS-stimulated TNF-alpha ex vivo. *J Clin Pharmacol* 2002; **42**: 297–303.

25. Bundschuh DS, Eltze M, Barsig J, Wollin L, Hatzelmann A, Beume R. In vivo efficacy in airway disease models of roflumilast, a novel orally active PDE4 inhibitor. *J Pharmacol Exp Ther* 2001; **297**: 280–90.

26. Lamas AM, Leon OG, Schleimer RP. Glucocorticoids inhibit eosinophil responses to granulocyte-macrophage colony-stimulating factor. *J Immunol* 1991; **147**: 254–9.

27. Schimmer BP, Parker KL. Adrenocorticotrophic hormone; adrenocortical steroids and their synthetic analogs; inhibitors of the synthesis and action of adrenocortical hormones. In: Hardman JG, Limbird LE (eds). *Goodman and Gilman's The pharmacological basis of therapeutics*, 9th edn. New York: McGraw Hill, 1996; pp 1459–87.

28. Schleimer RP. Effects of glucocorticoids on inflammatory cells relevant to their therapeutic application in asthma. *Am Rev Respir Dis* 1990; **141**(2 Pt 2): S59–S69.

29. Wallen N, Kita H, Weiler D, Gleich GJ. Glucocorticoids inhibit cytokine-mediated eosinophil survival. *J Immunol* 1991; **147**: 3490–5.

30. Ohnishi T, Kita H, Mayeno AN, Okada S, Sur S, Broide DH, Gleich GJ. Lidocaine in bronchoalveolar lavage fluid (BALF) is an inhibitor of eosinophil-active cytokines. *Clin Exp Immunol* 1996; **104**: 325–31.

31. Okada S, Hagan JB, Kato M, Bankers-Fulbright JL, Hunt LW, Gleich GJ, Kita H. Lidocaine and its analogues inhibit IL-5-mediated survival and activation of human eosinophils. *J Immunol* 1998; **160**: 4010–17.

32. Hunt LW, Swedlund HA, Gleich GJ. Effect of nebulized lidocaine on severe glucocorticoid-dependent asthma. *Mayo Clin Proc* 1996; **71**: 361–8.

33. Decco ML, Neeno TA, Hunt LW, O'Connell EJ, Yunginger JW, Sachs MI. Nebulized lidocaine in the treatment of severe asthma in children: a pilot study. *Ann Allergy Asthma Immunol* 1999; **82**: 29–32.

34. Rosario NA, Riedi CA, Farias L. Lidocaine nebulization for treatment of asthma. *Ann Allergy Asthma Immunol* 2000; **85**: 245–6.

35. Joos GF, Germonpre PR, Pauwels RA. Role of tachykinins in asthma. *Allergy* 2000; **55**: 321–37.

36. Naline E, Devillier P, Drapeau G, Toty L, Bakdach H, Regoli D, Advenier C. Characterization of neurokinin effects and receptor selectivity in human isolated bronchi. *Am Rev Respir Dis* 1989; **140**: 679–86.

37. Maggi CA, Patacchini R, Rovero P, Giachetti A. Tachykinin receptors and tachykinin receptor antagonists. *J Auton Pharmacol* 1993; **13**: 23–93.

38. Advenier C, Lagente V, Boichot E. The role of tachykinin receptor antagonists in the prevention of bronchial hyper-responsiveness, airway inflammation and cough. *Eur Respir J* 1997; **10**: 1892–906.

39. Joos GF, Van Schoor J, Kips JC, Pauwels RA. The effect of inhaled FK224, a tachykinin NK-1 and NK-2 receptor antagonist, on neurokinin A-induced bronchoconstriction in asthmatics. *Am J Respir Crit Care Med* 1996; **153**: 1781–4.

40. Van Schoor J, Joos GF, Chasson BL, Brouard RJ, Pauwels RA. The effect of the NK2 tachykinin receptor antagonist SR 48968 (saredutant) on neurokinin A-induced bronchoconstriction in asthmatics. *Eur Respir J* 1998; **12**: 17–23.

41. Joos G, Schelfhout V, Van De Velde V, Pauwels R. The effect of the tachykinin NK2 receptor antagonist MEN 11420 (nepadutant) on neurokinin A-induced bronchoconstriction in patients with asthma. *Am J Respir Crit Care Med* 2001; **163**: A628.

42. Gerspacher M, La Vecchia L, Mah R, von Sprecher A, Anderson GP, Subramanian N, Hauser K, Bammerlin H, Kimmel S, Pawelzik V, Ryffel K, Ball HA. Dual neurokinin NK(1)/NK(2) antagonists: N-[(R,R)-(E)-1-arylmethyl-3-(2-oxo-azepan-3-yl)carbamoyl]allyl-N-methyl-3, 5-bis(trifluoromethyl)benzamides and 3-[N′-3, 5-bis(trifluoromethyl)benzoyl-N-arylmethyl-N′-methylhydrazino]-N-[(R)-2-oxo-azepan-3-yl]propionamides. *Bioorg Med Chem Lett* 2001; **11**: 3081–4.

43. Tough IR, Lewis CA, Fozard J, Cox HM. Dual and selective antagonism of neurokinin NK(1) and NK(2) receptor-mediated responses in human colon mucosa. *Naunyn Schmiedebergs Arch Pharmacol* 2003; **367**: 104–8.

44. Fozard JR, Mazzoni L, Hoshiko K. Effects of DNK333, a dual NK1/NK2 neurokinin receptor antagonist, on airway responsiveness induced by lipopolysaccharide or allergen challenge in guinea-pig. *Am J Respir Crit Care Med* 2001; **163**: A627.

45. Sanderson CJ. Interleukin-5, eosinophils, and disease. *Blood* 1992; **79**: 3101–9.

46. Collins PD, Marleau S, Griffiths-Johnson DA, Jose PJ, Williams TJ. Cooperation between interleukin-5 and the chemokine eotaxin to induce eosinophil accumulation *in vivo. J Exp Med* 1995; **182**: 1169–74.

47. Oldhoff JM, Darsow U, Werfel T, Katzer K, Wulf A, Laifaoui J, Hijnen DJ, Plotz S, Knol EF, Kapp A, Bruijnzeel-Koomen CA, Ring J, de Bruin-Weller MS. Anti-IL-5 recombinant humanized monoclonal antibody (mepolizumab) for the treatment of atopic dermatitis. *Allergy* 2005; **60**: 693–6.

48. Leckie MJ, ten Brinke A, Khan J, Diamant Z, O'Connor BJ, Walls CM, Mathur AK, Cowley HC, Chung KF, Djukanovic R, Hansel TT, Holgate ST, Sterk PJ, Barnes PJ. Effects of an interleukin-5 blocking monoclonal antibody on eosinophils, airway hyper-responsiveness, and the late asthmatic response. *Lancet* 2000; **356**: 2144–8.

49. Flood-Page PT, Menzies-Gow AN, Kay AB, Robinson DS. Eosinophil's role remains uncertain as anti-interleukin-5 only partially depletes numbers in asthmatic airway. *Am J Respir Crit Care Med* 2003; **167**: 199–204.

50. Gnanakumaran G, Babu KS. Technology evaluation: mepolizumab, GlaxoSmithKline. *Curr Opin Mol Ther* 2003; **5**: 321–5.

51. Allergen immunotherapy: therapeutic vaccines for allergic diseases. Geneva: January 27–29 1997. *Allergy* 1998; **53**(44 Suppl): 1–42.

52. Echechipia S, Tabar AI, Lobera T, Munoz D, Rodriguez A, Blasco A, Olaguibel JM, Casanovas M, Fernandez de Corres L. Immunotherapy with a standardized Dermatophagoides pteronyssinus glutaraldehyde-modified extract against an unmodified extract: a comparative study of efficacy, tolerance and *in vivo* and *in vitro* modification of parameters. *J Investig Allergol Clin Immunol* 1995; **5**: 325–32.

53. Ferrer A, Garcia-Selles J. Significant improvement in symptoms, skin test, and specific bronchial reactivity after 6 months of treatment with a depigmented, polymerized extract of Dermatophagoides pteronyssinus and D. farinae. *J Investig Allergol Clin Immunol* 2003; **13**: 244–51.

54. Guerra F, Daza JC, Almeda E. Immunotherapy with a depigmented, polymerized vaccine of Olea europaea pollen allergens. Significantly reduces specific bronchial and skin test reactivity in sensitized patients after one year of treatment. *J Investig Allergol Clin Immunol* 2003; **13**: 108–17.

55. Malet A, Lluch M, Valero AL, Casanovas M. Clinical and immunological effects of immunotherapy with glutaraldehyde modified house dust mite extract. *Allergol Immunopathol (Madr)* 1994; **22**: 226–32.

56. Corne J, Djukanovic R, Thomas L, Warner J, Botta L, Grandordy B, Gygax D, Heusser C, Patalano F, Richardson W, Kilchherr E, Staehelin T, Davis F, Gordon W, Sun L, Liou R, Wang G, Chang TW, Holgate S. The effect of intravenous administration of a chimeric anti-IgE antibody on serum IgE levels in atopic subjects: efficacy, safety, and pharmacokinetics. *J Clin Invest* 1997; **99**: 879–87.

15

Other therapies (antihistamines, leukotriene modifiers, calcineurin inhibitors, anti-IgE)

BRETT PEREIRA

Antihistamines and leukotriene receptor antagonists

Antihistamines have been shown to be effective in seasonal allergic rhinitis and chronic idiopathic urticaria [1]. They improve quality of life scores [2], inflammatory markers in atopic asthma [3] and symptom scores [4]. Newer histamine H_1-receptor antagonists may also have an antiplatelet-activating factor effect and are equally effective in seasonal allergic rhinitis [5]. The antileukotrienes were developed in the 1980s. The first compounds of this novel class of anti-asthma drugs were registered in the second half of the 1990s. The mechanism of action of the cysteinyl leukotriene receptor antagonists (LTRAs) is based on counteracting the effects of cysteinyl leukotrienes at their receptor site (CysLT1 receptor) within the airways. This results in a dual effect: (i) suppression of airway inflammation and, as a result, (ii) mild bronchodilator properties. LTRAs have been shown to be effective in asthma, including cough-variant asthma [6], as monotherapy and in combination with inhaled corticosteroids in improving asthma control [7,8] and reducing exacerbations [9,10].

The early asthmatic response to inhaled allergen is thought to be due to contraction of airway smooth muscle, from immunoglobulin (Ig) E-mediated release of multiple mast-cell mediators, including leukotrienes and histamine, both of which cause bronchoconstriction. The idea that a mechanism involving multiple mediators might require multiple interventions continues to attract interest in the role of combination therapies for the treatment of atopic asthma, as blocking the activity of these mediators might prevent bronchoconstriction. Combination therapy directed at blocking the effects of histamine and leukotriene mediators might protect against the early asthmatic response better than either therapy alone. In a recent study of the combination of desloratadine and montelukast, the early response to inhaled allergen was unchanged after desloratadine therapy and

© Atlas Medical Publishing Ltd

partially inhibited with montelukast therapy, but the combination of desloratadine and montelukast provided superior efficacy to either blocker administered alone [11].

Efficacy of montelukast during the allergy season in patients with chronic asthma and seasonal aeroallergen sensitivity

Busse WW, Casale TB, Dykewicz MS, *et al. Ann Allergy Asthma Immunol* 2006; **96**: 60–8

BACKGROUND. Montelukast has proven efficacy in the treatment of chronic asthma and seasonal allergic rhinitis, but it has not been evaluated in the subpopulation of asthmatic patients with seasonal asthma symptoms.

INTERPRETATION. In patients with chronic asthma and seasonal aeroallergen sensitivity, montelukast treatment provided significant asthma control during the allergy season compared with placebo.

Comment

In order to determine the effectiveness of montelukast treatment in improving the control of asthma symptoms during the allergy season in patients with active asthma and seasonal aeroallergen sensitivity, the authors of this study enrolled adults with a history of chronic asthma who were also symptomatic during the allergy season and with skin-test sensitivity to seasonal aeroallergens. Patients were randomized to a parallel-group, multicentre study with a 1-week, single-blind, placebo run-in period followed by 3 weeks of double-blind treatment with either oral montelukast (10 mg) or placebo. Daytime and night-time asthma symptom scores, β-agonist use and morning and evening peak expiratory flow rates were recorded daily using an electronic diary. The primary end-point was mean change from baseline to week 3 in the daytime asthma symptom score. Of 455 randomized patients, 433 completed the study. Compared with placebo, treatment with montelukast resulted in significant improvements from baseline in the daytime asthma symptom score (–0.54 vs –0.34; $P = 0.002$), β-agonist use, night-time symptoms and peak expiratory flow rates.

This study suggests that the addition of an LTRA may improve asthma control in patients who are symptomatic to relevant aeroallergens causing seasonal allergic rhinitis. Unfortunately, this study was only conducted for a short period and hence we cannot evaluate whether this effect would be sustained throughout the relevant season. There were some dropouts in both groups in this short period, and again this may take on relevance if the study were prolonged to reflect real-life practice. Allergic rhinitis is known to affect asthma control significantly and montelukast has been shown to be effective in treating rhinitis. It is likely that it is because of this effect that the patients in this group showed better control of asthma. This may pave the way for more aggressive treatment of concomitant disease routinely in the future.

Repeated dosing effects of mediator antagonists in inhaled corticosteroid-treated atopic asthmatic patients

Lee DKC, Jackson CM, Haggart K, Lipworth BJ. *Chest* 2004; **125**: 1372–7

BACKGROUND. Treating allergic rhinitis may have a downstream effect on concomitant asthma and this may be due to attenuation of the underlying inflammatory process.

INTERPRETATION. Fexofenadine and montelukast exhibited additive effects to moderately high doses of inhaled corticosteroids when used as add-on therapy in the treatment of patients with persistent atopic asthma.

Comment

While H_1 antihistamines have an established role in the treatment of allergic rhinitis, they are not currently recommended in the treatment of asthma. The authors evaluated the effects of repeated dosing with fexofenadine and montelukast at clinically recommended doses as add-on therapy in patients with atopic asthma who had been treated with inhaled corticosteroids using bronchial challenge with adenosine monophosphate (AMP) as the primary outcome. They also evaluated secondary outcomes, including the exhaled nitric oxide level, peripheral blood eosinophil count, forced expiratory volume in 1 s (FEV_1), domiciliary peak expiratory flow rate, asthma symptom score and use of rescue medication. Twenty patients with stable atopic asthma who had had mild to moderate persistent asthma for at least 3 months prior to the study, who were on inhaled corticosteroids at a daily dose up to 2000 μg for beclomethasone dipropionate/budesonide or 1000 μg for fluticasone propionate, and who had not received a course of therapy with oral corticosteroids or antibiotics during this period were recruited from an asthma database. Patients were randomized to receive either fexofenadine 180 mg, montelukast 10 mg or placebo for 1 week with a washout period of 1 week prior to each randomized treatment. Mean morning and evening peak expiratory flow values were significantly higher (P<0.05) when comparing fexofenadine (442 ± 23 and 440 ± 23 l/min respectively) and montelukast (444 ± 22 and 445 ± 22 l/min respectively) with placebo (425 ± 25 and 424 ± 25 l/min respectively). Mean morning asthma symptom scores improved significantly (P<0.05) with montelukast (0.2 ± 0.1) but not fexofenadine (0.3 ± 0.1) compared with placebo (0.4 ± 0.1). Salbutamol rescue use in the morning and evening was significantly reduced (P<0.05) with fexofenadine (0.4 ± 0.2 and 0.8 ± 0.2 puffs respectively) and montelukast (0.4 ± 0.2 and 0.8 ± 0.2 puffs respectively) compared with placebo (0.8 ± 0.2 and 1.4 ± 0.6 puffs respectively). Repeated dosing with fexofenadine and montelukast as add-on therapy also significantly improved AMP PC_{20} (the concentration of methacholine required to produce a 20% drop in FEV_1) and other surrogate inflammatory markers, such as exhaled nitric oxide and peripheral blood eosinophil count. This is the first study to demonstrate that H_1 antihistamines improve AMP PC_{20} as add-on therapy to inhaled corticosteroids.

Limitations of this study include the small numbers and its short duration. The authors tried to remove bias towards treating concomitant rhinitis by conducting the study outside the pollen season, but as all their patients were sensitized to house dust mite, a significant number could have had perennial rhinitis. The washout periods for long-acting β_2-agonists (LABAs) and LTRAs at the beginning of the study and the 1-week washouts between treatments may also have been insufficient to prevent carryover effects of previous treatment affecting results. Nevertheless, this study does show improvement in bronchial reactivity with antihistamines as measured by AMP PC_{20}.

This should encourage further studies in both atopic and non-atopic subjects with asthma to see if the bronchoprotective effect is indeed reproducible and sustained, and has clinical impact in the longer term.

Section conclusion

The potential for inhaled corticosteroids to cause dose-related adverse systemic effects has driven the asthma guidelines toward the use of corticosteroid-sparing, second-line controller agents such as LABAs and LTRAs. LTRAs have an established role in the guidelines for asthma treatment, and in a recent retrospective, cross-sectional, observational study of clinical outcomes in patients prescribed montelukast for asthma, montelukast was well tolerated and no new adverse events were recorded |**12**|.

LTRAs have already been prescribed to over 25 million patients with asthma worldwide, including 6.4 million young children, and few adverse events related to their use have been reported |**13**|. Montelukast has been studied extensively, although other LTRAs, such as pranlukast, have also been shown to be safe and effective |**14,15**|.

LTRAs appear to provide beneficial effects in patients using inhaled corticosteroids, perhaps by suppressive effects on airway hyper-responsiveness and the underlying inflammatory pathway. Further data are required to confirm whether this in turn has a positive effect on parameters of airway remodelling in the long term.

Evidence is gradually accumulating that the addition of antihistamines may benefit a select group of patients with asthma and may further improve symptom scores and asthma control. This effect may well be seen in the large numbers of patients who also have concomitant allergic rhinitis. Further studies should be conducted to see which patients will benefit the most from these combination therapies.

Anti IgE

Omalizumab, a recombinant humanized monoclonal antibody, is the first therapeutic agent specifically targeting IgE. It has been investigated in the treatment of patients with allergic diseases and is approved in the USA for the treatment of patients with moderate to severe persistent asthma. In the studies pertaining to this, omalizumab reduced the frequency and incidence of asthma exacerbations and asthma control was well maintained, even though patients reduced their dose of inhaled corticosteroid. Importantly, omalizumab has been shown to reduce asthma exacerbations in high-risk patients (e.g. patients with previous intubation and hospitalization) and to reduce the level of severe asthma exacerbations (those resulting in emergency treatment and hospitalization). Omalizumab also proved to be effective in patients with seasonal and perennial allergic rhinitis and to improve quality of life for patients with asthma or rhinitis. As expected with a systemic anti-IgE agent, omalizumab was shown to be effective in the treatment of patients with concomitant asthma and allergic rhinitis. The efficacy of omalizumab in a range of allergic diseases reaffirms the importance of IgE in the pathogenesis of these conditions and establishes the potential benefit to be obtained by inhibiting IgE, especially in patients with more severe and comorbid allergic diseases.

Omalizumab is a recombinant humanized monoclonal antibody comprising a human IgG framework onto which is grafted the complementarity-determining region from an anti-IgE antibody raised in mice, such that less than 5% of the resulting product consists of residues of murine origin, minimizing the potential for an immune response to the non-self protein. It recognizes the binding site of IgE for its high-affinity Fc receptor and inhibits the attachment of free serum IgE onto mast cells and other effector cells. Theoretically, mouse sensitivity, which occurs in up to 13% of people in a US population [16], could play a part in adverse reactions to this product. Eight randomized controlled trials that had registered 2037 patients with mild to severe allergic asthma (children and adults) with high serum IgE levels were recently meta-analysed. Treatment with omalizumab significantly reduced serum IgE levels compared with placebo. Omalizumab administration led to significant reduction in inhaled steroid consumption compared with placebo and to significant increases in the numbers of patients able to reduce steroid dosages by greater than 50%, as well as in those who were able to totally discontinue daily steroids. Patients receiving omalizumab and steroids experienced fewer disease exacerbations than those treated with steroids alone.

Omalizumab appears to provide the greatest benefit in patients with more severe asthma, and this has been confirmed by recent studies establishing the efficacy of omalizumab in patients whose asthma is poorly controlled despite their receiving the best standard care in medication.

Effects of treatment with anti-immunoglobulin E antibody omalizumab on airway inflammation in allergic asthma

Djukanovic R, Wilson SJ, Kraft M, *et al. Am J Respir Crit Care Med* 2004; **170**: 583–93

BACKGROUND. IgE plays an important role in allergic asthma. Reducing IgE in the airway mucosa should reduce airway inflammation.

INTERPRETATION. Omalizumab has significant anti-inflammatory effect and reduces serum and airway IgE, but IgE or eosinophils may not be causally linked to airway hyper-responsiveness to methacholine in mild to moderate asthma.

Comment

This 4-month, randomized, double-blind, placebo-controlled, parallel group study was conducted in five centres. Forty-five patients with mild to moderate persistent asthma and with sputum eosinophilia of 2% or more were treated with humanized monoclonal antibody against IgE (omalizumab) ($n = 22$) or placebo ($n = 23$) for 16 weeks. Outcomes included inflammatory cells in induced sputum and bronchial biopsies, and methacholine responsiveness. Treatment with omalizumab resulted in marked reduction in serum IgE and a reduction in IgE^+ cells in the airway mucosa. The mean percentage sputum eosinophil count decreased significantly ($P < 0.001$) from 6.6 to 1.7% in the omalizumab group, a reduction significantly ($P = 0.05$) greater than with placebo (8.5 to 7.0%). This was associated with a significant reduction in tissue eosinophils; cells positive for the high-affinity Fc receptor for IgE; $CD3^+$, $CD4^+$ and $CD8^+$ T lymphocytes; B lymphocytes; and cells staining for interleukin-4, but not with improvement in airway hyper-responsiveness to methacholine. Treatment led to almost complete eradication of sputum eosinophils, which was mirrored by a similar reduction in eosinophils in bronchial biopsies, when treatment caused near depletion of eosinophils within the bronchial submucosa in all but two subjects. This study shows anti-inflammatory effects of omalizumab treatment and may explain the outcome of reducing asthma exacerbations and other asthma outcomes in more severe asthma. The findings of the present study are, therefore, significant in that they show omalizumab to be the first non-steroidal agent with major anti-inflammatory activity in the airways of individuals with allergic asthma. The lack of effect of omalizumab on methacholine responsiveness suggests that IgE may not be causal in airway hyper-responsiveness, although methacholine challenge may not have been the best way to assess this. Methacholine is a direct bronchoconstrictor stimulus which acts upon effector cells such as smooth muscle, causing contraction and narrowing of the airway. Bronchoprovocation with indirect stimuli such as AMP and mannitol is considered to be more relevant to real-life situations causing bronchoconstriction, such as cold air, exercise and allergens, which act in a similar fashion in terms of the release of proinflammatory mediators, such as histamine and leukotrienes, from primed mast cells. Further studies with alternative challenge methods might help clarify this issue.

Benefits of omalizumab as add-on therapy in patients with severe persistent asthma who are inadequately controlled despite best available therapy (GINA 2002 step 4 treatment): INNOVATE

Humbert M, Beasley R, Ayres J, *et al. Allergy* 2005; **60**: 309–16

BACKGROUND. Patients with severe persistent asthma who are inadequately controlled despite Global Initiative for Asthma (GINA) 2002 step 4 therapy are a challenging population with a significant unmet medical need.

INTERPRETATION. In patients with inadequately controlled severe persistent asthma despite high-dose inhaled corticosteroid and LABA therapy, and often additional therapy, omalizumab significantly reduced the rate of clinically significant asthma exacerbations, severe exacerbations and emergency visits.

Comment

The effect of omalizumab on clinically significant asthma exacerbations (requiring systemic corticosteroids) was studied in the first omalizumab study to exclusively enrol patients from this difficult-to-treat patient population. This was a randomized, placebo-controlled, double-blind study with a 28-week treatment phase to determine the efficacy, safety and tolerability of omalizumab. Following a run-in phase, patients (aged 12–75 years) whose asthma was inadequately controlled despite therapy with high-dose inhaled corticosteroids and LABAs, with reduced lung function and a recent history of clinically significant exacerbations, were randomized to receive omalizumab or placebo for 28 weeks. All patients were receiving inhaled corticosteroid and LABA, and two-thirds of the patients were receiving additional controller medications (22% were receiving maintenance oral corticosteroids). Patients were recruited at 108 centres in 14 countries. The study comprised four phases: a 7-day screening period (for evaluating eligibility); an 8-week run-in phase; the 28-week drug add-on treatment phase; and a 16-week follow-up phase. Patients were seen at screening, every 2 weeks during the run-in, at weeks 0, 1, 2, 4, 12, 20 and 28 of the treatment phase, and at weeks 4 and 16 of the follow-up. The primary efficacy variable was the rate of clinically significant asthma exacerbations (defined as a worsening of asthma symptoms requiring treatment with systemic corticosteroids) during the 28-week double-blind treatment phase.

A total of 419 patients were included in the efficacy analyses. The clinically significant asthma exacerbation rate (primary efficacy variable), adjusted for an observed relevant imbalance in history of clinically significant asthma exacerbations, was 0.68 with omalizumab and 0.91 with placebo (26% reduction) during the

28-week treatment phase ($P = 0.042$) (Fig. 15.1). Without adjustment, a similar magnitude of effect was seen (19% reduction), but this did not reach statistical significance. Omalizumab significantly reduced the severe asthma exacerbation rate (0.24 vs 0.48; $P = 0.002$) and emergency visit rate (0.24 vs 0.43; $P = 0.038$) (Table 15.1). Omalizumab significantly improved asthma-related quality of life, morning peak expiratory flow and asthma symptom scores. The incidence of adverse events was similar between treatment groups. The number needed to treat for 1 year to save one clinically significant exacerbation requiring oral steroids was 2.2. This was a well-conducted study in patients with severe asthma who were on appropriate treatment but remained inadequately controlled. The main impact of omalizumab

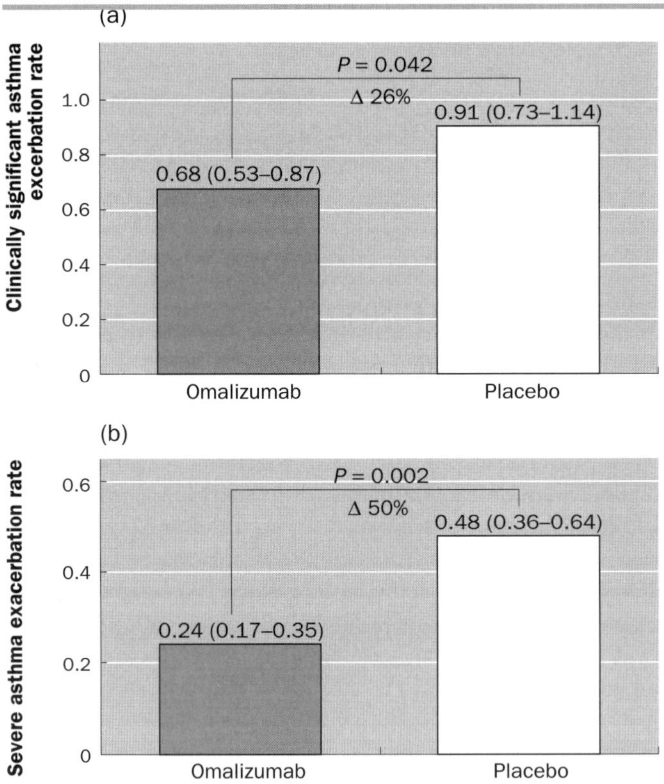

Fig. 15.1 (a) Effect of omalizumab treatment on the rate of clinically significant asthma exacerbations (adjusted for baseline exacerbation history) during the 28-week treatment period (primary intent-to-treat [PITT] population); mean (95% confidence interval). (b) Effect of omalizumab treatment on severe exacerbations (peak expiratory flow [PEF] or forced expiratory volume in 1 s [FEV_1] <60% of personal best) during the 28-week treatment period (PITT population). Source: Humbert *et al.* (2005).

Table 15.1 Frequency of emergency visits for asthma using Poisson regression (primary intent-to-treat population)

Type of visit	Statistic	Omalizumab (*n* = 209)	Placebo (*n* = 210)
Total emergency visits	Number	50	93
	Rate per treatment period	0.24	0.43
	Ratio of rates (95% CI)	0.561 (0.325–0.968)	
	P-value for ratio	0.038	
Hospital admissions	Number	13	25
	Rate per treatment period	0.06	0.12
	Ratio of rates (95% CI)	0.540 (0.250–1.166)	
	P-value for ratio	0.117	
Emergency room visits	Number	9	14
	Rate per treatment period	0.04	0.06
	Ratio of rates (95% CI)	0.659 (0.208–2.094)	
	P-value for ratio	0.480	
Unscheduled doctor visits	Number	28	54
	Rate per treatment period	0.13	0.24
	Ratio of rates (95% CI)	0.546 (0.271–1.100)	
	P-value for ratio	0.090	

CI, confidence interval.
Source: Humbert *et al.* (2005).

treatment seemed to be on exacerbations and improved quality of life scores, as in other studies, but this is especially relevant in this group of patients.

Efficacy and tolerability of anti-immunoglobulin E therapy with omalizumab in patients with concomitant allergic asthma and persistent allergic rhinitis: SOLAR

Vignola AM, Humbert M, Bousquet J, *et al.* *Allergy* 2004; **59**: 709–17

BACKGROUND. Anti-IgE therapy could be particularly beneficial for patients with concomitant asthma and rhinitis as it targets a common factor in the two diseases.

INTERPRETATION. Omalizumab is significantly more efficacious than placebo in preventing asthma exacerbations and in improving disease-related quality of life scores when added to standard asthma and rhinitis therapies.

Comment

Asthma and rhinitis frequently coexist, most patients with allergic asthma experiencing concomitant rhinitis. Both diseases are associated with elevated serum IgE levels and they share similar inflammatory pathophysiology. IgE is a common factor in both allergic asthma and rhinitis, and clinical studies have found anti-IgE therapy with omalizumab to be efficacious in both diseases.

This multicentre, randomized, double-blind, parallel-group, placebo-controlled trial evaluated the safety and efficacy of omalizumab. The primary efficacy variables were the incidence of asthma exacerbations and the proportion of patients showing a response in both asthma and rhinitis quality of life assessments. The authors enrolled a total of 405 patients (aged 12–74 years) with a history of allergic asthma for at least 1 year with an increase of at least 12% in FEV_1 after 400 μg salbutamol on stable treatment (≥400 μg budesonide via a Turbuhaler) and with two or more unscheduled medical visits for asthma during the past year or three or more visits during the past 2 years. At baseline, fewer than half of the patients in this study were on a LABA, despite having moderate to severe asthma by the GINA classification. An IgE level between ≥30 and ≤1300 IU/ml was required, together with a positive skin-prick test to at least one indoor allergen. The positively testing allergen had to be one to which the patient would be exposed daily for the duration of the study, thus helping ensure that it was clinically relevant to the patient's disease. Patients received omalizumab (≥0.016 mg/kg/ per IU/ml of IgE per 4 weeks) or placebo for 28 weeks. Fewer patients treated with omalizumab experienced asthma exacerbations (20.6%) than placebo-treated patients (30.1%) ($P=0.02$). Omalizumab reduced symptom scores for asthma ($P=0.023$), rhinitis ($P<0.001$) and the composite asthma/rhinitis scores ($P<0.001$) compared with placebo. Serious adverse events were observed in 1.4% of omalizumab-treated patients and 1.5% of placebo-treated patients. Both primary end-points (asthma exacerbations and disease-related quality of life) were significantly in favour of omalizumab. Omalizumab treatment resulted in more responders (an improvement of at least 1.0 point in both AQLQ (Asthma Quality of Life Questionnaire) and RQLQ (Rhinitis Quality of life Questionnaire) than placebo (57.7% [120/208] vs 40.6% [78/192]; $P<0.001$), although the response rate in the placebo group in this study is particularly high. Omalizumab was more effective than placebo for all RQLQ domains (activities, sleep, non-nose/eye symptoms, practical problems, nasal symptoms, eye symptoms and emotional). This study shows that omalizumab is well tolerated and effective in preventing asthma exacerbations and improving quality of life in patients with concomitant asthma and persistent allergic rhinitis.

Section conclusion

Anti IgE holds promise in the treatment of the patient with severe and difficult-to-control asthma and has been conclusively shown to reduce exacerbations and hospitalizations in this important group. It has significant anti-inflammatory effects and causes eosinophil depletion, which may be of great relevance to the exacerbations and release of cytokines in the tissues. As more studies become available, the role that omalizumab has in the treatment of allergic diseases such as rhinitis, asthma and even eczema is likely to expand. There is already a school of thought that it may be of benefit in treating IgE-mediated food allergy and at the start of rush immunotherapy schedules. It has a favourable risk/benefit ratio and its pharmacological and clinical efficacy make it a valuable therapy for allergic diseases.

Calcineurin inhibitors

For more than five decades, topical corticosteroids and emollients have been the mainstay of therapy for atopic dermatitis. However, the potential for side effects limits the clinical utility of corticosteroids in providing long-term disease control. The two steroid-sparing calcineurin inhibitors tacrolimus and pimicrolimus cream are useful new drugs for topical eczema treatment. They have been shown to be effective against placebo and corticosteroids in clinical trials and appear to have a good safety record [17]. In contrast to topical steroids, they do not induce skin atrophy, allowing their use on delicate areas such as eyelids, perioral skin and genital areas. The most frequently reported side effect has been a transient sensation of warmth or burning at the site of application. Both tacrolimus and pimecrolimus prevent disease flares and provide progressive and sustained disease improvement with long-term therapy.

Their long-term efficacy continues to be validated in both adults and children [18–20].

These agents are potent immunosuppressive agents because of their inhibitory actions on lymphocyte gene transcription. Lymphocytes are important in the pathogenesis of many skin disorders and the role of these drugs will expand in time as reports of their efficacy in other skin conditions continue to encourage further studies.

The oral calcineurin inhibitor cyclosporin is associated with photocarcinogenicity and hence topical UV protection with sunscreens is recommended with the topical calcineurin inhibitors. Some concern has also been raised about their implication in the development of lentigines, which would require close follow-up to ensure there is no progression to melanocytic transformation [21].

Calcineurin inhibitors hold the promise of providing long-term treatment and control of a chronic skin disease that may persist for years. Both topical calcineurin inhibitors are approved in the European Union from 2 years of age and above [22]. Further studies of combination treatment of calcineurin inhibitors with corticosteroid, better delivery methods of the drugs and long-term efficacy and safety are being conducted.

A multicentre, randomized, double-blind, controlled study of long-term treatment with 0.1% tacrolimus ointment in adults with moderate to severe atopic dermatitis

Reitamo S, Ortonne JP, Sand C, *et al.*; European Tacrolimus Ointment Study Group. *Br J Dermatol* 2005; **152**: 1282–9

BACKGROUND. Topical corticosteroids are the usual therapy for patients with atopic dermatitis, but prolonged use can result in skin atrophy and other side effects. The long-term safety and efficacy of tacrolimus would prove an attractive alternative.

INTERPRETATION. Long-term treatment with 0.1% tacrolimus ointment is significantly more efficacious than a corticosteroid ointment regimen in adults with moderate to severe atopic dermatitis.

Comment

This study was a 6-month, randomized, double-blind, comparative phase III study conducted in 57 centres in twelve European countries with 0.1% tacrolimus ointment compared with a corticosteroid ointment regimen in adults with moderate to severe atopic dermatitis. Patients applied either a thin layer of 0.1% tacrolimus ointment twice daily to all affected body areas ($n = 487$) or 1% hydrocortisone acetate ointment twice daily to the head and neck and 0.1% hydrocortisone butyrate ointment ($n = 485$) twice daily to the trunk and extremities. After clearance, the lesions were to be treated for an additional 7 days. In the event of flare, ointment application was to resume twice daily until the lesion cleared. The primary end-point of the study was the response rate, i.e. the proportion of patients with at least 60% improvement in the modified Eczema Area and Severity Index (mEASI) between baseline and month 3. Secondary end-points included the response rate at time-points other than month 3, mEASI, EASI, the physician's global evaluation of clinical response, the patient's assessment of global response, the physician's assessment of individual signs, affected total body surface area, the patient's assessment of itch and quality of sleep, and the number of days on treatment as a percentage of days in the study.

By month 3, more patients in the 0.1% tacrolimus group responded to treatment (72.6 vs 52.3% in the corticosteroid group, $P < 0.001$). The patients treated with 0.1% tacrolimus also showed greater improvement in mEASI, EASI, affected body surface area, and physician and patient assessments of global response. The reduction in the individual signs of atopic dermatitis throughout the study was greater for the patients in the 0.1% tacrolimus group, and more patients treated with 0.1% tacrolimus experienced clearance or excellent improvement (≥90%) compared with the corticosteroid treatment group. Patients applying 0.1% tacrolimus ointment experienced more skin burning (52.4 vs 13.8% in the corticosteroid group; $P < 0.001$). In most patients, skin burning was mild to moderate in severity and decreased rapidly after the first week of treatment. These data show that, in adults with moderate to severe atopic dermatitis, 0.1% tacrolimus ointment is significantly better in reducing the signs and symptoms of atopic dermatitis regardless of the body area to which the ointment is applied. Treatment efficacy was sustained and no increased risk of infection or cumulative side effects were observed during the prolonged application of 0.1% tacrolimus ointment.

Long-term safety and tolerability of pimecrolimus cream 1% and topical corticosteroids in adults with moderate to severe atopic dermatitis

Luger T, Lahfa M, Fölster-Holst R, *et al. J Dermatolog Treatment* 2004; **15**: 169–78

BACKGROUND. The long-term safety and tolerability of pimecrolimus is not well known.

INTERPRETATION. Pimecrolimus demonstrated a favourable safety profile when used to treat adult patients with moderate to severe atopic dermatitis for up to 1 year. A significant proportion of patients could be maintained without topical corticosteroids (TCS) for a year.

Comment

This randomized, double-blind, multicentre study in 35 centres in nine countries compared the long-term safety and tolerability of pimecrolimus cream 1% and TCS in 658 adults aged 18–79 years, with moderate to severe atopic dermatitis affecting at least 5% of the body surface area. Patients applied either pimecrolimus or TCS (i.e. 0.1% triamcinolone acetonide cream and/or 1% hydrocortisone acetate cream) twice daily to all affected areas until complete clearance or for up to 1 year. The primary objective was to evaluate the tolerability and safety of pimicrolimus in comparison with TCS. The majority of patients treated with either pimecrolimus or TCS tolerated the drug on a continuous basis over 1 year. In patients who had more than 30% of the body surface involved by atopic dermatitis, the incidence rate of all skin infections was significantly lower in the pimecrolimus group than in the TCS group (95% confidence interval [CI] of the treatment difference, –25.3 to –3.4%). The most frequent application site reaction was burning (25.9% of patients on pimecrolimus and 10.9% on TCS), which was transient and mild to moderate in most cases. Three TCS-treated patients reported skin striae. There were no treatment-related serious or clinically significant systemic adverse events. Efficacy was better in patients on continuous TCS therapy, although patients completing the study were similarly well controlled in the two groups. About 42% of the pimecrolimus-treated patients were maintained for 1 year without TCS. There was no difference between treatment groups in median time to first remission or recurrence.

Pimecrolimus demonstrated a favourable safety profile when used to treat adult patients with moderate to severe atopic dermatitis for up to 1 year. In contrast to steroids, which act on a broad range of cells, pimicrolimus acts on T cells and mast cells in the skin, which may limit its side effects. Patients with moderate to severe atopic dermatitis are particularly difficult to treat and are often corticosteroid-dependent. In this study a significant proportion of patients could be maintained without TCS for a year. This is especially important as almost 90% of patients in both treatment groups had head and neck involvement, which would limit the use of TCS.

Pharmacokinetics of topical calcineurin inhibitors in adult atopic dermatitis: a randomized, investigator-blind comparison

Draelos Z, Nayak A, Pariser D, *et al.* *J Am Acad Dermatol* 2005; **53**: 602–9

BACKGROUND. The pharmacokinetics of pimecrolimus cream 1% and tacrolimus ointment 0.1% in adults with extensive, moderate to severe atopic dermatitis, including systemic absorption, has relevance to patient safety and drug efficacy. Past pharmacokinetic studies have demonstrated that most patients with atopic dermatitis treated with topical calcineurin inhibitors experience negligible systemic absorption, resulting in low or undetectable blood concentrations of the active compound, but have not compared these two agents directly.

INTERPRETATION. Pimecrolimus appears to be associated with lower systemic drug exposure than tacrolimus.

Comment

This study was a randomized, investigator-blind, parallel-group, multicentre trial. Adult patients with moderate to severe atopic dermatitis (Investigators' Global Assessment score of 3–5) affecting at least 30% of the total body surface area received twice-daily treatment with either pimecrolimus or tacrolimus for 13 days.

Patients received twice-daily treatment for 13 days. Blood concentrations of pimecrolimus and tacrolimus were measured at days 1, 5 and 13. Treatment success was defined as an Investigators' Global Assessment score of 0 (clear) or 1 (almost clear). Thirty-seven patients were randomized at six centres in the USA to receive either pimecrolimus ($n = 18$) or tacrolimus ($n = 19$). A greater proportion of patients treated with tacrolimus had detectable levels of drug in their blood compared with those treated with pimecrolimus (36 vs 12%). Blood concentrations of tacrolimus were higher than those of pimecrolimus in both men and women. Tacrolimus is currently indicated for patients with moderate to severe AD, whereas pimecrolimus is indicated for patients with mild to moderate disease.

In patients with measurable blood drug concentrations, systemic exposure to tacrolimus (mean area under the curve$_{0\text{–}10h}$ <9.7 ng/h/ml; $n = 7$) was higher than to pimecrolimus (mean area under the curve$_{0\text{–}10h}$ <2.5 ng/h/ml; $n = 2$). Whole-body treatment success (day 13) was achieved in 1 of 18 (5.6%) and 2 of 19 (10.5%)

patients treated with pimecrolimus and tacrolimus respectively, and face/neck treatment success in 5 of 18 (27.8%) and 5 of 19 (26.3%) patients respectively. Patients included in the study were adult patients with severe atopic dermatitis. The results and conclusions drawn from this study population may not be applicable to the majority of patients with atopic dermatitis, who have mild to moderate disease.

Pimecrolimus is highly lipophilic, and systemic absorption is negligible even in patients with extensive areas treated. As a non-steroidal drug, pimecrolimus does not induce skin atrophy and can be used for extended periods to control early manifestations of atopic dermatitis. This study was conducted over a relatively short period and longer-term studies of patients with severe disease are warranted.

Section conclusion

The topical calcineurin inhibitors were introduced in Japan in 1999 for the treatment of moderate to severe atopic dermatitis and have proved that they are valuable in treating both children and adults in the long term without major side effects. They appear to decrease the need for other therapies, including topical and oral corticosteroids, and avoid the potential side effect of skin atrophy; hence they would be especially useful for atopic dermatitis of the head and neck, for which limiting the use of topical corticosteroids is desirable. They reduce the time to first exacerbation of atopic dermatitis and seem to have a relatively good safety profile. Further studies, including head-to-head comparisons of tacrolimus and pimicrolimus, should clarify their place in the therapy of atopic dermatitis and, in the future, other inflammatory diseases of the skin.

Other therapies

Magnesium sulphate in asthma

The use of magnesium sulphate is one of numerous treatment options available during acute exacerbations and has been incorporated into various treatment guidelines for acute asthma. While the efficacy of intravenous magnesium sulphate has been demonstrated, little is known about inhaled/nebulized magnesium sulphate. In the few studies that relate to nebulized magnesium in the reversal of bronchospasm, samples remain small and conflicting results persist regarding the optimal dose of magnesium and the efficacy of magnesium as the sole agent. In a recent Cochrane review of six trials involving 296 patients, comparing magnesium sulphate with or without a nebulized β_2-agonist in adults or paediatric patients with asthma, there was a non-significant improvement in pulmonary function in patients whose treatments included nebulized magnesium sulphate in addition to a β_2-agonist (standardized mean differences [SMD] 0.23; 95% CI –0.03 to 0.50; four studies) [23]. Hospitalizations were similar between the groups (relative risks [RR] 0.69; 95% CI 0.42–1.12; three studies). Subgroup analyses did not demonstrate significant differences in lung function improvement between adults and children, but in patients with severe asthma the lung function difference was significant (SMD 0.55; 95% CI 0.12–0.98). The authors concluded that nebulized inhaled magnesium sulphate in addition to β_2-agonist in the treatment of an acute asthma exacerbation appears to improve pulmonary function in patients with severe asthma and that there is a trend towards benefit in terms of hospital admission.

Further evidence of the efficacy of magnesium in nebulized form is needed before any firm recommendations for its use in acute asthma can be made.

Corticosteroid sparing effects of vitamin C and magnesium in asthma: a randomised trial

Fogarty A, Lewis SA, Scrivener SL, *et al. Respir Med* 2006; **100**: 174–9

BACKGROUND. Epidemiological evidence suggests that dietary factors may have an important influence on the incidence and severity of asthma, and both vitamin C and magnesium are nutrients that have been particularly implicated in this respect. Several studies using short-term supplementation with these agents have indicated that they may be effective as therapies for asthma. However, there is little evidence on the effects of longer-term supplementation with either magnesium or vitamin C.

INTERPRETATION. Vitamin C supplements may have modest corticosteroid-sparing effects and hence the potential to reduce exposure to their side effects, while magnesium supplements have no effect on the inhaled corticosteroid dose required to maintain asthma control.

Comment

This study aimed to assess the hypothesis that regular supplementation with vitamin C or magnesium will permit a reduction in the corticosteroid dose required to maintain asthma control in adults. Men and women aged 18–60 with a physician diagnosis of asthma who had been using at least one dose of an inhaled corticosteroid daily for 6 months or more were identified from computerized records in 24 general practices in the Nottingham area. The participants had stable asthma and were excluded if they were using dietary supplements. The intervention study used a double-blind, randomized, parallel-group, placebo-controlled design in a two-phase study over a total of 26 weeks. In the first phase the authors compared the effects of 16 weeks of daily supplements of magnesium (450 mg), vitamin C (1 g) or placebo, given in addition to regular asthma medication, on the clinical control of asthma. All participants completing the first phase were invited to continue with their allocated blinded supplement and enter a protocol of staged reduction of inhaled corticosteroid. A total of 234 participants completed 16 weeks of supplementation, and 92 of these (29 randomized to vitamin C, 31 to magnesium and 32 to placebo) consented to continue taking their allocated supplements and enter the inhaled corticosteroid reduction protocol. Assuming no reduction in corticosteroid dose in the ten subjects who subsequently withdrew, the geometric mean reductions in inhaled corticosteroid dose achieved with vitamin C, magnesium and placebo were 49, 13 and 11 μg respectively. Relative to placebo, the unadjusted effect of vitamin C was significant, and remained at borderline significance after adjustment for baseline corticosteroid dose (relative reduction ratio 4.03; 95% CI 0.95–17.1; $P = 0.06$). Although this effect was of borderline statistical significance, its relevance to clinical practice is uncertain.

This study was conducted over a period of 26 weeks in patients with well-controlled asthma but lacked power because of the low numbers. The intrinsic variability of asthma, together with seasonal factors, may not allow firm conclusions to be drawn regarding longer-term control. Patients with well-controlled asthma are often reluctant to take regular inhaled corticosteroids and hence the ability to maintain control by other means, including dietary supplementation, is attractive. A study with larger numbers of participants and for a greater length of time would be useful in this context.

Comparison of nebulized magnesium sulfate plus albuterol to nebulized albuterol plus saline in children with acute exacerbations of mild to moderate asthma

Mahajan P, Haritos D, Rosenberg N, Thomas R. *J Emerg Med* 2004; **27**: 21–5

BACKGROUND. There are only a few studies using magnesium sulphate together with nebulized albuterol in adults and very few studies comparing the effects of nebulized magnesium sulphate with that of albuterol in the paediatric population.

INTERPRETATION. The addition of magnesium to albuterol seems to provide short-term benefits in children with acute exacerbations of mild to moderate asthma.

Comment

Patients presenting to the emergency department between the ages of 5 and 17 years and with a known history of asthma (defined as three or more episodes of wheezing) with an acute exacerbation of mild to moderate asthma (defined as resting FEV_1 between 45 and 75% of the predicted value for age) took part in a prospective, randomized, double-blinded study to determine whether a combination of nebulized magnesium sulphate and albuterol as a single dose adds any benefit in management when compared with nebulized albuterol with saline. The intervention involved administering a single dose of 2.5 mg (0.5 ml) of albuterol mixed with 2.5 ml of normal saline (A+S group) or 2.5 mg (0.5 ml) of albuterol mixed with 2.5 ml of isotonic magnesium sulphate 6.3% (A+M group) nebulized via 8–10 l of oxygen. The study medications were provided in identical syringes and both the pharmacy and the investigator were blinded to their contents. All patients received 2 mg/kg of prednisone for asthma after their first dose of inhalation medication. A total of 62 patients took part in the study and were randomized to the two groups (31 in each group). The primary outcome measure was change in FEV_1, both absolute and percentage of predicted. There was a statistically significant improvement in FEV_1 (absolute) in the magnesium-treated group (A+M) at 10 min when compared with the saline-treated (A+S) group (1.41 ± 0.53 vs 1.13 ± 0.34 l respectively; $P = 0.03$). This improvement was sustained at 20 min but was not statistically significant (1.44 ± 0.62 vs 1.18 ± 0.33 l, respectively; $P = 0.06$). This is the first study that has looked at the use of a combination of magnesium with albuterol in children with asthma exacerbation. The results show that the improvement in FEV_1 in children who received magnesium together with albuterol was more than in those who received albuterol alone. The peak effect of magnesium seemed to be at 10 min and was sustained to 20 min, compared with patients who received albuterol alone (in whom the peak effect was seen at 20 min).

This study has the advantage of objective measurement in the form of FEV_1 rather than peak flow, which is dependent on effort and less reliable in children. It is uncertain whether the bronchodilation seen with the combination of albuterol and magnesium sulphate persists beyond 20 min or translates into a better clinical outcome or a shorter duration of hospitalization. The difference between the two groups in this study had lost its statistical significance by 20 min, which suggests that the effect would not be sustained. The authors did not comment on the total length of stay in the emergency department and whether repeated or further therapy was instituted subsequently.

References

1. Kaplan AP, Spector SL, Meeves S, Liao Y, Varghese ST, Georges G. Once-daily fexofenadine treatment for chronic idiopathic urticaria: a multicenter, randomized, double-blind, placebo-controlled study. *Ann Allergy Asthma Immunol* 2005; **94**: 662–9.
2. Potter PC; Paediatric Levocetirizine Study Group. Efficacy and safety of levocetirizine on symptoms and health-related quality of life of children with perennial allergic rhinitis: a double-blind, placebo-controlled randomized clinical trial. *Ann Allergy Asthma Immunol* 2005; **95**: 175–80.
3. Fardon TC, Lee DK, Hodge MR, Lipworth BJ. Addition of fexofenadine to inhaled corticosteroid therapy to reduce inflammatory biomarkers in atopic asthma. *Ann Allergy Asthma Immunol* 2005; **95**: 259–65.

4. Horak F, Zieglmayer PU, Zieglmayer R, Kavina A, Lemell P. Levocetirizine has a longer duration of action on improving total nasal symptoms score than fexofenadine after single administration. *Br J Clin Pharmacol* 2005; **60**: 24–31.
5. Saint-Martin F, Dumur JP, Perez I, Izquierdo I; French Rupatadine–Rhinitis Study Group. A randomized, double-blind, parallel-group study, comparing the efficacy and safety of rupatadine (20 and 10 mg), a new PAF and H1 receptor-specific histamine antagonist, to loratadine 10 mg in the treatment of seasonal allergic rhinitis. *J Investig Allergol Clin Immunol* 2004; **14**: 34–40.
6. Spector SL, Tan RA. Effectiveness of montelukast in the treatment of cough variant asthma. *Ann Allergy Asthma Immunol* 2004; **93**: 232–6.
7. Price DB, Hernandez D, Magyar P, Fiterman J, Beeh KM, James IG, Konstantopoulos S, Rojas R, van Noord JA, Pons M, Gilles L, Leff JA; Clinical Outcomes with Montelukast as a Partner Agent to Corticosteroid Therapy (COMPACT) International Study Group. Randomised controlled trial of montelukast plus inhaled budesonide versus double dose inhaled budesonide in adult patients with asthma. *Thorax* 2003; **58**: 211–16.
8. Vaquerizo MJ, Casan P, Castillo J, Perpina M, Sanchis J, Sobradillo V, Valencia A, Verea H, Viejo JL, Villasante C, Gonzalez-Esteban J, Picado C; CASIOPEA (Capacidad de Singulair Oral en la Prevencion de Exacerbaciones Asmaticas) Study Group. Effect of montelukast added to inhaled budesonide on control of mild to moderate asthma. *Thorax* 2003; **58**: 204–10.
9. Bisgaard H, Zielen S, Garcia-Garcia ML, Johnston SL, Gilles L, Menten J, Tozzi CA, Polos P. Montelukast reduces asthma exacerbations in 2- to 5-year-old children with intermittent asthma. *Am J Respir Crit Care Med* 2005; **171**: 315–22.
10. Ostrom NK, Decotiis BA, Lincourt WR, Edwards LD, Hanson KM, Carranza Rosenzweig JR, Crim C. Comparative efficacy and safety of low-dose fluticasone propionate and montelukast in children with persistent asthma. *J Paediatr* 2005; **147**: 213–20.
11. Davis BE, Todd DC, Cockcroft DW. Effect of combined montelukast and desloratadine on the early asthmatic response to inhaled allergen. *J Allergy Clin Immunol* 2005; **116**: 768–72.
12. Barnes N, Thomas M, Price D, Tate H. The national montelukast survey. *J Allergy Clin Immunol* 2005; **115**: 47–54.
13. Diamant Z, van der Molen T. Treating asthma: is there a place for leukotriene receptor antagonists? *Respir Med* 2005; **99**: 655–62.
14. Niitsuma T, Izawa J, Maruoka N, Nukaga M, Tsuji A, Okita M, Sakurai K, Morita S, Tsuyuguchi M, Matsumura Y, Hayashi T. Clinical evaluation of response to long-term treatment with Pranlukast in patients with bronchial asthma. *J Invest Allergol Clin Immunol* 2004; **14**: 284–91.
15. Tsuchida T, Matsuse H, Machida I, Kondo Y, Saeki S, Tomari S, Obase Y, Matsuo N, Shimoda T, Kohno S. Evaluation of theophylline or pranlukast, a cysteinyl leukotriene receptor 1 antagonist, as add-on therapy in uncontrolled asthmatic patients with a medium dose of inhaled corticosteroids. *Allergy Asthma Proc* 2005; **26**: 287–91.
16. Matsui EC, Wood RA, Rand C, Kanchanaraksa S, Swartz L, Eggleston PA. Mouse allergen exposure and mouse skin test sensitivity in suburban, middle-class children with asthma. *J Allergy Clin Immunol* 2004; **113**: 910–15.

17. Reitamo S, Rustin M, Ruzicka T, Cambazard F, Kalimo K, Friedmann PS, Schoepf E, Lahfa M, Diepgen TL, Judodihardjo H, Wollenberg A, Berth-Jones J, Bieber T; European Tacrolimus Ointment Study Group. Efficacy and safety of tacrolimus ointment compared with that of hydrocortisone butyrate ointment in adult patients with atopic dermatitis. *J Allergy Clin Immunol* 2002; **109**: 547–55.

18. Reitamo S, Wollenberg A, Schopf E, Perrot JL, Marks R, Ruzicka T, Christophers E, Kapp A, Lahfa M, Rubins A, Jablonska S, Rustin M. Safety and efficacy of 1 year of tacrolimus ointment monotherapy in adults with atopic dermatitis. The European Tacrolimus Ointment Study Group. *Arch Dermatol* 2000; **136**: 999–1006.

19. Wahn U, Bos JD, Goodfield M, Caputo R, Papp K, Manjra A, Dobozy A, Paul C, Molloy S, Hultsch T, Graeber M, Cherill R, de Prost Y; Flare Reduction in Eczema with Elidel (Children) Multicenter Investigator Study Group. Efficacy and safety of pimicrolimus cream in the long-term management of atopic dermatitis in children. *Pediatrics* 2002; **110**(1 Pt 1): e2.

20. Patel RR, Vander Straten MR, Korman NJ. The safety and efficacy of tacrolimus therapy in patients younger than two years with atopic dermatitis. *Arch Dermatol* 2003; **139**: 1184–6.

21. Hickey JR, Robson A, Barker JN, Smith CH. Does topical tacrolimus induce lentigines in children with atopic dermatitis? A report of three cases. *Br J Dermatol* 2005; **152**: 152–4.

22. Darsow U, Lubbe J, Taieb A, Seidenari S, Wollenberg A, Calza AM, Giusti F, Ring J; European Task Force on Atopic Dermatitis. European Task Force on Atopic Dermatitis. Position paper on diagnosis and treatment of atopic dermatitis. *J Eur Acad Dermatol Venereol* 2005; **19**: 286–95.

23. Blitz M, Blitz S, Beasely R, Diner B, Hughes R, Knopp J, Rowe B, Blitz M. Inhaled magnesium sulfate in the treatment of acute asthma. *Cochrane Database Syst Rev* 2005; (**4**): CD003898.

Abbreviations

AAAAI	American Academy of Asthma, Allergy and Immunology
ACQ	Asthma Control Questionnaire
AD	atopic dermatitis
AEDS	atopic eczema/dermatitis syndrome
AHR	airway hyper-responsiveness
AM	ampicillin
AMP	adenosine monophosphate
AMP	antimicrobial peptide
anti-PnPs	anti-pneumococcal polysaccharide
APC	antigen-presenting cell
APT	atopy patch test
AQLQ	Asthma Quality of Life Questionnaire
AR	allergic rhinitis
ARIA	Allergic Rhinitis and its Impact on Asthma (workgroup)
AU	allergen unit
AUC	area under the curve
AX	amoxicillin
BAL	bronchoalveolar lavage
BEAS-28	bronchial epithelial cells
BHR	bronchial hyper-responsiveness
BLT1	gene for leukotriene B4 receptor 1
BMI	body mass index
BrdU	5-bromo-2-deoxyuridine
CAMP	Childhood Asthma Management Program
cAMP	cyclic adenosine monophosphate
CCR7	CC chemokine receptor 7
CHQ-PF50	Child Health Questionnaire Patient Form 50
CI	confidence interval
CLA	cutaneous lymphocyte antigen
COAST	Childhood Onset of Asthma study
COPD	chronic obstructive pulmonary disease
COX-1	cyclooxygenase
cPLA2	cellular PLA2
CT	computed tomography
CVID	common variable immunodeficiency
DBPCFC	double-blind, placebo-controlled food challenge
DC	dendritic cell
DDE	dichlorodiphenyldich-loroethylene
EAACI	European Academy of Allergy and Clinical Immunology
EAD	extrinsic atopic dermatitis
EAR	early allergen reaction
EASI	Eczema Area and Severity Index
EBC	exhaled breath condensate
EBV	Epstein–Barr virus
EGEA	Epidemiological Study on the Genetics and Environment of Asthma

© Atlas Medical Publishing Ltd

ELISA	enzyme-linked immunosorbent assay
ERK	extracellular signal regulated kinase
ESID	European Society for Immunodeficiencies
ETS	environmental tobacco smoke
FAQL-PB	Food Allergy Quality of Life–PB
FENO	nitric oxide fraction
FEF	forced expiratory flow
FEV1	forced expiratory volume in 1 s
FVC	forced vital capacity
GC/MS	gas chromatography/ mass spectrometry
GINA	Global Initiative for Asthma
GM-CSF	granulocyte-macrophage colony stimulating factor
GPRD	General Practice Research Database
HDM	house dust mite
HEPA	high-efficiency particulate air filter
HES	hypereosinophilic syndromes
HFA	hydro fluro alkane
HLA	human lymphocyte antigen
HPA	hypothalamic–pituitary–adrenal (axis)
HRQOL	Health-Related Quality of Life
IAD	intrinsic atopic dermatitis
ICAM-1	intercellular adhesion molecule 1
ICOS	inducible costimulator
ICS	inhaled corticosteroid
IFN-β	interferon-β
IFN-γ	interferon-γ
Ig	immunoglobulin
IgE	immunoglobulin E
IgM	immunoglobulin M
IL	interleukin
IL1ra	IL1 receptor antagonist
iNOS	inducible nitric oxide synthase
IRAK-4	interleukin receptor-associated kinase 4
ISAAC	International Study of Asthma and Allergies in Childhood
IVIG	intravenous immunoglobulin
LABA	long-acting b2-agonist
LAR	late allergen reaction
5-LO	5-LO-activating protein
5-LO	5-lipoxygenase
LOD	log of the odds
LPS	lipopolysaccharide
LT	leukotriene (e.g. LTC4)
LTB4	leukotriene B4
LTRA	leukotriene receptor antagonist
MAP	mitogen-activated protein
mEASI	modified Eczema Area and Severity Index
MEF	maximum expiratory flow
MgSO4	magnesium sulphate
MMP	matrix metalloproteinase
NEMO	NFκB essential modulator
NFκB	nuclear factor κB
NKA	neurokinin A
NMR	nuclear magnetic resonance
NNH	number needed to harm
NO	nitric oxide
NO2	nitrogen dioxide
NS	not significant
NSAID	non-steroidal anti-inflammatory drug

OAS	oral allergy syndrome
OME	otitis media with effusion
OR	odds ratio
PAD	primary antibody deficiency
PAR	perennial allergic rhinitis
PBMC	peripheral blood mononuclear cell
PC	provocative concentration
PC20	dose of metacholine that causes a 20% decrease in the patient's baseline FEV1 forced expiratory volume in 1 second
PCR	polymerase chain reaction
PDE	phosphodiesterase
PDGF	platelet-derived growth factor
PED4	phosphodiesterase type 4
PEF	peak expiratory flow
PHA	phytohaemagglutin
PI3K	phosphoinositide 3-kinase
PITT	primary intent-to-treat
PnPS	pneumococcal polysaccharide
ppb	parts per billion
prn	as and when required
RAST	radioallergosorbent test
RBM	reticular basement membrane
RCT	randomized controlled trial
RQLQ	Rhinitis Quality of Life Questionnaire
RQLQ	Rhinoconjunctivitis Quality of Life Questionnaire
RR	relative risk/risk ratio
RV16	rhinovirus 16
SABA	short acting b-agonist
SAR	seasonal allergic rhinitis
sCD14	soluble CD14
SCID	severe combined immunodeficiency
SCIG	subcutaneous immunoglobulin
SCIT	specific subcutaneous immunotherapy
SCORAD	Scoring Atopic Dermatitis
SEB	staphylococcal enterotoxin B
sGAW	specific airway conductance
sIgE	serum immuno-globulin E
sIgE	specific IgE
SIT	specific immunotherapy
SLAM	signalling lymphocyte activation molecule
SLIT	sublingual immunotherapy
SMD	standardized mean difference
SNP	single-nucleotide polymorphism
SPACE	Study on the Prevention of Allergy in Children in Europe
sPLA2	secretory phospholipase A2
SPT	skin-prick test
sGaw	specific airway conductance
sRaw	specific airway resistance
START	Steroid Treatment as Regular Therapy
Syk	spenic tyrosine kinase
TACE	TNF-α converting enzyme
TCS	topical corticosteroids
TGFβ	transforming growth factor β
Th	T-helper

TIM	T-cell immunoglobulin domain and mucin domain
TIMP	tissue inhibitor of metalloproteinase
TLR	toll-like receptor
TNF-α	tumour necrosis factor α
TNRFR	TNF receptor
Treg	T-regulatory
TSS	total symptom score
UTR	untranslated region
VEGF	vascular endothelial cell growth factor
VCAM-1	vascular endothelial cell adhesion molecule 1
VEGF	vascular endothelial growth factor
VIT	venom immunotherapy
WHO	World Health Organization
XLP	X-linked lympho-proliferative disease

Index of papers reviewed

© Atlas Medical Publishing Ltd

General index

© Atlas Medical Publishing Ltd

T

KEEPING UP TO DATE IN ONE SERIES

"THE YEAR IN ..."

EXISTING AND FUTURE VOLUMES

The Year in Allergy 2003	ISBN 1 904392 05 9
The Year in Allergy 2004	ISBN 1 904392 25 3
The Year in Allergy Volume 3	ISBN 1 904392 60 1
The Year in Anaesthesia and Critical Care Volume 1	ISBN 1 904392 47 4
The Year in Diabetes 2004	ISBN 1 904392 20 2
The Year in Gastroenterology and Hepatology Volume 1	ISBN 1 904392 48 2
The Year in Gastroenterology and Hepatology Volume 2	ISBN 1 904392 81 4
The Year in Gynaecology 2003	ISBN 1 904392 10 5
The Year in Heart Failure Volume 1	ISBN 1 904392 38 5
The Year in Hypertension 2004	ISBN 1 904392 28 8
The Year in Hypertension Volume 6	ISBN 1 904392 56 3
The Year in Infection Volume 2	ISBN 1 904392 32 6
The Year in Infection Volume 3	ISBN 1 904392 72 5
The Year in Interventional Cardiology 2003	ISBN 1 904392 14 8
The Year in Interventional Cardiology Volume 3	ISBN 1 904392 33 4
The Year in Neurology 2004	ISBN 1 904392 22 9
The Year in Osteoporosis Volume 1	ISBN 1 904392 27 X
The Year in Osteoporosis Volume 2	ISBN 1 904392 62 8
The Year in Post-Menopausal Health 2004	ISBN 1 904392 23 7
The Year in Renal Medicine Volume 1	ISBN 1 904392 39 3
The Year in Respiratory Medicine 2003	ISBN 0 9537339 8 X
The Year in Respiratory Medicine 2004	ISBN 1 904392 31 8
The Year in Respiratory Medicine Volume 3	ISBN 1 904392 53 9
The Year in Rheumatic Disorders Volume 4	ISBN 1 904392 29 6
The Year in Rheumatic Disorders Volume 5	ISBN 1 904392 57 1
The Year in Schizophrenia Volume 1	ISBN 1 904392 04 0
The Year in Therapeutics Volume 1	ISBN 1 904392 50 4
The Year in Urology Volume 2	ISBN 1 904392 30 X
The Year in Urology Volume 3	ISBN 1 904392 82 2

To receive more information about these books and future volumes,
or to order copies,
please contact us at the address below:

Clinical Publishing
Oxford Centre for Innovation
Mill Street
Oxford OX2 0JX, UK

T: +44 1865 811116
F: +44 1865 251550
E: info@clinicalpublishing.co.uk
W: www.clinicalpublishing.co.uk

KEEPING UP TO DATE IN ONE VOLUME
THE YEAR IN ALLERGY VOLUME 3

SUBJECT MATTERS DEALT WITH IN PREVIOUS VOLUME

Epidemiology and prevention
- Prevalence and natural history
- Risk factors for allergy
- Early origins of allergy
- Prevention of allergy

Mechanisms of allergic disease
- Allergic asthma and allergic trinities
- Atopic dermatitis

Food allergy/intolerance
- Immunological reactions involved in food allergy
- Diagnosis and management
- Nut allergies
- Food intolerances

Treatment modalities for allergic diseases
- Conventional treatments for asthma
- Anti-leukotrienes in the treatment of allergic disorders
- Immunotherapy for allergic disorders
- Treatment of allergic diseases with Omalizumab
- Treatment of atopic dermatitis
- Management of asthma in emergencies
- Newer therapies for allergic diseases
- Health economics of allergic disorders

Clinical Publishing
Oxford Centre for Innovation
Mill Street
Oxford OX2 0JX, UK

T: +44 1865 811116
F: +44 1865 251550
E: info@clinicalpublishing.co.uk
W: www.clinicalpublishing.co.uk